Physicians at Work, Patients in Pain: Biomedical Practice and Patient Response in Mexico

Physicians at Work, Patients in Pain: Biomedical Practice and Patient Response in Mexico

Kaja Finkler

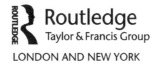

Routledge
Taylor & Francis Group

LONDON AND NEW YORK

First published 1991 by Westview Press

Published 2019 by Routledge
52 Vanderbilt Avenue, New York, NY 10017
2 Park Square, Milton Park, Abingdon, Oxon OX14 4RN

Routledge is an imprint of the Taylor & Francis Group, an informa business

Library of Congress Cataloging-in-Publication Data
Finkler, Kaja.
    Physicians at work, patients in pain : biomedical practice and
patient response in Mexico / Kaja Finkler.
        p. cm.
    Includes bibliographical references.
    Includes index.
    ISBN 0-8133-1154-3—ISBN 0-8133-1155-1 (if published as a paperback)
    1. Social medicine—Mexico. 2. Medical care—Mexico.
3. Physician and patient—Mexico. 4. Patients—Mexico—Attitudes.
I. Title.
    [DNLM: 1. Anthropology, Cultural—Mexico. 2. Health Services,
Indigenous—Mexico. 3. Medicine, Traditional—Mexico. 4. Patient
Acceptance of Health Care—ethnology—Mexico. 5. Physician-Patient
Relations. WB 50 DM4 F4p]
RA418.3.M6F56 1991
610′.972—dc20
DLC
for Library of Congress   90-12902
                                                                         CIP

ISBN 13: 978-0-367-28290-5 (hbk)
ISBN 13: 978-0-367-29836-4 (pbk)

Contents

List of Tables   ix
Preface   xi
Acknowledgments   xix

1   **Introduction**   1

PART ONE: THE SETTING

2   **The Mexican Context**   17

3   **Sickness: A Mexican View**   31

         Typical Symptoms, 32
         Etiological Beliefs, 35

4   **Health Care Delivery in Mexico**   45

         Biomedicine in the Public Sector: Institutional
              Health Care Delivery, 45
         Biomedicine in the Private Sector, 47
         Salud Hospital, 48
         Nonbiomedical Treatment Options, 50
         Patients' Trajectories Within Health
              Delivery Options, 52

PART TWO: BIOMEDICAL PRACTICE IN MEXICO

5   History of Medicine in Mexico   59

The Preconquest Period, 59
The Colonial Period, 60
Independence, 63
Contemporary Biomedicine, 65
Psychiatry, 66
Recruitment into the Profession
    and Medical Education, 67
Physicians' Social Status, 70

6   Biomedical Beliefs and Practices   75

General Considerations, 75
Biomedicine in Mexico, 78
Etiological Beliefs, 78
The Diagnostic Process, 84
Treatment Management, 86
A Model of the Cultural Transformation
    of Biomedicine, 88

**7   Variations in Biomedical Beliefs
and Practices**   91

Description of Individual Physicians, 91
Individual Variations in Physicians' Practice, 95
Jose, 98
Sharon, 101
Nomi, 108

8   The Medical Consultation   123

Arthur, 129
Serge, 138
Esperanza, 143
Thelma, 149

PART THREE: PATIENTS' RESPONSES TO
BIOMEDICAL PRACTICE

9   **Patients and Their Complaints**   163

    Sociodemographic Profile, 163
    Health Characteristics and Patient Complaints, 165

10   **Patient-Perceived Therapeutic Outcomes:**
    An Aggregate Analysis   171

    Response to Treatment, 171
    Patients' Diagnosed Conditions and
        Characteristics as Related to
        Recovery, 173
    The Medical Consultation and Patients'
        Perceived Recovery, 177
    Sickness Management, 184
    Sociodemographic and Socioeconomic Variability, 186
    Social Supports and Life Events, 187
    Attributions for Recovery, 189

11   **Patient-Perceived Therapeutic Outcomes:**
    A Phenomenological Perspective   197

    Jose, 198
    Arthur, 199
    Serge, 202
    Esperanza, 205
    Thelma, 208
    Nomi, 210

PART FOUR: TWO SYSTEMS OF HEALING

12   **A Comparison Between Sacred**
    Healing and Biomedicine   219

13   **Conclusion**   229

Appendix: Methodology   235
References   237
Glossary   261
Index   263

Tables

2.1	Persons Considered Closest to the Subject	28
3.1	Most Common Attributions of Illness by Sex of Patient	43
4.1	Type of Treatment Sought by Patients Prior to Hospital Treatment by Sex of Patient	53
7.1	Number of Patients and Diagnoses by Physician	96
7.2	Diagnoses by Individual Physician	96
9.1	Selected Characteristics of Sample Group by Sex	164
9.2	Economic Status as Measured by Dwelling and Material Possessions	165
9.3	Medical Diagnoses for the Study Group	166
9.4	Patients' Expectations of Treatment Before and After Medical Consultation	169
10.1	Patients' Perceived Recovery Along Sex Lines	172
10.2	Patients' Perceived Recovery by Condition at Time of First Follow-up Interview	173
10.3	Patients' Perceived Recovery by Diagnosis Category	174
10.4	Patients' Perceived Recovery by Number of Diagnoses	175
10.5	Patients' Perceived Recovery by Results of Laboratory Analyses	176
10.6	Patients' Perceived Recovery by Whether or Not Physicians Explained to the Patients What Was Wrong	179
10.7	Patients' Perceived Recovery by Physician Providing a Diagnosis	179
10.8	Patients' Perceived Recovery by Whether or Not Patients Agreed with Physicians' Diagnoses at Time of First Follow-up Interview	180

10.9   Patients' Perceived Recovery by Whether or Not
           Patient Posed Questions to the Physician   180
10.10   Patients' Perceived Recovery by Whether or Not
           Patients' Expectations Were Met   181
10.11   Patients' Perceived Recovery by Whether Medication
           Was or Was Not Prescribed   183
10.12   Patients' Perceived Recovery by Whether or Not They
           Reported Taking Prescribed Medication   183
10.13   Patients' Perceived Recovery by Other Treatment Sought
           Between 30 and 50 Days Following Hospital Visit
           Before First Follow-up Home Visit   185
10.14   Patients' Perceived Recovery by Number of Days Patients
           Had Been Sick Before Seeking Treatment at
           Salud Hospital   186
10.15   Patients' Perceived Recovery by Ranking of
           Socioeconomic Status   187
10.16   Patients' Perceived Recovery by Life Events   188
10.17   Patients' Stated Condition of How They Were Feeling
           at Time of Second Home Follow-up by
           Attribution and Treatment Sought   191

Preface

This book has its roots in eight years of my professional life in Mexico, from the first time when I visited the country as a novice "to discover the world" to my subsequent returns as a professional anthropologist beginning in 1970. During this period I addressed anthropological concerns bearing on the socioeconomic and political life of the peasant population.[1] Living with people in their homes and participating in their lives, I was drawn into their experiences of affliction and was often called upon to assist in its management when I was asked to drive a member of the community to a physician or, if that failed, to a Spiritualist healer. By 1975 I became immersed in matters related to sickness and its alleviation. This concern led me to carry out a study in 1977-1979 of Spiritualist healing, a predominant mode of alternative healing in rural and urban Mexico.

Spiritualist healing was a propitious subject through which to address theoretical concerns relevant to sickness and to the healing process from the patient's perspective. I therefore systematically examined the therapeutic outcomes of Spiritualist healing, a type of investigation that had not been carried out before in Latin America.

In doing the study of Spiritualist therapeutics, I discovered that all newcomers to a Spiritualist temple had already sought outpatient care from a variety of biophysicians who failed to alleviate their ailments. Since Spiritualist healers drew such a large clientele, I asked, "Why does biomedicine fail to alleviate patients' afflictions?" This question led me to return to the field for another investigation, this time to study biomedicine and its patients.

I chose to address this question in Mexico City rather than in the rural region for methodological reasons: In the rural towns where I had previously worked there was no one medical center that brought together sufficient numbers of ambulatory patients to allow for a large sample within a limited research period. Conversely, in Mexico City I was given access to an outpatient clinic of a large hospital where numerous first-time patients were seen daily.

While the patient population in both the rural and urban settings originated from similar social strata of Mexican society, doing fieldwork in Mexico City using traditional anthropological techniques of participation and observation was difficult. Unlike the countryside, where I was incorporated into the community and encompassed by it, Mexico City limited community participation because of the amorphous boundaries of city neighborhoods. Full participation in the daily rhythm of life with the same people is not usually feasible, as it had been in a rural village, because of the extensive size of the city and its many neighborhoods. Moreover, unlike the rural communities, where I found people, especially women, at home most of the time, in the city the daily rhythm of life is tied to an endless round of errands and petty commerce. So it was a special treat, rather than a daily routine, to share a meal with a family.

During this field stay, much of what I learned was from people's narratives about their existence rather than by direct observation of their daily activities, as in my previous studies. Nevertheless, individuals repeated the same narratives often enough that I was satisfied that I was getting at the realities of subjects' lives as they perceived them.

Before my study of Spiritualism, I was unfamiliar with its healing techniques and specialized vocabulary. In contrast, I was conversant with biomedicine and its practices and vocabularies as part of my own cultural heritage and from a previous study in the United States.[2] During my sojourn in the Spiritualist temple I was invited to participate in the rituals and recruited to train as a healer; in the hospital in which I did this study, however, I was not spurred to become a physician. Rather, my role was one of a welcomed observer. I was received at the hospital with utmost graciousness and encouragement by most of the physicians and administrators. The findings bearing on biomedical practice I present are based on my direct observations.

Despite my overt familiarity with biomedicine and its vocabularies, I wondered whether it was practiced in the same way I knew it as a European-American. Could I assume that what appeared the same was the same? Or do practices ostensibly international in scope become transformed and reinterpreted by practitioners in other cultures? To address this and other questions of theoretical and practical importance, including patients' responses to biomedical therapeutics, I spent two years (1986-1988) in Mexico City at one of the oldest and largest metropolitan hospitals. There, I was privileged to observe physicians in their day-to-day activities and their dealings with patients.

Upon exiting from the subway in the heart of the city, where the hospital is situated, I would pass a series of food vendors, some hawking traditional Mexican foods that they prepared there on coal burners, others selling sundry articles such as candy, cigarettes, pens, creams, newspapers, tissues, cassette tapes, and numerous other easily portable goods. On Tuesdays and Fridays, I made my way through a small market set up by vendors selling chickens, cheeses, and other foodstuffs. At least twice a year stalls with used books line the street paralleling the hospital entrance.

At least four times a week, a group of ten to fifteen men were usually assembled at the hospital entrance. I later met them inside interrupting medical consultations to present their prepared speeches to physicians, and plugging the newest drugs produced by their respective companies.[3] The pharmaceutical salesmen, dressed in expensive suits and carrying elegant leather briefcases laden with drug samples that they readily distributed to the physicians, provided a startling contrast to the predominantly indigent, poorly dressed patients lined up for a consultation in the outpatient clinics, some holding young children in their arms, others Xrays in their hands; some accompanied by relatives or friends and others by themselves. Some had European faces, but the majority were clearly a mixture of European and Indian ancestry typical of the population dominating the Mexican human landscape.

Some patients arrived at 5 a.m. to form the line. Many came from far-off states, while others lived in Mexico City and its environs. Some days the long lines inside the hospital extended to where the pharmaceutical salesmen congregated and on other days the lines were contained within the confines of the hospital's waiting room. The lines moved slowly as people were processed for admission. Many of those waiting patiently were first-time patients who required identity cards (IDs) issued by the hospital, while others with their IDs in hand came for follow-up visits.

Patients were processed inside a poorly lit waiting room with rows of chairs surrounded by little booths where, upon paying a minuscule fee, they received the IDs entitling them to medical services at the hospital. The line began moving around 7:30 a.m., when clerical staff in charge of admissions arrived. Patients milled around after they received their cards until they saw one of several physicians who, on the basis of a few presenting symptoms, channeled them to the various medical specialties, including Internal Medicine, which subsequently was renamed General Medicine. Once directed to the proper medical department, those assigned to Internal/General Medicine sat waiting for the doctors who trickled in between 8 and 10 a.m. to attend to their patients.

My own day began at the hospital at 7:30 a.m., when I would select patients for the study, participate in the interviews conducted by my assistant, and then observe the physicians as they conducted consultations with new and old patients, including those interviewed by my assistant for the study. The morning shift with its frantic pace ended around noon. The physicians working the first shift quickly dispersed to other jobs, to their private practices, or to other government medical institutions.

In order to randomize the sample population, I and my assistant waited for the afternoon shift to interview patients seen by a new crew of doctors, nurses, and clerical staff. I welcomed the afternoon shift when a calm befell the outpatient service. Fewer patients sought treatment then and the pharmaceutical representatives were gone. The physicians began arriving between 2 and 3 p.m. and saw patients until 6 p.m.

At first we interviewed patients both during the morning and afternoon shifts; later, I rotated the interviews between morning and afternoon, which left the remainder of the day and weekends to follow up on patients in their homes dispersed in various districts of Mexico City. After having interviewed 267 first-time patients at the hospital, I and my assistant spent longer and longer periods in the homes and neighborhoods of the people interviewed in the hospital to gain a better understanding of life's rhythm in the megalopolis.

Unlike in laboratory work, methodological requisites in anthropological fieldwork are intertwined with the realities of the field site. Doing fieldwork in a city of 20 million people and immense geographical expanse presented various personal hardships despite the availability of conveniences such as a toilet, a shower, a telephone, and other modern amenities that I lacked in earlier field stays. Finding appropriate living quarters was very difficult; after the 1985 earthquake housing became especially scarce. In addition, the polluted air, the sheer logistics of getting around a city the size of Mexico City to meet with the study participants within a time stipulated by methodological criteria, and the constant reminder by the local inhabitants of dangers and their apprehensions that another devastating earthquake was imminent took their toll. But perhaps most draining on me was witnessing the drama of the medical consultation and the squalor in which participants of the study lived, some even lacking food to eat, and becoming involved in the suffering of so many of the people as they unfolded their lives to me during the course of the study. The voice of the mother of one twenty-year-old patient who had recently lost her first baby resonates especially in my ears as I hear her recounting how her husband had violated this daughter, asking me, "How can I live with this pain?" I encountered various ethical dilemmas that gnawed at me, as when I witnessed what I regarded an inappropriate management of one woman's sickness or when patients asked my advice about how to deal with problematic relationships with a spouse or child. I believe that my role as researcher is incompatible with that of a personal advisor.

Regardless of the numerous hardships, fieldwork was extraordinarily rewarding because I got to know many valiant people, both patients and physicians, who maintain their dignity despite the numerous insults to their being sparked by their distresses. Amid untold hustle and bustle and personal anguish, the study was, nevertheless, carried out with methodological rigor. Each admissions clerk had a specific task: One was charged with distributing the newly created files for new patients to the attending physicians. When a patient's file indicated that he or she resided within a radius of approximately ten miles of the hospital, the clerk gave the name of the patient to my assistant, who would then seek out the patient from the large crowd waiting for a consultation. After giving a detailed explanation of the study and its purpose, my assistant inquired whether the selected patient was willing to participate and be visited in his or her home. The doctor was then informed that one of the new patients assigned to him or her was being interviewed for the study.

Patients were interviewed while they waited to be seen by the physicians in a cubicle assigned to me by the hospital. Physicians usually saw new patients after they had attended to their regular ones, allowing for the one and a half hours necessary to carry out the initial interview before the patient received the medical consultation. The majority of patients were interviewed by my assistant; I was present at the initial phase of the interview, when I engaged patients in open-ended discussion. Then the assistant administered a specially constructed 122-item interview schedule that incorporated Kleinman's explanatory model (1980) and a standardized health questionnaire, the Cornell Medical Index (CMI), while I sat with the physician to whom the subject in the study was randomly assigned during all of his or her medical consultations for that given day. When the participant in the study was called in by the nurse, I was present during the consultation. Many people indicated to me that they were reassured by my presence. At first my presence affected the physicians' comportment. Once the doctors became accustomed to my being there, I was accepted by them and the patients as one of the various people present during a consultation.

Depending on the time of day, various other people were usually present during a consultation. Two physicians almost always had second-year medical students in their cubicles. Nurses routinely came in and out, and during the morning shift, the pharmaceutical salesmen entered at will, one after the other, to present their monologues.

Generally speaking, sickness is not usually regarded as a private matter in Mexican popular culture, and the need for privacy is not a paramount concern. In fact, when I questioned patients about how they perceived the presence of strangers during the medical consultation, they indicated that to them it signified that the people present were concerned about them and this was the reason they were there.

The unresolvable dilemma of anthropological fieldwork is, of course, the degree to which the presence of the anthropologist defines the situation and affects the aims of the study. Some people, in fact, reported that they had felt better after the initial interview, even before they saw the physician. Undoubtedly, my presence may have influenced one of the study's aims: to assess patients' responses to biomedical practice. Nevertheless, the variability in patient perceived recovery suggests that my intervention may have had a minimal effect. Otherwise, patients would have uniformly reported positive recovery.

Both the initial interviews and the consultations were tape-recorded with the patients' and physicians' permission. After the consultation, the physicians furnished me with their diagnoses and assessment as to the condition's etiology, whether they considered the disorder grave or not grave, and the expected recovery time following treatment. I recorded the date of the patients' next appointment so that I could be present during each patient's follow-up hospital visit. I engaged the physicians in lengthy open-ended discussion about how they established the diagnosis in order to give me insight into the clinical reasoning of each of the doctors.

If I was absent from the hospital for a few days, the physicians and clerks inquired about my whereabouts, and on various occasions physicians contacted me at home if they knew that one of the patients we had interviewed requested an unanticipated appointment.

I followed up on patients at the hospital, on return visits, and in their homes. Usually two or three patients were interviewed at the hospital each day. One or two were followed up at home during a day, depending on the length of each visit. Sometimes I spent eight hours with a subject and his or her family, sitting on an uncomfortable chair, and in some homes water dripped down on us from the tin roofs during the rainy season. The visitation schedule was the most difficult to maintain in a standardized manner. Each patient was scheduled to be followed up on at home between thirty and forty days after the initial medical consultation.[4] Prearranging appointments even a few days in advance was impossible in almost all cases because patients lacked telephones. As a result I often spent one or two hours traveling by subway and then by a collective van that squeezed thirteen people in space normally designed to accommodate six, then spent another half hour finding the house, to discover that the person was not at home.

Even visiting patients who lived in the same general vicinity (for example, those residing in Nezahualcóyotl) was extraordinarily time consuming because the district is so extensive. When a person was not home on the first attempt, one or two weeks sometimes elapsed before I could visit him or her again. Thus, while methodologically it was important to follow up on subjects within the exact same time interval, logistically this could not be accomplished.

The reader ought not expect descriptions of exotic customs, as one might have come to anticipate from anthropological studies. To most readers biomedical practice is familiar from their own experience. But we will learn about subtle distinctions between ourselves and the people of Mexico, including differences in biomedical practice. It is not my aim to establish the correctness of any one medical system, to glorify or to demean biomedicine. As an anthropologist, my aim is to describe and interpret my observations, using anthropologically informed theories about sickness, healing regimes, and the healing process. I posed four basic and simple questions: Why do people get sick? What makes them well? How and why does biomedicine in Mexico succeed or fail to heal patients with non-life-threatening, non-acute conditions? Is biomedicine a universal system of healing or is it culturally shaped? The answers to these questions are complex, however. In this book I attempt to shed light, if only a minimal amount, on these issues, and I can only hope that it will stimulate others to build upon it.

Kaja Finkler

Notes

1. See Finkler 1974.

2. I carried out a pilot study using similar methodologies in a university hospital in the American South. See Finkler 1989.

3. For a discussion of the pharmaceutical industry in Mexico, see Gereffi 1983.

4. I will note the reason for this timing in Chapter 10, note 2.

Acknowledgments

This research was made possible by grants from the National Science Foundation (1986-1987), #BNS8607543, and the Department of Health and Human Services (1987-1989), #BSR1RO1MH42309-1 and #BSBRO1MH42309-2. I am grateful for the support of those institutions. A project of this scope benefits from contact and assistance with countless numbers of people. First and foremost I am grateful to all the participants in the study for receiving me in their homes and for their trust and cooperation. The study could not have been carried out without the aid of many people in the public hospital in Mexico City where much of the study was done. The study was facilitated by the support of the hospital authorities. I especially wish to thank Dr. Raul Cicero and Dr. Carlos Garcia Calderas of the Hospital's research department for their kind assistance. Maria Cristina Plata L. graciously facilitated the space for carrying out the interviews. I am especially grateful to the many physicians who aided the project, including Drs. Jose Luis Bonilla R., P. Cadeza, Luis Cruz B., Jesus Hernandez N., Daniel Medina M., Trinella Flores G., and Luis Martin A. I benefited from participation in the seminar "La Medicina del Hombre en su Totalidad" led by Dr. Fernando Martinez Cortes who was supportive and inspiring, and also from discussions with Dr. Carlos Viesca T. I am especially grateful to Dr. Luis Martin Armendariz for the diagnostic classification, for the many insights I gained about biomedicine in Mexico from our numerous lengthy discussions, and for his ongoing interest in this project. My appreciation to Norma Jara for assistance in data collection. I owe a very special debt for Patricia Ryan's close reading of the entire manuscript and for her and Bruce Warren's assistance with the statistical analysis. I greatly appreciate Bernard Ortiz de Montellano's close reading of Chapter 5. My thanks to Richard Vonk for carrying out part of the statistical analysis. My thanks also to Mark Venburen for his assistance with the computer analysis. I very much appreciate Carol M. Sanks' dedicated assistance in processing parts of the data base and in bibliographic work, and Bonita Samuels' competent help in preparing the manuscript.

K. F.

1

Introduction

This book presents a theoretical and an empirical study of biomedical practice in Mexico and patients' responses to it. The research is based upon intensive and extensive fieldwork in the Internal Medicine outpatient clinic of a public hospital in Mexico that, for this study, I will call Salud Hospital. By focusing on biomedicine as practiced in Mexico, I explore three interrelated theoretical issues: the ways in which a system of knowledge developed in one society translates in another; the ways in which patients respond to biomedical treatment received in a public hospital; and the nature of sickness and recovery requisites that illuminate patients' differential responses to treatment.

This work is a direct outgrowth of my previous extensive investigations in Mexico, including my last study of *Spiritualist Healers in Mexico* (Finkler 1985). The reader may wonder what Spiritualist healing, whose footing rests on sacred revelations, and whose practitioners have little formal education and no medical training, has in common with biomedicine, which is predicated on a scientific epistemology and dependent on complex technologies and highly professional personnel with numerous years of training. The answer is found in the recognition that the history of biomedicine and its practices has undergone numerous transformations, reflecting societal transformations in Western society (Foucault 1975). Thus, contemporary biomedicine, like science itself (Kuhn 1970; Latour and Woolgar 1979; Richter 1972), is not an objective, acultural system of knowledge but one that emerged out of a particular historical moment in the social formation of Western society in much the same way as Spiritualism has.

Contemporary biomedical practice had its beginnings in seventeenth- and eighteenth-century Europe[1] and like any other system of knowledge is socially and culturally constructed (Ingleby 1982; Young 1981; Wright and Treacher 1982) and reflects themes of the society and culture of which it forms part. For example, biomedicine's model of the human body as a standardized machine and sickness as the breaking down of its component parts (Berliner 1975;

Osherson and Amara Singham 1981; Turner 1984) mirrors the predominance of machines in modern society.

In 1800 sickness was conceived chiefly in individual terms (Jewson 1976). According to Rosenberg, "Even epidemic disease was understood to be an unbalanced state in a particular individual, imbalance resulting from the sum of interactions between an individual's constitutional endowment and his environment"(1986:40). "In the first third of the nineteenth century physicians through the Paris clinical school began to consider disease as a specific, ordinarily lesion-based entity that reenacted itself in every individual sufferer. Lesions discernible at post-mortem could be correlated with symptoms exhibited during the patient's life" (Rosenberg 1986:42).

Because biomedical knowledge and practices form part of a cultural system, they are subject to anthropological scrutiny in much the same way as any other cultural practices the world over. Focus on biomedical activities allows us to address profound issues pertaining to the nature of medical systems in general, and to health, sickness, and the healing process.

In my previous work I focused on patients' responses to treatment in order to gain an understanding of the requisites of recovery and the healing process, of the beneficial components of a medical system, and of patients' expectations of treatment. In this book I continue to pose similar questions concerning the healing processes by focusing on biomedical treatment in Mexico. By addressing the question of patient- perceived therapeutic outcome, the study underscores various components of biomedicine that differentially influence patients' responses to it, including specific constituent aspects of the medical encounter, and permits us to identify universal and culturally molded aspects of biomedical practice. By examining how patients perceive biomedical treatment we also gain a better understanding of how human beings deal with and explain the existential human dilemma of sickness and the requisites for recovery. To understand the healing process is to understand the web of interconnections between sickness and recovery, as well as the therapeutic regimens that people select to alleviate their sickness.

There was a time when medicine was purely a theoretical science (Pellegrino and Thomasma 1981), when the patient's perspective was unimportant. But medicine is no longer a theoretical discipline; it has become goal oriented, and its goals are to cure the patients. As a goal-oriented profession, the patient's perception is the essence of medicine's realization of its goals, and "the prized objectivity of the physician must yield somewhat to the patient's report. However objective he may wish to be, the physician has always to rely on the history, the story really, which is largely the patient's subjective report" (Spiro 1986:3).

To understand how people comprehend and manage their illness and what makes them well has practical consequences as well. Human beings relinquish sickness when they perceive themselves recovered, irrespective of objective medical measures. Until then they continue to engage in a quest for a cure by "doctor shopping" at great expense to themselves and the nation (Calnan 1988, 1988a; Finkler 1985; Fitzpatrick et al. 1983; Trostle et al. 1983; Tuckett et al. 1985).

Elsewhere (Finkler 1985) I discussed at great length the difficulties of assessing therapeutic outcomes of any type of healing system including biomedicine. While there is an extensive literature dealing with issues pertaining to the feasibility of assessing biomedical treatment outcomes,[2] any measure of medical treatment has its pitfalls, not the least of which is the obvious fact that diseases are self-limiting and that in some measure the body heals itself with or without ministration. For these and other technical reasons it is difficult to establish the efficacy of any type of therapy. According to Pellegrino (1979) therapeutic efficacy is defined as "the capability of an agent to alter the statistically predictable natural course of the disease" (256). At present with the exception of antimicrobial agents, there are no therapeutic agents capable of removing the causes of most diseases (Pellegrino 1979). A large array of impairments, including many chronic conditions, lack a cure comparable to that for microbial disease (Thomas 1977). If the underlying causes of most pathologies cannot be eliminated, how then can effective treatment be assessed?

In fact, researchers have been locked in a controversy as to what, if anything, ought to be measured. Some have argued that inasmuch as it is impossible to define efficacy, owing to a host of intervening variables, medical interventions can be assessed only by determining whether standard therapeutic procedures have been followed.[3] Such procedures include the use of medical histories, physical examinations, laboratory tests, and other technical diagnostic interventions. Alternatively, others have failed to find any relationship (Lindsay et al. 1976) or only a tenuous one (Nobrega et al. 1977) between performance of medical procedures and outcomes; still others have found that therapeutic outcomes are dependent on psychosocial variables unrelated to the care received by patients (Cay et al. 1975).

In this study my aim is not to seek objective measures of outcome of the treatment patients received in the hospital. The measures in this study are subjective, as assessed by the patients themselves. In the words of Spiro (1986), "Relief of symptoms is important even when the physician is not sure what is wrong with a patient" (6). Concomitantly, recovery attributions open a window to the nature of the sickness and its etiology. My findings suggest that differentially perceived responses to biomedical treatment are associated with a concatenation of factors encompassing certain objective conditions of a person's existence, distinct aspects of the medical encounter, and what I identify as *life's lesions*, by which I mean embodied, perceived adverse existence that is also linked to the onset of the sickness itself.

Therapeutic outcomes and the healing process are, in fact, tied to the nature of the sickness, and as we come to understand what makes people well, we also gain new insights into what makes people sick. From this vantage point, the book is concerned with the anthropology of sickness: the various individual, social, and cultural factors that are linked with an episodic disorder and its resolution.

In my previous work I found that people uniformly resort to biomedicine as their initial treatment option. While there is an extensive body of literature on folk-curing cross-culturally, including folk healing in Mexico,[4] little is known about how patients perceive, respond to and interpret biomedical treatment in other cultures (Helman 1981) or in the developing nations, including Mexico (Pendleton and Hasler 1983). My study of biomedical practice generated questions that had not arisen in my study of Spiritualist therapeutics, however. While Spiritualist healing is a widespread religious and healing movement in Mexico and Latin America, it is a folk rather than professional medical regimen (Kleinman 1978) not formally sanctioned by the Mexican state.

Biomedicine, on the other hand, is the reigning health care delivery system in both the private and public sectors supported by the state apparatus. It was introduced into Mexico following Mexico's independence from Spain in the nineteenth century. Its development parallels that in Europe and the United States. Contemporary biomedicine was spawned in Western Europe and the United States, and it has become the prevailing international system of health care. Our goal as anthropologists is not only to identify biomedicine's roots in Western Europe's cultural past but to examine its specific cultural underpinnings, and to assess its invariant and its changing aspects, those features of practice that remain international in scope and those that are shaped and transformed by cultural comprehensions and social conditions. How does biomedicine become constructed in a society in which it was introduced after it had already taken root in Europe?

We are beginning to learn more and more about how biomedicine is disparately practiced in different cultures.[5] In her study of Asian medicine, Lock (1980) observed that while biomedical practice in Japan shows American influences, beneath its Western appearance are traditional Japanese values. Thus, upon closer inspection Western medicine is "modernized in a uniquely Japanese way" (225). Cross-cultural studies have attended chiefly to patients' choices among treatment options, between folk healing and biomedicine.[6] More recently biomedicine has become a central concern for study in Western settings[7] and, perhaps more significantly, outside Western industrial societies. With few exceptions[8] there is a dearth of anthropological studies of contemporary biomedicine and its practice in Latin America in general and Mexico in particular.

We need to assess how Mexican social and cultural realities influence biomedical practice and how day-to-day biomedical therapeutic practices, gleaned from observations and open-ended discussions with physicians, contribute to emerging sociocultural forms and ideologies (Cicourel 1983) and to sustaining and restructuring the social order, what Giddens identified as the structuration process (Giddens 1979, 1981; Waitzkin 1983). We must probe the ways in which biomedicine exercises its dominance and penetrates the consciousness of the society in which it is practiced. In short, we must explore the interplay between micro- and macrophenomena in order to reveal the intertwining of social processes and individual human behavior.

In the process of examining the transformations of a system of knowledge from one society to another, we gain a glimpse of how biomedical beliefs and practices have seeped down to the folk level of understanding by a process analogous to that of sixteenth-century Spanish medicine, which came to influence contemporary folk medicine (Fabrega and Silver 1973). Consider, for example, that biomedically prescribed medications have become incorporated into folk pharmacopoeia and various pharmaceutical drugs are routinely self-prescribed by patients and folk healers alike, in much the same way as herbal teas and other traditional remedies are (Finkler 1985). Neumelubrina, Enteroveoforma, and Terremicine are routinely sold in every corner grocery store.

But on a more profound level, the biomedical model has introduced etiological understandings that have been incorporated into the pool of folk attributions. Two that merit consideration are the inheritability of sickness, whether transmitted by an ancestor or by the mother during pregnancy, and the concept of nerves. Concepts of the inheritability of sickness were absent in Prehispanic America (Ortiz de Montellano 1989, 1989a) and they did not prevail in Spanish medicine. During the Colonial period it was believed that humors were altered but not necessarily passed on from father to son (McVaugh 1989). However, scholars have demonstrated that the concept of heredity found its way into medical prominence when medicine became wedded to science (Yoxen 1982) during the second half of the nineteenth century. Moreover, the notion that a mother transmitted dangerous substances to her offspring became current during this period (Rosenberg 1974). "It was in France, indeed, rather than the United States that the application of broad hereditarian schemata to the explanation of social realities first became important in academic circles" (Rosenberg 1974:217). It was a "product of mid-century French psychiatry and appeared in the guise of what later came to be called the 'degeneration thesis'" (Rosenberg 1974:217). As Rosenberg showed concepts of inheritability survived in the twentieth century and they helped lend scientific legitimacy to "all those marginal conditions--migraine headache, hysteria, obsessional states, anxiety, depression, homosexuality, which were gradually becoming part of the newly specialized neurologist's clinical world" (218). These were accepted as true disease states and not mere impostors or evils; they were given a physical foundation through inheritance. Not surprisingly, states of anxiety and headaches became tied to neurology as they currently are in Mexican biomedical practice, since Mexican biomedicine was greatly influenced by French medicine.

The notion of the inheritability of disease is transmitted to patients at every medical consultation with the taking of a medical history of the family, as virtually all physicians question patients about the family diseases. Thus, the taking of a medical history imposes a genetic model on one's experience of the body. The attribution of sickness to heredity imposes order on a chaotic world, on disturbances a physician cannot explain, concomitantly absolving the individual for his sickness; it suggests a certain inevitability to the diagnosis and reinforces the patient's continuity with his or her ancestors.

The belief in familial transmission of disease engages the Mexican in a profound contradiction, however. On the one hand, it affirms the continuity of the family in which he or she is embedded; on the other, it afflicts the familial unit, the source of a Mexican's identity, with pathology.

This contradiction may come into consciousness at a time when a person experiences symptoms and suspects having a serious disease, including heart failure or cancer, that is held in popular belief to be inherited from one's family. It is not surprising that when patients were questioned about what they feared most about their presenting symptoms, they often cited mental illness, cancer, heart disease, or other life-threatening conditions experienced by family members. Thus, not uncommonly Mexicans associate their symptomatology with that of a member of the family who has experienced a similar condition as, for example, Serge, who was afraid he was going mad because his uncle had gone crazy.

Significantly, too, "nerves" is an important folk etiological explanation for illness, as well as an illness state (Finkler 1985, 1989).[9] It is quite likely that the folk concept of nerves has its roots in nineteenth-century biomedical beliefs when neurologists widened the categories of ailments they chose to treat to include phobias, anxieties, and depression (Rosenberg 1986:44). "Emphasis of the weakness of nerves coincided with the rise of neurology as a medical speciality" (Sicherman 1977:39) in the mid-nineteenth century. "Knowledge of the brain and nervous system advanced rapidly in Europe after 1860 as experimental physiologists demonstrated that fixed parts of the brain controlled specific motor activities" (39). "By the late 1860s, important teaching and hospital positions in neurology had been established in England, France, and the German-speaking world, a sign that the specialty had come of age" (Sicherman 1977:40). Mexican physicians reinforce the folk concept by attributing many of the ills patients experience to nerves, and they often situate their cause in the nervous system.

To reiterate an assertion made earlier, the anthropological scrutiny of biomedical practice rests on the assumption that biomedicine is neither asocial nor acultural but that it is molded by and molds the society of which it forms part. "Modern medicine, it seems, is not simply a body of instrumental knowledge but serves as a set of categories that we use both to filter and construct our experience" (Wright and Treacher 1982:6). It is shaped by nonscientific factors (Gaines 1979; Gordon 1988), including cultural and idiosyncratic ones.

I examine the medical encounter from the vantage point of a dramaturgical event because of the doctor's and patient's disparate experiences of suffering, and because the medical model guiding physicians incorporates a temporal dimension while the patient's sickness experience transcends time. The drama also emanates from the struggle between Mexico's historical tradition of clinical practice and contemporary technological medicine, which subordinates the physicians and their clinical skills to technological management. The inherent drama and struggles are not unique to Mexican biomedical practice, but they take on a uniquely Mexican cast.

A casual visitor to the Salud Hospital would detect little difference between it and a hospital with scarce resources in a large metropolitan city in the United States. The lighting is poor, the sparse furniture old, the wooden chairs in the waiting rooms uncomfortable, and the cubicles where doctors attend their patients are small and congested. On first glance, a foreign visitor would find the architectural outlay, the technological apparatus, the personnel dressed in white, the directories to the various medical services, and the encounter between doctor and patient familiar. Upon closer scrutiny we begin to glean its distinctively Mexican character when we listen to the physicians' etiological explanations or attend to the idiosyncracies of the physicians' diagnoses.

I opted to carry out the study in Mexico for several reasons. First, I had extensive experience in both rural and urban Mexico. Second, it is a propitious site for exploring several important theoretical issues that bear on the diffusion of systems of knowledge, especially biomedicine. Third, Mexico is especially interesting for the American reader because of the extensive border we share. More important, as an advanced developing nation it possesses all the modern medical technological accoutrements, and contemporary medical education there is nourished through North American textbooks and teachings. I therefore hypothesized that because of Mexico's cultural affinity and geographic proximity to the United States, biomedical practice would retain its international cast there, a hypothesis that is only partially borne out. The findings of this study illuminate those aspects of biomedical practice that are subject to cultural transformations and those that remain invariant. Fourth, my extensive experience with alternative medical systems in Mexico, especially Spiritualist healing, enabled me to compare two disparate therapeutic regimes and patients' responses to them using similar methodologies to assess the universal and specific nature of sickness and recovery requisites. Few studies have been done in developing nations that address these issues in tandem.

While this book examines sickness and recovery as mediated biomedically, these human experiences are separated only for analytical purposes. These phenomena are, in fact, embedded in Mexican lived experience and are not independent of one another. The study of sickness and recovery concomitant with therapeutic modalities is a window to and reverberates on social and cultural processes in general and on ideology and social relations in particular. In the course of the presentation, we learn about daily life, especially about Mexican ideologies and the contradictions and conflicts they create as they relate to the spheres of work, male-female and parent-child relations, morality marked by emotional discharges, and beliefs about witchcraft.

Individual crises expressed symptomatologically may be embedded in the contradictions between the realities of social class differences and socioculturally produced ideologies of equality, in differential power relations between males and females, and between hegemonic and folk ideologies. These are the types of conditions that intrude on one's sense of coherence (Antonovsky 1980). People are caught up in unresolved contradictions that become imprinted on the body and that not only contribute to sickness (Helman 1987; Turner 1984) but also militate against its resolution.

The ascendency of positivism and the ideology of "progress" in the nineteenth century have imbued Mexicans with a hegemonic theme that everybody can progress, which in contemporary times means, advance economically. Industrial development gives a thrust to expanding wants and aspirations and a thirst for economic goods to which the people in this study have limited access.

Wolf (1982), describing capitalist society in general, could have been speaking about Mexico when he stated, "In the capitalist mode the regnant ideology assumes the equality of all participants in the market, in the face of basic distinctions in political and economic power between capitalists and workers. While all social actors are defined as participants in commodity exchange, the mode is structurally dependent upon the 'unequal factor endowment' of owners of capital and sellers of labor power. Ideology-making thus transmutes the distinction between classes into distinctions of virtue and merit. Success is demonstrated by the ability to acquire valued commodities; hence, inability to consume signals social defeat" (389-90). The differential access to economic resources (Felix 1977) conflicts with the prevailing ideology, and "social defeat" brings indignation and anger, encapsulated in one patient's question, "Why is it that I work so hard and I get nowhere, and I have nothing?"

Moreover, Catholicism, and later positivism, with its attendant emphasis on modernity and the ethos of progress, have denigrated beliefs in witchcraft, beliefs that embroil people in ambiguities and inner conflicts of believing and not believing. On the one hand, only "ignorant" people believe in witchcraft. On the other, to believe that one's illness was produced by malfeasance removes the responsibility for the sickness from the sick person; denial of etiological belief in witchcraft requires assumptions of culpability and a search for exculpation. Beliefs in witchcraft engage the individual in yet another moral dilemma. It is believed that when one has a strong character, meaning that one is "an angry person," one is protected from witchcraft; yet anger is, in the Mexican view, the singularly most important source of illness (Fabrega and Manning 1979).

Male-female and parent-child relations generate powerful emotions, especially anger, and when one "makes an anger" and one "gets nerves," one also risks getting sick. The experience encircles the individual in a contradiction produced in response to social interaction and moral evaluations between what ought to be and what is respecting these relations. More and more scholars have come to recognize that emotions such as anger are culturally constructed moral evaluations of the life world (Bedford 1986; Harre 1986a; Lutz 1985; Solomon 1984). "The concept of emotion defined here as culturally constructed and socially negotiated about such situations, remains useful therefore, given the assumption that human groups universally find certain types of events to be especially problematic and that they attempt to make sense of them variously as biological, social, moral, psychological, or otherworldly dilemmas" (Lutz 1985:92).

Anger is in direct relation to the action of the body: One experiences the emotion through the body (Rosaldo 1984). In the words of one informant, "I feel anger in my body." It is not that the mind influences the body and crafts its sickness; it is that the mind and body are experienced as one, that anger is felt physically and expressed symptomatologically. Emotions such as anger are interpretations of the world (Solomon 1984) involving social relationships that have gone awry (Levy 1984). The study of emotions such as anger "require[s] careful attention to the details of local systems of rights and obligations, of criteria of value and so on. In short, these emotions cannot seriously be studied without attention to the local moral order" (Harre 1986: 6). The expression of emotions involves an understanding of moral rules (Armon-Jones 1986).

It is my contention that the emotional discharges resulting from conflicts in which people are engaged and that are singularly significant etiologically in Mexico are instrumental not only in producing sickness but also in impeding perceived recovery. Individual patients are wrapped in contradictions whose template is economic deficits, concepts of social justice, and cultural under-standings of proper human conduct, including obligations of men to women and parents to children; in short, how men and women *ought* to behave under given circumstances.

More women than men are engaged in conflicts and dilemmas that produce anger and nerves. Not surprisingly, almost six times more women (261) than men (44) comprise our sample of sick individuals with *non-life-threatening, sub-acute* ailments, as was the case in my previous study (Finkler 1985). More women than men experience anger and nerves to which they attribute a sickness. Women's differential structural positions promote emotional discharges and generate contradictions stemming from situations that are morally reprehensible and contrary to what one knows ought to be--the kind that produce anger, nerves, and sickness. While this book is not specifically about women, we gain insight into women's lives and issues concerning women because they, more than men, are enmeshed in dilemmas that elicit the anger and nerves that subjectively make people sick.

It has been suggested that all our knowledge is embodied knowledge, that all our experience becomes part of our bodies, but not all our experiences produce sickness. Numerous distinctions have been made between disease, illness, and sickness. In my previous work I distinguished between disease and illness, with disease referring to a biological and biochemical malfunction and illness as impaired functioning as perceived by the patient within a cultural context (Eisenberg 1977; Finkler 1985; Kleinman 1980; Young 1983). Disease refers to "patterns of causes correlated with clusters of signs and symptoms which constitute the illness at hand" (Englehard 1975:135), while illness pertains to self-perceived states of ill health. In this study I employ the term "sickness" to encompass both disease and illness.

Sickness, as Brody (1987) pointed out, is an ontological assault affecting our very being within the context of our existence; it also speaks to the suffering of anatomical and life's lesions. By sickness I mean an assault on the very being of the human body as it is embedded in an inimical ecological environment, and in day-to-day existence played out in a given social and cultural milieu (Kleinman 1988). Sickness embraces suffering carved by life's lesions, and its alleviation requires concomitantly a transformation of both anatomical and life's lesions.

Sickness signifies the embodiment of generalized adversity and contradictions and re-creates in the internal world of the body the perceived contradictions and disorder of the external world. Informed by Merleau-Ponty (1963), who proposed that the body communicates to the world and the world becomes expressed by the body, Kleinman (1986) observed, "The body feels and expresses social problems" (194). "The body mediates structure and cultural meaning making them part of the physiology" (195).

An individual's health and sickness states are interconnected with other people and the milieu in which he or she exists (Dossey 1982). Consider, for a moment, human beings evolved as social sentient beings, whose very day-to-day existences are embedded in a social as well as physical environment which is an extension of the human body. Or, "Contrary to Objectivism, we are not merely mirrors of a nature that determines our concepts in one and only one way. Instead, our structured experience is an organism-environment interaction in which both poles are altered and transformed through ongoing historical process" (Johnson 1987: 207). The lived body affects and is being affected by the world (Gadow 1980; Spicker 1984). An assault on the day-to-day existence which forms our environment and the attendant contradictions produces life's lesions in tandem with anatomical lesions, in much the same way as an insult to the body inscribes its lesion on the person's life. In keeping within a phenomenological framework, I propose that sickness is the embodiment (Leder 1985, 1990) of adverse existential, environmental, and bodily conditions. If we accept the Merleau-Pontian premise, as I believe we ought, then sickness is as much the embodiment of adverse environmental social and existential conditions, with their ensuing experiences of suffering, as it is the embodiment of pathogens.

Adversity often becomes condensed in contradictions and expressed by culturally constructed emotional discharges, especially anger, revealing moral indignation about how the world ought to be and is not that in Mexican cultural understandings is illness producing. While sickness is universally embodied adversity and embodied contradictions (Turner 1984), each culture gives specific meanings to its expression and its attribution. Symptomatologies and their attendant meanings and attributions become culturally molded (Good and Good 1981; Helman 1985a; Zborowski 1952). Similarly, the resolution of a sickness, the perceived therapeutic outcome, is linked to ministrations by health providers and to the provider's adroitness in transforming the patient's existence and resolving the paradoxes that had enmeshed the individual.

Biomedicine's focus is on the body that is defined by the clinical interaction (Pellegrino and Thomasma 1981). When patients seek treatment from the physician, they cease to take their bodies for granted, and they seek ministration for sensations newly felt or of which they were not mindful before (Leder 1990). Physicians usually regard patients' presenting symptoms in literal and physical terms. Doctors are innocent of the fact that patients' presenting symptoms are conduits encapsulating the social, cultural, and moral order in which the body plays out its existence. Given the prevailing medical model, the physician's armamentarium lacks a cure to transform the patients' existence, to heal concurrently anatomical and life's lesions. The requisite transformations require societal changes above and beyond the capacities of any one physician or even of a healing system (also Waitzkin 1983).

In recent years biomedicine has attended to extrasomatic factors of disease by implicating sociological and psychological factors (Rosenberg 1986), attributes of the individual, in the production of "illegitimate" illness or somatized conditions (Barsky 1979, 1981; Quill 1985). Behavioral medicine, on the other hand, has adopted the "stress" model for explaining disease and illness. The former places the blame on psychodynamic aspects of the patient's being, the latter on external, amorphous societal pressures with which the individual cannot cope (also Kirmayer 1988). Behavioral medicine has become as reductionist as the biomedical model itself (Engel 1977). Whenever a condition eludes a physician's diagnosis, it is attributed either to the failings of the patient's psyche or to an impassive and incompetent individual lacking moral and judgmental abilities, unable to deal with daily pressures.

While both the psychosomatic and the stress models attempt a holistic view of human beings, these paradigms remove the individual from his or her embodied self and the flux of sickness that transcends time and is anchored in the rhythm of day-to-day actualities. These assessments strip the patient of the capacity to judge and to evaluate his or her existence. While we have all experienced stress at some point in our lives, and the people of this study live under ongoing stressful environmental and economic conditions, the exploration of such stressors must be fine-tuned to take into consideration nuances of meaning of specific life events coupled with each actor's perceived life conditions. Individuals, as thinking and evaluating beings, differentially perceive their familial and social interactions within the parameters of their cultural pool of understandings. Esperanza lives in dire poverty and her suffering is as much connected with it as it is to her husband's abandonment of her, along with her belief that the husband's mistress is bewitching her. Another woman had conflicting relationships with her neighbor which she held led her to "make angers" that produced her sickness rather than her miserable poverty.

It is important to reassert the proposition advanced earlier that patients seek to alleviate symptoms that embody the physical, social, and cultural circumstances, the evaluations they make of their existence, and their moral sensibilities. The symptoms cannot be reduced to any one life event or to any one stressor but must be viewed within the context of the life of each individual, his or her social relations, and the contradictions in which he or she is entwined.

The interpretation of the empirical data is informed by concepts developed in phenomenology, in the anthropology of knowledge, and in critical theory. But most of all, the interpretations are guided by the physicians and patients themselves and the rich ethnographic and quantitative materials I gathered during the field stay coupled with my previous extensive sojourns in Mexico. I combine an interpretative approach with the folk view to make sense of all that I observed and heard. While from the "native's point of view" (Geertz 1973) people are intuitively aware that their sickness embodies their existence, they are not always cognizant of the specific aspects of their lives that are implicated in their condition, be they residential structural arrangements, moral evaluations, or other factors that impede recovery. It is the anthropologist's task to interpret the flow of patients' experience and understandings within the context of their lives.

The empirical data are based upon over 400 taped observations of doctor-patient encounters, 267 in-depth interviews with patients in the hospital, lengthy open-ended discussions and narratives, and guided interview schedules administered to 205 patients in their homes located throughout metropolitan Mexico. I also maintained an ongoing contact with many of the patients. While only a small fraction of the case materials and doctor-patient encounters can be presented in this book, the in-depth observations at the hospital and contacts with patients in their homes deepened my understanding of biomedicine, patients' sickness, and its resolution within the context of each patient's life. This invaluable experience illuminated not only patients' responses to treatment but also the intracultural variability extant in complex societies such as Mexico City, and the caution we must exercise in generalizing about cultural behaviors in urban environments the size of Mexico City. I realized that while behavior is often guided by cultural understandings, many dilemmas that human beings face are probably universal, especially those bearing on male-female relations, generational conflicts between parents and children, and some produced by a recently developed universal economic culture dominated by consumerism and expanding wants for material possessions.

It is not the intention of this endeavor to either glorify or demean biomedicine or its practitioners. There are no heroes or villains in this book. Both physicians and patients are people who must deal with and resolve contradictions that emerge out of the world in which they live. While the patients of the study share common cultural understandings, for the most part they are inheritors of great poverty and blatant inequalities, and they reside in an inimical physical environment that adversely affects their health. Nevertheless, they are not simply passive beings lacking moral judgments and abilities to evaluate their lives under harsh conditions. To the contrary, they are people with great dignity, mindful of the complexities of their lives and active in the struggle to resolve the disorder of their existence; each faces decisive dilemmas that must be located within the context of their existence. These illuminate differential responses to treatment.

The physicians discussed in this study are competent, well-meaning, and themselves caught in binds over which they lack control, especially those generated by the biomedical model which guides their ministrations and sets them in conflict with their intuitive understandings as bearers of Mexican culture. Modern medicine and its technology has dazzled the imagination with its spectacular achievements. Biomedicine as a primary health care delivery system has its strengths as well as its limitations, however. The limitations are as much due to the narrowness of its model as to adversities experienced by patients over which individual physicians have no control. Physicians are caught in dilemmas that limit their ability to maneuver non-life-threatening, sub-acute conditions because they are encompassed by a powerful state bureaucracy to whose vagaries they, like their patients, are subject.

In sum, it is my conviction that biomedicine must be considered from a multidimensional perspective in order to gain an understanding of it as a culturally constituted health care delivery system. Similarly, patients' responses to its ministrations cannot simply be measured by any single criterion of efficacy, such as medication prescribed, the technology employed, patient compliance, or even the doctor-patient relationship. We must consider these in relation to the lived experience of the patient and his or her suffering. Only in this manner will we begin to get at the roots of sickness and the healing process. This contention is developed in the following chapters.

The study is situated in a particular, historical context (shortly following the cataclysmic earthquake in Mexico City in 1985, and in the midst of an especially harsh economic crisis), but the theoretical issues it addresses rest outside of time and place. The book will be of interest to Latin America scholars in general and Mexicanists in particular, to scholars concerned with sickness and health care delivery from a cross-cultural perspective, especially those interested in biomedicine and its practices cross-culturally, and to health professionals concerned with the healing process and international health in developing nations.

Each of the chapters presents empirical data relevant to specific theoretical issues touched upon in these introductory remarks. Part I highlights aspects of Mexican society and culture that bear on the discussion in Part II. Chapter 2 describes the cultural landscape of Mexico City to situate the patients and their lives in context. By way of additional background, Chapter 3 furnishes Mexican cultural etiological understandings and cultural conceptions of symptomatologies that are relevant to the understanding of biomedical practices. Chapter 4 furnishes a synoptic view of Mexico's health care delivery system, including the variety of health options such as homeopathy available to the people when confronted by sickness.

In Part II attention is turned to biomedicine and its practice in Mexico from a historical perspective. Here we observe the permutations of biomedicine as defined by cultural forms. Chapter 5 provides a historical overview of the reciprocal developments in medicine and Mexico's political history, with a brief discussion of medical practices during the Preconquest and Colonial periods and their legacies in contemporary medicine. The central focus is, however, on biomedicine when it was introduced into Mexico from France in the nineteenth century.

Chapter 6 explores how biomedicine is practiced in contemporary Mexico based upon my field observations in one hospital. In this chapter I identify and furnish a model of the international, the culturally specific, and the idiosyncratic aspects of routine biomedical practice of non-life-threatening, sub-acute sickness. Chapter 7 reveals the variability of biomedical practices as we meet eight physicians and learn about their backgrounds.

Chapter 8 focuses on the medical consultation as a dramaturgical event by providing a glimpse of biomedical practice, using verbatim transcriptions. In this chapter we meet the individual patients during the medical encounter, learn how patients present symptoms and how physicians deal with similar symptoms presented by different patients. The verbatim transcriptions of entire consultations, rarely provided in such detail, are presented to allow the reader to make his or her interpretations as well.

In Part III our concern turns to the patients and their responses to the treatments they received during the consultations. In Chapter 9 I present sociodemographic profiles of the 205 patients and their medical conditions as diagnosed by the attending physicians we met in Chapter 7. In Chapter 10 I present patient-perceived treatment outcomes in aggregated terms and identify statistically significant variables relevant to the medical consultation that influence differential perceptions of recovery. Here we learn of specific constituents of the doctor-patient encounter that influence patients' perceived recovery.

In Chapter 11 I return to the patients we first met in Chapters 7 and 8 during the medical consultation to learn about the outcomes of their treatments and to analyze in depth those aspects of patients' lives that illuminate their differential recovery responses. Chapter 12 of Part IV compares biomedical and sacred healing of the Spiritualist kind along several dimensions to shed light on the similarities and dissimilarities between the two types of health care delivery systems and the allure of each. By way of conclusion Chapter 13 reflects on the major contribution of these findings to the anthropology of medical knowledge, sickness, and recovery. The methodology is briefly described in the Appendix.

Notes

1. Sess Ackerknecht 1967; Berliner 1975; Foucault 1975; Reiser 1978; Shryock 1979; Starr 1982.

2. See Chapter 8 in Finkler 1985 for a detailed discussion of this issue.

3. See, for example, McAuliffe 1978, 1979; Starfield 1974, 1979; Starfield and Scheff 1972.

4. See the bibliography in Finkler 1985.

5. See Dunlop and Inch 1972; Field 1976; Henderson and Cohen 1984; Jennette 1986; Jordan 1983; Kleinman 1980, 1986; Lock 1977, 1980, 1988; Low 1985; Maretzki 1989; O'Brien,1984; Townsend 1978; Unschuld 1980; Vander Geest and Whyte 1988; Maretzki 1985, 1988, 1989; Weisberg 1984. For an overview of biomedicine and anthropology, see Hahn and Kleinman 1983.

6. See, for example, Finkler 1981; Lieban 1976; Nichter 1980; Sussman 1981; Young 1981; and numerous others.

7. See, Comaroff and Maguire 1981; Hahn and Gaines 1985; Helman 1985; Lock 1986; Lock and Gordon 1988; Plough 1981.

8. Ordonez Plaja et al. 1968; Low 1982, 1985; Selwyn and Ruiz de Chávez 1985; Stebbins 1986.

9. Nerves, in fact, is not a uniquely Mexican phenomenon. See, for example, Davis and Low (1989) for discussion of nerves in other cultural settings; also Low 1981.

PART ONE

The Setting

2

The Mexican Context

This chapter highlights aspects of life in Mexico City that are relevant to our understanding of physicians and patients and to sickness and recovery.

Prior to World War II Mexico was predominantly a rural society, but within the decades that followed a great demographic shift took place favoring the cities, especially Mexico City, the capital.[1] Mexico City, the political and industrial capital of contemporary Mexico, bedazzles the casual visitor, as it did the Spanish conquerors (Díaz de Castillo 1963), with its broad avenues, its lush parks, its modern luxury houses, its shopping malls, as well as its pulsating tempo, traffic congestions, and polluted air. The people's faces and the architecture attest to a confluence of cultures delineated by three predominant historical periods: the Preconquest, when great Indian civilizations flourished, followed by 300 years of Spanish Colonial domination, and the contemporary period that was launched with Mexico's independence from Spain in 1810. Contemporary Mexico City, as other capital cities in Latin America (Perlman 1976), discloses glitter and great wealth, as well as great poverty. The subjects of our concern, the inheritors and producers of a rich convergent culture, do not reside in the elegant houses or shop in the shimmering shopping centers, however. The people of this study inhabit metropolitan Mexico City, encompassing the Federal District and its environs. Some of the neighborhoods in which the people reside are situated on the slopes of the surrounding mountains; others are vecindades, rooms built around courtyards and with shared facilities.

Mexico City is renowned for its untoward physical environment. Its geographical location in a valley a mile above sea level, combined with several million motor vehicles and unenforced emission control laws, renders the capital one of the world's most polluted environments.[2] While the adverse environment affects all social segments of Mexican society, the people in this study are subject to environmental hardships because the neighborhoods in which they live are especially affected by the inimical environmental and public health conditions (Córdova 1988; Evans et al. 1981; López Acuña 1976, 1978). The smog is differentially distributed in the vastness of the city; the impoverished neighborhoods are located near the industrial zones and the air there is especially polluted. Some neighborhoods are situated on sandy terrains that produce dust storms during the dry winter season. According to some physicians, the dust storms transmit parasitic infection, as do the impoverished sanitary facilities, which contaminate the food and water. Mexico City residents are cognizant of the fact that the inimical habitat in which they live reverberates upon their health. Not uncommonly they complain of "anginas" or sore throats, respiratory problems, and a variety of other conditions that they invariably attribute to the environment in general and the smog in particular.

Twenty-six percent of the sample population and most of those I followed on a regular basis reside in Nezahualcoyótl (Neza), separated from Mexico City by a wide avenue, and connected to it by a network of private minibuses and a subway. On one side Neza borders the Federal District, and on the other it is flanked by a garbage heap more than a mile long. In Neza, unlike in the capital, only the major avenues are paved. During the rainy season torrential rains stagnate to form lagoons (also Velez-Ibañez 1983) and the unpaved side streets are littered with infrequently collected garbage and loitering dogs.

Most dwellings in Neza are constructed of cinder block and are enclosed by courtyards and iron gates. The dwellings are equipped with electricity and drainage; each courtyard contains a cistern into which drinking water is piped. In many courtyards one also encounters pigs, chickens, and occasionally a sheep. The dwellings often house extended families, and like similar compounds in villages throughout Mexico, the dwellings "grow" commensurate with the growth of the family. Hence, most dwellings appear unfinished, as they expand to accommodate married children, parents, or siblings who migrate into the city. In older communities parents and married children often live on the same block, if not in the same compound.

There are many government-supported local health clinics and hospitals providing tertiary care throughout the city, but many patients living in Neza seek treatment in Salud Hospital, which can be reached by subway and busses. There are permanently enclosed and weekly rotating markets in most neighborhoods. These sell fresh produce and portable merchandise. In Neza the major avenues house grocery stores, bakeries, liquor stores, small appliance and furniture stores, car repair shops, and a variety of other small service businesses. Not uncommonly a woman may sit on the side streets in front of a little table adjacent to her dwelling, selling chewing gum, shoelaces, candy, and tissues.

In Neza there is no industry to speak of. Of the 3 million inhabitants, the majority of those who are employed travel to work to Mexico City.

Consequently, the vast stretches of wide avenues are usually devoid of people in the streets during the day.[3] As one walks down the streets of Neza, one experiences a sense of outward tranquility reminiscent of a village community writ large, as if the migrants that started settling there in the 1940s replicated their natal villages.

Streets are paved in neighborhoods within the Federal District, and the dwellings contain running water, but the people live mainly in congested rented housing. Those who were displaced by the earthquake were living in windowless barracks with as many as fifteen people crammed into a ten by fifteen foot space, and as many as fifty families sharing washing, cooking, and toilet facilities.

From a macro perspective, the people in this study are known to belong to the poorest sector of Mexican society, and ample evidence shows the relationship between poverty and overall health status (Ingman and Thomas 1975; McKeown 1979). Nevertheless, the poor sector does not comprise an undifferentiated mass of people, as is evidenced from the differential amenities of the houses in the sample population. Most of the people residing in Neza own their dwellings and the land on which they stand.[4] Disparities exist between dwellings with respect to the number of people who reside in each, the overall construction, furnishings, and other comforts that differentiate families along economic lines. Some domiciles are covered with tin roofs, lack floors, and have outdoor facilities. Others have asbestos roofs and cement floors. Still others have cement roofing and floors, indoor toilets, and even a shower. The numerous people I got to know during this study differentially appraise and respond to the conditions of their lives, which reflects back on their health and recovery. In spite of their abject poverty, and hopes stifled by societal conditions, they experience joy when they watch their children grow, when they celebrate birthdays and baptisms, and when they attend Sunday family gatherings.

Although outwardly the communities appear tranquil, Marcel, a twenty-five-year-old male, voiced a prevailing view when, after indicating his desire to migrate to the United States, he stated, "I want to go there because look at the disorder I live in here, I live in chaos." As it happens, Marcel's statement pertains to the inhabitants' lack of legal protection from the police, from common criminals, and from drug traffickers in marijuana. Marcel implicated the police themselves for perpetrating an attack on him and other young men. Similarly, Alice, who lives in a vecindad in the heart of the city, noted that "there is no law" in Mexico City and that she had in fact gone to a renowned pilgrimage center to pray to the Virgin "to protect her against assaults by the police." Indeed, the dangers people feel resonate on their health. When a member of the family has not arrived at an expected time, mothers become submerged in worry, the kind of experience that causes one to get "nerves" and become sick.

Generally speaking, Mexican society views all inhabitants residing in Neza and in the other poor neighborhoods as dirty and ignorant. Many poor neighborhoods are reputed to be dangerous. Some physicians share these prejudicial beliefs about the poor, as is demonstrated by their questions about the frequency with which patients bathe, whether they can tell time, or why they came to live in congested Mexico City. Indeed, various men in the sample reported having been assaulted at one time or another, often by the police, and parents with teenage boys fear most that their sons will join a neighborhood gang. Only a small segment of the poor population, some of whom may be policemen,[5] engage in crime and drug trafficking. For the most part the people, including those of the study, work hard to eke out a meager subsistence and are themselves victims of crime.

No discussion of Mexico City's physical environment in the 1980s can fail to refer to the earthquake of 1985, which proved to be a cataclysmic event both literally and metaphorically in Mexican history. Earthquakes are not uncommon and there are many references to them in Precolumbian myths and histories, as in the Codex Vaticanus 3778 or Codex Rios (Ortiz de Montellano 1989). Because of the city's high population density and contemporary architectural construction, the 1985 earthquake had a particularly devastating effect on the city and its inhabitants. Two earthquakes occurred in succession, and the second one proved to be even more frightening than the first. It destroyed thousands of lives and it affected the health of the survivors. Many thought the "end of the earth" had come.

In the wake of this destruction, hospitals[6] and dwellings were devastated and thousands of people were dislocated from their homes, separated from their families, and lost their jobs. People were left homeless, living on the streets and in barracks under untold hardships. Many of those living in Neza remained without water for several months. Moreover, people were left profoundly fearful of another occurrence in the future.

This earthquake has become a marker of time; people speak about their lives before and after the earthquake. It has taken on etiological significance as well, and it had a profound effect on people's health. Sixty-three percent of the men and 82 percent of the women in the study reported that they had been adversely affected by the earthquake. The majority developed a state of nerves or experienced a sudden fright, a *susto*, a condition that left people still "trembling" two years later. In the words of one woman, "the other day I trembled and I thought it was an earthquake, but it wasn't, it was me trembling." One man reported that his hands had not stopped trembling a year later. Quintessential, an eighteen-year-old girl, stated that the "earthquake passed through my body and has made me tremble since."

But while the earthquake generated fright and sickness, it also gave rise to acts of valor. Stories of heroism abound telling of how people's lives were saved in Salud Hospital, one of several that had been partially damaged. The disaster mobilized the populace to concerted action such as obtaining housing from the government and the Red Cross. Vecindades were destroyed, and a few families benefited from the disaster by having been relocated from the vecindades to better housing.

The earthquake became symbolic of the destabilization of the country by the economic crisis. In fact, the economy was the dominant, if not the sole, topic of all conversations among most sectors of Mexican society. It brought misfortune to the poor and the middle class. Many patients associated their sickness directly or indirectly with their day-to-day economic worries. The state of the economy had an impact on both physicians and patients and on the public sector of health care delivery. In fact, since the crisis began there was more than a 40 percent decrease in government expenditures on health care (Báez 1988).

Because of its significance in people's lives, the economy merits a brief overview without my making any attempt to elucidate its perplexities. Mexico is usually characterized as an industrially developing nation tied to the international market economy with its attendant economic disparities (Bizzarro 1981; Felix 1977; Gonzales Casanova 1980). With the oil boom of the 1970s the country enjoyed accelerated development on a national level, differentially beneficial to the elite and middle-class sectors. Rapid economic development coupled with an increase in the national debt was followed by a decrease in oil prices on the international market. This resulted in decreased revenues, leading to an economic crisis in 1982, at which time the government nationalized the banks and devalued the currency.[7] In a high-inflation market economy, wages failed to rise commensurate with daily price increases. People could not meet their minimal daily subsistence needs.[8] Despite the resiliency of the people, there exists great animosity towards the government. The people attributed the crisis to the foreign debt, to the patronage system, and to government corruption.

The economic crisis has severely affected the permanently employed, including physicians in the public sector who are government employees. In fact, physicians usually hold more than one post to maintain themselves and their families. Not only has the purchasing power of their governmental salaries diminished, but they have partially lost their private clientele. In the past, many people eligible for government health care services sought private physicians to avoid bureaucratic altercations. As a result of the economic crisis they have turned to the public health care sector.[9]

The economic crisis has been devastating to the urban poor. In the rural area where I had done fieldwork previously among the peasants (Finkler 1974, 1978, 1980), families were less affected economically by the economic crisis. Rural people are usually less dependent upon the cash economy and wage work. To illustrate, during the course of the study, the minimum wage in Mexico City increased by about 3,000 pesos, but the dollar equivalent and purchasing power decreased by 150 percent. Unlike urban dwellers, the peasantry is not solely dependent on wage labor for subsistence, nor is age a factor of employment. In the city many people, specially women above the age of forty, complained that they lacked employment. Almost 90 percent of the study population was impermanently employed and subsisted on petty commerce, odd jobs, and self-employment, which provided only a minimum wage. Families that kept animals supplemented their incomes by selling eggs or a pig. Carmen's husband, a street vendor selling plastic book covers, earned about 8,000 pesos a day (about $4), about half the amount Carmen said she required for daily subsistence to feed, dress, house, and pay for school supplies for her family of seven.

For those employed in factories, not only were wages very low but working conditions were also harsh. People remembered the ten-hour working days, airless and dark rooms, and filthy toilets. Roselind, who had worked in a dress factory destroyed by the earthquake, which killed most of the employees, recalled how she used to sneak out to run home to the bathroom because of the rats and cockroaches roaming around in the factory toilets and how she was not permitted to take a break to eat.

The industrialization of Mexico created a demand for an educated work force. To give one's children an education is to progress and participate in modern mainstream society. Whereas at one time primary school was a sufficient qualification for any job, at present not only high school, but preparatory school has become the sine qua non to gain entry to any job. The economic crisis has frustrated people's aspirations to educate their children in two ways. Fewer jobs are available and competition for work has increased. Concurrently, while the government provides education on all levels at very low tuition costs, it has become more and more difficult for parents to meet other requirements, such as uniforms and school supplies, and to continue supporting their children during the additional years of schooling. When daughters attend school the women are left without help at home, increasing their daily chores.

Against a background of an ideology of parental sacrifice for one's children, people decidedly make extraordinary efforts to educate their offspring despite the hardships it imposes upon them. Parents would apologize for being able to provide their children with only a "short career" rather than a "long" one, meaning a vocational rather than professional education. Parental pressure to study places enormous burdens on children, which become manifested in various symptomatologies among young people, especially "high and low blood" pressure and chest pains.

While gaining an education as an avenue for economic mobility is a dominant ideology among the poor, extant economic realities mitigate against its realization. Some of the women lamented that they lacked the opportunity to study to become secretaries due to their parents' poverty. Instead they became pregnant and suffered abuse from drunken husbands.

People whose children finished vocational schools but who were unable to find jobs blamed the failures on themselves or on their children. A child's failure in school or in finding a job is not uncommonly seen as the failure of the entire family, especially the parents. In Mexico the family is prior to the individual. The individual is embedded in a family that is the basic unit of human existence across all class lines (Lomnitz and Perez-Lizaur 1987). The family encompasses a bilateral group that includes one's parents, siblings, and grandparents, as well as collateral relatives such as aunts, uncles, and cousins. One looks to one's family, especially to one's mother, for social, moral, and economic support throughout one's life. Consanguinity is emphasized, and stepchildren are not looked upon with favor by a stepparent. In fact, widows and abandoned women with young children have difficulty remarrying, and they must either leave their children with their parents or risk losing a potential mate. Generally speaking, children, especially unmarried ones, are expected to obey and respect their parents. When such expectations are not met, they may produce anger and sickness.

Children invariably reside with their parents until marriage and often after. But even when married children live apart from their parents, many live within the same neighborhood, even on the same block, and there is weekly visiting. Customarily, when a couple could not afford to live apart from their parents, the women moved to their husbands' parents' home to form an extended family, if only temporarily until the couple was economically able to rent separate lodgings.

When the man's parents are deceased or live outside the city, the couple may establish residence with the wife's parents. This situation is contrary to cultural norms and reflects poorly on a man. Several young men in the study sample, including Arthur and Jose, resided with their in-laws. This fact is significant in understanding their sickness and its resolution. While conflicts may exist in almost all families the world over, the extended family in Mexico is burdened by dissensions among sisters-in-law, between mothers-in-law and daughters-in-law, or, in the case of Arthur, among brothers-in-law. Family frictions also often result from ambiguities that revolve around financial matters, including expenditures and proportionate contributions by different family members.

Forty-two percent of the study population lived in nuclear families, 18 percent in extended families, and 17 percent in female-headed households. Of the remaining 23 percent of the sample, 8 percent lived with married siblings or cousins and 15 percent worked as live-in maids. Female- headed households lack economic security until the children are grown. However, many women living without a spouse experience a sense of independence from conflicts with a mate.

There is great variability in the relationships between women and their sons' wives. While a mother-in-law may exacerbate the marital relationship, senior members of the family may also cushion hostilities between husband and wife (Finkler 1985a). A woman who was married twice, and who was experiencing an illness which she attributed to her problems with her current mother-in-law, musingly noted that when the husband was terrible, the mother-in-law was nice, but when the husband was nice, the mother-in-law was terrible. An individual is often torn between allegiance to his or her natal family and conjugal roles and obligations and the dissonance may become embodied and expressed symptomatologically. For example, sons are frequently caught between financial obligations they owe to their mothers and to their wives and children. In these situations, the mothers usually win out, leaving the wives angry.

To state that male-female, husband-wife interpersonal relationships are problematic in Mexico, as elsewhere, is to state the obvious. But more than any other aspect of existence, phenomenologically these relations form a template in which sickness is played out in Mexico, because people get caught up in emotional discharges of the kind that in Mexican cultural comprehensions are illness producing. Patients may refer to their interpersonal relationships during medical consultations. Importantly, these relationships influence sickness resolutions too. Because the majority of the study sample are women, it is essential to give some consideration to contemporary Mexican cultural beliefs and practices relevant to male- female interactions before and after marriage and to gender roles.[10] While clearly there exists individual variability in male-female relations, the study sample reveals in broad terms a pattern of combative conjugal relationships.

Romantic love and monogamy are the ideal norms, both for physicians and patients in the sample population. A woman is expected to be a virgin at marriage and many young women are tortured by conflicts between pressures from their fiances, or *novios*, for sexual intercourse and the accepted moral standards and parental wishes. Young women frequently seek medical treatment when their periods are even a week late because they fear parental accusations and suspicions. Male physicians usually support the prevailing ideology concerning female virginity.

Young women do get pregnant, however, before the couple establishes a formal union, and the girl becomes isolated from her family. She is in a liminal state, no longer a virgin, but also not a wife or mother, the legitimate roles for a woman. Not until the birth of the child, when she becomes a mother, is the girl reincorporated into the family. Not uncommonly, the child is raised by the grandparents. In one instance, a patient's daughter ran off with a boy who claimed that not only was his bride not a virgin but she was also pregnant. To the mother's anguish, the boy returned the girl to her natal family. The mother attributed her sickness to the daughter's return.

Ideally, a woman aspires to be formally asked for her hand in marriage and to be married in both civil and religious ceremonies. A religious ceremony is a highly desired affirmation of the marriage bond, but a civil ceremony bestows legal protection on the woman and access to social security health benefits. Women announce with great pride that they have been married by "both laws," meaning in civil and religious ceremonies. Women are especially outraged when they are abandoned by a man to whom they were married under both laws.

The common view is that all poor people live in free unions. Physicians in the study tended to frown upon patients living in common law arrangements, and one doctor regularly lectured her patients about its evils. Contrary to the commonly held view that such unions are typical among the poor, the majority of men (56.4 percent) and women (49.0 percent) were married in both civil and religious ceremonies. Only 23.1 percent of the men and 28.3 percent of the women were living in common law unions (also Velez-Ibañez 1983). The remainder (20.5 percent of the men and 17.2 percent of the women) were married in a civil ceremony only and 5.5 percent of the women were married in church only. The latter are especially interesting, because in these cases the men were married, unbeknown to the wives, to other women by civil ceremony.

While monogamy is the cultural norm, it is very common for men not only to have casual affairs, but also to establish families with more than one woman. Having more than one woman is one of the characteristics of being a macho male, along with drinking alcoholic beverages and ordering people around, especially women. In the words of Nomi, speaking of her husband, "Machos are people who don't reason." A man who possesses only one woman may be regarded a homosexual, and when he resists going out to drink, he may also lose his male friends. These powerful cultural pressures on men exert their toll on women and on those men who are not cut out to fulfill the macho role (Finkler 1981). Although women, including female physicians, accept the cultural view of powerful male sexuality, not all women learn to acquiesce to the fact that their husbands possess other women, especially when the men fail to support them financially. When a woman realizes but fails to resolve for herself these realities, she experiences emotional discharges that she associates with her sickness.

In the sample population conjugal relations are marked by male domination and physical coercion that includes wife-battering, especially when the man is drunk. This was the case of Esperanza, whose husband kicked her in the vagina. With few exceptions, when women spoke about their husbands, they cried. Of the numerous married women whom I followed and with whom I had spent considerable time, only a handful reported having "good husbands" and happy marriages. According to one woman, a "good marriage is subject to envy and possible accusations of witchcraft." Generally speaking, from the woman's perspective a good husband is one who provides her and her children with her economic needs and treats her well, meaning that he does not beat her.

A young married woman's movements are usually circumscribed by her husband; she generally requires permission to leave the house. Women say that because of their husbands' jealousies, their husbands prohibit them from seeking employment outside the household. In one extreme case, Margaret was locked up in the house behind iron bars for five years, after which she finally managed to escape. Margaret, like many of the other women in this study, experienced her first illness when she got married. Many women reported that when they claimed they were sick, their husbands accused them of being crazy.

Women disclosed that they remained with their husbands because their children needed their father. Occasionally a woman may desert her husband, as in the case of one young man who fell ill when his wife left him, taking their child. A woman may even abandon a child to escape from an oppressive mate.

In Mexico extraordinary value is placed on children, and children are desired by both men and women. Men often pressure women to bear many children. Sometimes, a husband may threaten a barren woman, or one who has only one or two children, with abandonment. One woman did not question the husband's right to leave her because she could not bear more than one child. In another instance, a barren woman was taunted by her sister-in-law, who told her she was useless. However, in this instance the husband refused to leave the woman, even though she encouraged him to do so because of her infertility.

The woman's procreative power--to have or not to have children--is governed by the man's desire for children. A woman needs her husband's permission to have a tubal ligation, and several women reported that their husbands would not permit them to use contraceptives. Under such circumstances, women induce abortions, illegal in Mexico, by various means, including self-injection, ingestion of a concoction, and by lifting and carrying heavy things. When asked how they were affected by self-induced abortions, all the women reported that it was simply an inconvenience because they had felt sick for a few days.

While a man's self-esteem is attained by being a macho, a sexual being, a woman's self-esteem emanates from her being a mother. Typically, both men and women, physicians and patients, accept the commonly held notion that men are governed by powerful sexual urges that women must endure. If the woman cannot meet the man's sexual demands, she may even be blamed by her parents for the resulting difficulties with her husband. It is also believed that sexual intercourse is curative for a woman. Two women reported that they were advised that their symptomatologies issued from lack of sexual relations. The curative power of sexual intercourse was also voiced by one physician, who believed that abstinence most assuredly led to a mental institution. One physician, instructing medical students on sexuality, reflected a common stance that women require sexual intercourse at most weekly to satisfy them; more frequent sexual intercourse and orgasms may be dangerous to their health. Men, however, require frequent sexual intercourse and orgasms to avoid falling ill. This physician pointed out to the students that they must question patients about their sexual relations with their husbands because they affect women's health. The doctor noted that a man may desire to have sex with his wife fifteen times a day in order to exhaust her so that she could not betray him.[11] According to this physician sexually related diseases include divorce, gonorrhea, and odd sexual practices. Conflicts revolving around sexuality emerged for some women in the study group. Notably, Margaret refused to accept a passive sexual role, which she related to her illness. For Alice the role of mother resulting from a brief liaison conflicted with her role as mistress of a man with whom she was extremely happy, a contradiction she was unable to resolve except through her long-lasting symptomatology.

Women often blame other women for their husbands' sexual or other transgressions by accusing the "other woman" of bewitching the husband. In one case the wife was blamed by her female neighbors for her husband's drinking behavior. While women are subject to marital strains and denunciations by other women, men too are subject to perturbations, though they can more easily dissipate their angers by removing themselves from the situation, an option usually unavailable to women (Finkler 1985a). Men are vulnerable to pressures external to the household from which women are shielded, especially if the women remain housewives. Aside from cultural pressures to demonstrate machismo, embroiling men in machinations they are not always able to handle and risking being bewitched by a jilted woman, men are subject to harassments by the authorities, assaults, arrests, exploitation by unconscionable employers, and joblessness, that assail the core of their beings and thus their health. Rafael fell sick when he was dismissed from his job because he turned fifty years old, which also led to loss of authority at home, causing him great anger.

Although both parents have great authority over their children, mothers are venerated by both their sons and daughters. A woman's source of strength and support is her mother and her siblings, especially her sisters. Men usually look to their mothers or siblings. Indeed, social support is more likely to come from one's mother and siblings rather than spouse. The mother-child bond persists throughout a human being's life. For those who must live away from their parents, as, for example, the live-in maids who usually come from the provinces, separation from the natal family adds to their overall hardships. Although approximately 60 percent of the patients in the sample had a spouse, when they were asked whom they regarded as persons closest to them, the common response was one or several members of the natal family, as can be seen in Table 2.1.

Table 2.1: Persons Considered Closest to the Subject
(in percent)

	Men (N=44)	Women (N=161)
Mother	24.1	22.9
Father	3.2	1.0
Both father and mother	9.6	10.7
Brothers	22.5	13.6
Sisters	6.4	13.1
Children	6.4	16.0
Spouse	6.4	2.9
Other relatives	8.0	7.8
Friends	6.4	1.0
None	1.6	2.5
Other (e.g., *compadres* or neighbors)	5.4	8.5
	100.0	100.0

Some respondents selected more than one person as being closest to them. Only the first person mentioned by a respondent was tabulated here. It must, however, be stressed that the most common response was mother and sister or brother, or sister, brother, mother.[12]

The central role of the family in Mexican life assumes that most people do not lack social support although subjectively some people expressed a sense of solitude. Nevertheless, over 72 percent of the sample population indicated that a family member was concerned about their current health state, with social support being embedded in the natal family rather than in the conjugal unit. Day-to-day existence is played out in the vicissitudes of family interrelations and in the routines of daily activities that for many women impose a heavy burden. Normally, the daily rhythm involves the women in a round of household chores that many associate with specific symptomatologies. A woman's day may begin at 5 a.m. when she lines up to purchase tortillas that can only be eaten freshly prepared, and when she prepares the morning meal and takes her children to school. The main meal is eaten at about 3 or 4 p.m. and until that time, a woman is engaged not only in its preparation but in washing and ironing. Most men are not usually home during the day, irrespective of their employment status.

To conclude the depiction of Mexican life relevant to our subject population, some remarks need to be made regarding religious beliefs and practices. Whereas there was a time when to be Mexican was to be Catholic, Protestant and other dissident groups have been encroaching upon Catholicism

(Finkler 1983; Willems 1975). The Catholic religious calendar, of course, continues to structure people's religious activities. Passion plays are performed during Easter and the traditional Christmas festivities are celebrated in most neighborhoods of the city. Yet, while 82 percent of the men and 88 percent of the women identified their religion as Catholic, less than 40 percent of the people in the study indicated that they attended church with any regularity, and 8 percent of the men and 4 percent of the women professed no religious beliefs.

A wide variety of Protestant, Spiritualist, and charismatic groups have flourished in the city and especially in Neza. In fact, approximately 10 percent of the sample group belong to an evangelical Protestant denomination. All such sectarian groups advocate strict monogamy and sobriety, traits especially attractive to women married to macho men. Like Spiritualism (Finkler 1981), these religious groups transform men's behavior to be more like that of the women: sober and monogamous. The women who succeed in converting their husbands benefit from a less turbulent conjugal relationship (Finkler 1981). Most of these groups also deny the existence of witchcraft and by so doing promote more harmonious interpersonal relationships. Norma, for example, stopped believing in witchcraft when she converted to an Evangelical sect. She remarked that since her conversion, God personally watched over her and therefore she could no longer be harmed by other people through witchcraft.

In fact, I have found that in this sector of the population the more a person professed to Catholic orthodoxy, the more likely he or she was to draw on witchcraft beliefs when all other explanations for a sickness failed. This proposition is based upon my observation of individuals who purported to attend Catholic church regularly and who usually had shrines in their homes. Those who indicated that they rarely frequented church services and did not have religious icons in their homes also denied believing in witchcraft. Adherence to a witchcraft ideology is especially significant in relation to illness resolution, as well as to etiological beliefs, to which our attention is turned in the next chapter.

Notes

1. A recent report anticipated that by the year 2000, 80 percent of Mexico's population will live in its major cities (*Unomasuno*, December 24, 1987). The report estimates that of Mexico's 75 million people, 20 million, or 26, percent reside in Mexico City.

2. See *Newsweek* article, June 13, 1988, on the pollution of Mexico City. *La Jornada* (January 4, 1988) reported a 129 point ozone content. According to the article, an ozone count of between 101 and 200 concomitant with the thermal inversions during the winter months is dangerous to health.

3. Based on 1984 statistics obtained from the authorities in the community, 7 percent of the population of Neza was unemployed.

4. Land prices in Neza, as in all the other communities, are relatively prohibitive given the people's economic resources. One hundred square meters may cost as much as $700.

5. According to one informant who was a policeman for a brief period, the police confiscated drugs, which they themselves may then use.

6. Hospital services were reduced because several hospitals had been destroyed by the earthquake (Marcos Mares, *Unomasuno*, September 19, 1986).

7. For a lucid summary overview of Mexico's economic crisis, see "Mexico" in *The Economist*, September 5, 1987, pp. 3-22.

8. During the field stay inflation was so high that when peso values are reported, the reader will note that the equivalent dollar values will vary, depending on the day on which the data were collected. For example, when the study was initiated, 1,000 pesos was equivalent to about $3. A year later it was equivalent to less than 50 cents.

9. Unemployment and underemployment among physicians are very high. In fact, when I began the project four physicians had asked me if they could work as research assistants. For methodological reasons I could not hire them.

10. For those conversant with the literature on gender cross-culturally (MacCormack and Strathern 1980; Rosaldo and Lamphere 1974; Sanday 1974, 1981), as well as in Mexico (Finkler 1974, 1981, 1985a), the discussion will have a familiar ring.

11. Parenthetically, it is noteworthy that in his discourse to the students, he informed them that in childhood girls have penis envy "because little girls see that boys have something girls do not. In adolescence girls begin to develop breasts and they may think it's a cancer."

12. In the sample of healthy people who were interviewed (N=85), only 8 percent responded that their spouses were the people closest to them, suggesting that both in healthy and sick populations consanguinity, rather than affinity, is a predominant cultural value.

3

Sickness: A Mexican View

In this chapter I put forth culturally patterned presenting symptoms that I call "typical symptoms" and shared etiological beliefs that reverberate on daily life in Mexico. Etiological beliefs form a core of medical knowledge (Foster 1976, 1978; Kleinman 1980). To know the cause of a sickness is to make sense of one's suffering. A people's etiological explanations shape their expression of sickness and sickness behavior. They are assertions about human behavior and human interaction, about moral failures, and about social relations gone sour. The typical symptoms people present and the explanations they give for their suffering are culturally molded[1] (Good and Good 1981; Kleinman 1988; Zborowsky 1952). These furnish a window to people's ideologies, morality, social interaction, and relations to themselves, their bodies, and their environment. Their corporeal pains are statements, made in a cultural way, of perceived existence and of unresolved contradictions by which they are confronted. Moreover, culturally shared etiological beliefs elucidate an important component of biomedical comprehensions in Mexico, for these beliefs are grounded and reinterpreted in biomedical practice. Physicians modify traditional sickness attributions and deal with typical symptoms in ways that illuminate the cultural nature of biomedical practice. "Nerves," for example, a culturally accepted etiological belief, becomes translated by physicians as a problem of the nervous system or of the spinal column because the spine is central to the nervous system.

Human beings take their bodies for granted until they begin to experience distress and discomfort, until they sense their bodies in ways they had not perceived them before. At such times the experience of one's body is intensified, in a personal way, as my body, demanding attention. "The sensory aversiveness and world disruptions effected by pain cry out for removal" (Leder 1990:77). In any culture there exists a pool of typical styles of sensing the body and presenting symptoms. People become aware of and draw upon these when they experience sickness. To describe this pool of styles and cultural beliefs is not to say that every member of a culture draws upon it at all times or that every presenting symptom is culturally molded. As we listen to patients in their attempt to make sense of their bodily sensations, extant patterns emerge. Importantly, while patients seek treatment for symptoms at a given point in time, time often is obliterated by a sickness event. Current pains become blended into pains of the past, transcending the temporal dimensions. To the frustration of physicians for whom presenting symptoms are discrete events, patients frequently cannot pinpoint the precise time of the onset of the symptoms. When Josefina spoke about pains in her lungs, she was also speaking about all the work she had done during her life and the pains she had experienced a decade ago when she had a caesarian.

Typical Symptoms

Typical symptoms express embodied adversity; they are a cry for help in a cultural way. Not all typical symptoms are similarly laden with meaning, however. Some presenting symptoms signify the embodiment of pathogens, or organic lesions, while others communicate generalized experience of distress. Some are charged with relative specificity such as high and low blood pressure, fallen ovaries, or a fallen womb, and pain in the kidneys or lungs. It is the anthropologist's and physician's task to sort out these meanings for theoretical as well as practical reasons to gain an understanding of people's ailments.

In the discussion that follows, my focus is on the most common typical symptoms that have specific assignations in the Mexican context. I describe only those typical symptoms presented by patients in the study. There are, of course, others that have been discussed in the literature, including *empacho*, *caida de mollera* (fallen fontanelle), and *ojo* (evil eye) (Finkler 1985) that usually refer to children's sicknesses.

Headaches. In Mexico patients distinguish between pain in the head and pain in the *cerebro*. Pain in the head refers to the frontal and central portion of the skull, while pain in the *cerebro* pertains to the occipital-medula region of the head down to the nuchal muscle. This distinction is important because unlike pain in the head, pain in the *cerebro* is often associated with having "made an anger," which I will discuss shortly. Physicians frequently minimize the distinction made by patients and usually diagnose the pain as "headaches" or migraine headaches.

Anginas. Anginas refers to sore throat in general and to the tonsils in particular. Some people whose tonsils have been removed may, nevertheless, refer to pains from anginas. Anginas is a common way of signaling a general feeling of discomfort analogous to "having a bug" or a "virus" in the United States. It is associated with environmental conditions, especially exposure to cold or dampness.

Boca del estomago. "Mouth of the stomach" refers to the area around the diaphragm between the lower front ribs and the upper abdomen. This typical presenting symptom is associated with digestive disorders. While the anatomical designation is not in the biomedical lexicon, physicians recognize it and usually diagnose it as a type of parasitosis or gastritis. It is a typical way of presenting embodied pathogens.

Pain in ovaries/Fallen womb. Women of all ages point to the abdominal region when they report pain in their ovaries or that they are experiencing "fallen womb." Some physicians attribute these symptoms to women who have given birth to many children, or who have used intrauterine devices or other contraceptives for a long time. But women report these symptoms whether they have had few or no children, or have given birth to fifteen children. Similarly, these symptoms are reported by women who have had intrauterine devices for lengthy periods and those who have never used contraceptive devices, by women who have had complete hysterectomies, and those who have had the uterus removed.

Pain in the ovaries or fallen womb is a typical symptom that revolves around generalized issues related to sexuality and/or motherhood. In specific terms it may signify a woman's exhaustion with having too many children, or with being unable to bear any children. In the case of Abigail, who had been experiencing pain in the ovaries since the birth of her first child, a five-year old, the symptom stemmed from the son, whom she feared because he watched her in the absence of her husband, reporting to him every time she left the house without his prior permission.

When physicians fail to address these symptoms or when they recommend removal of the uterus, women may seek a traditional specialist healer who treats only fallen wombs and ovarian pain. Such treatments may include massages, teas, and rest. Occasionally the patient is placed with her feet up and head down to reposition the womb in its place.

Not infrequently women may also equate pain in the ovaries with pain in the *cintura*, which is sometimes linked with pain in the kidneys. Occasionally, pain in the *cintura* is cited by both men and women in connection with urinary problems. *Cintura* refers to lower back pain and pain around the waist, when one cannot walk or bend. The condition is variously diagnosed medically as a general musculoskeletal dysfunction of the lower back, as a hernia, as scoliosis, and in women sometimes as pelvic congestion syndrome and cystitis. Significantly, patients frequently associate pain in the *cintura* with their dominant work activity to signify tiredness or exhaustion. Patients link pain in the *cintura* with having lifted heavy things, as in the case of Jose, and with having worked hard. A woman taxi driver associated it with sitting for a long time when she drove her taxi.

When physicians' ministrations fail to alleviate "*cintura abierta*," or "open waist," a traditional specialist may be required, such as a bone setter or a specialist in treating fallen ovaries and "*cintura abierta.*" One patient reported that it is preferable to see a traditional specialist for this condition because "when one tells a doctor that you have 'open *cintura*' they say you have a bad spinal column and immediately they want to put you in a cast and a cast is cold and then one will feel cold all one's life." Traditional specialists treat the condition with massage. One patient reported that she was also given three cupping treatments for which she was charged 6,000 pesos each ($10). They alleviated the pain and "closed" the *cintura*.

Kidneys. Patients often refer to their lower back when they report they have pain in the kidneys. Pain in the kidneys, like pain in the *cintura*, is a metaphor for hard work or its concomitants. For example, one thirty-five-year-old woman attributed the pains in her kidneys to the strenuous work she had done between the ages of ten and fifteen and to the fact that her parents took all the money she and her sister earned. Physicians usually equate patients' reports of pain in kidneys with lower back dysfunction. In Nomi's case, however, the physician reinterpreted her pain in the kidneys as lumbar spondylitis, and his cultural interpretation had deleterious results for the patient, as we will see in Chapter 11.

Pulmon. Pain in the "*pulmon*" or lung, like *cintura* and kidney, is associated with hard work. When women, not without some pride, describe pain in the *pulmon*, they speak of all the ironing and washing they have done or continue to do, affirming all the womanly tasks their bodies had carried out. For example, Joan lived in extraordinary squalor, spending her days washing laundry for others for 600 pesos (50 cents) per dozen pieces. With this money she maintained herself, her children, and a drunken husband who beat her all their married life. Joan insisted, in spite of the physician's denial, that the pain in her lungs was due to the hard work she did.

But while *pulmon* is a common complaint of women, men present it as well, similarly communicating the difficult work they had done. Occasionally physicians recognize the relation between a woman's presenting the complaint of "pain in the lung" and washing and ironing when they ask the patient whether she engages in these activities. When physicians deny there is anything wrong with the patient's "lungs," they disavow the hard work the woman had done, especially washing and ironing. At least one physician accepted the patient's self-diagnosis in its literal sense and concluded that the patient's pain in the *pulmon* was due to the dust in the factory where he worked rather than to the work itself.

Piquetes. *Piquetes*, or jabbing pain in the heart or chest, and "high and low" blood pressure are typical symptoms that signify specific adversities. Patients usually link *piquetes* with an experience of a strong emotion, such as anger, and nerves. *Piquetes* are presented by persons of all ages and not infrequently by young people between the ages of eighteen and twenty-five of both sexes. In fact, all patients in the study in this age range presented complaints of jabbing pain in the chest or heart, for which they expected to receive an Xray or an electrocardiogram. Among young people this presenting symptom may embody the contradictions they experience from the high parental expectations to study and to "progress" in the face of either limited societal possibilities or personal disinclinations, or both.

High and low blood pressure. Patients often present this condition together with jabbing pain. High and low blood pressure, or "pressure," serves in some instances as an etiological explanation for other presenting complaints. Pressure provides an especially good example of the structuration of typical symptoms that intertwine a biomedical construction with embodied day-to-day life experiences and emotional states. It is characterized by a wide variety of symptoms that incorporate the heart, eyes, head, and chest with faintness and/or feelings of dizziness and tiredness. Most important, it occurs when one feels either crestfallen or agitated and angry. In the words of Nomi, one knows one has high and low blood pressure "when things have gotten out of control."

High and low blood pressure describes the vicissitudes in one's daily life; when one is dejected one's pressure is low, and when one is agitated and angry one's pressure is high. People associate high and low blood pressure with familial conflicts, the death of a child, the loss of a spouse, economic problems, coming to live in Mexico City, and adversity that "brings down the sky." In the words of one patient, the pressure goes up "because I get desperate and I don't have any money, and it goes down when we don't have any money and we have many obligations and I feel desperate." One patient began experiencing "pressure" when her "womb was removed." Others developed high and low blood pressure after experiencing a fright or anger. Some physicians treat high and low blood pressure with medication, irrespective of the blood pressure monitor reading, while others ignore it or diagnose it as neurasthenia.

A point made earlier that merits repeating is that not all individuals express affliction by presenting their symptoms in a typical way. Among the typical symptoms I have described, some represent embodied life's lesions while others represent embodied pathogens and organic lesions.

Etiological Beliefs

The typical symptomatologies are closely linked with culturally constructed beliefs about their etiologies that also inform physicians' understandings of sickness. I have discussed Mexican traditional etiological beliefs elsewhere (Finkler 1985). As is the case with typical presenting symptoms, Mexicans draw upon a pool of shared etiological beliefs of which they become aware when struck by sickness. Generally speaking, these beliefs focus on environmental assaults, inappropriate diet and lack of vitamins, hard work and working conditions, heredity, parasites, infection, lack of hygiene, lack of education, and emotional discharges of anger and nerves frequently associated with conflicting social relations, life events, and lived day-to-day experience.

It must be stressed that some people cannot identify any reason for their sickness, for most sickness attributions are fluid. Individuals draw upon several causes concurrently or sequentially to explain a particular sickness episode. Moreover, I have found that explanations given for a sickness are not always the same as those for specific symptoms of any one part of the body. For example, when patients were questioned about what had brought on a particular symptom, for example, abdominal pain or headache, its attribution revolved around one or more reasons, including parasites, diet, environmental assaults, poor physiological condition resulting from tubal ligation, hysterectomy, use of contraceptive pills, overuse of medications, and so on. When the same person was asked to give a reason for his or her sickness, the explanations bore on existential conditions, including economic problems, an adverse life event, an emotional state such as sadness, or emotional discharges such as anger, nerves, or sudden fright.

In Mexican traditional beliefs the imputation of sickness to emotions is not based on a mind/body dualism. In fact, the culturally shared understanding is that the body is an extension of one's day-to-day experience; the state of being sick is commonly regarded as a continuance of day-to-day events embedded in adverse social interaction and in moral evaluations that become condensed in anger and nerves. The attributions require some elaboration.

Environmental Assaults and Diet

As we have seen earlier, people living in Mexico City are acutely aware of the deleterious effects of the environment on their health, especially polluted air, smog, dust, cold air, and getting wet from the rain. Physicians and patients agree that smog and polluted air affect people's eyes, throats, and overall state of health. Getting wet in the rain explains general discomforts, catarrhs, and grippes. Attributions related to diet bear on an inadequate diet, on an irregular eating schedule, and on eating the wrong foods, for instance, spicy foods or pork; food sold by street vendors is usually considered to be contaminated with parasites. Interestingly, in comparison with my previous studies in the countryside where few people attributed sickness to lack of food, in the Mexico City sample, a handful of people attributed their health state to an inadequate diet.

Diet and work become intertwined in illness attributions, as when a regular eating schedule could not be observed due to an erratic work schedule. Similarly, one patient attributed his pains in the right side of his abdomen and left side of his back to the fact that he was not allowed to eat or even go to the bathroom in the factory where he worked. As I noted previously, *hard work* in general and work conditions in particular are regarded as illness producing. For example, a young man suffering from dizziness, pain in the head, and blurred vision attributed his condition to his job, which entailed carrying heavy pipes.

It is not surprising that both hard work and working conditions become embodied in a large variety of symptoms, including abdominal pain, chest pain, back pains, and pains in the kidneys and lungs, when men and women in the sample worked at various jobs at home or in factories under abominable conditions only to eke out a very meager subsistence.

Anger

Negative emotional discharge of anger is probably the most widely attributed generalized explanation for sickness. Anger provokes sickness in general, but it can also cause facial paralysis, pain in the "mouth of the stomach," bloating, heart palpitations, jabbing in the heart, shortness of breath, and diabetes. Pain in the *cerebro* is almost always associated with anger, as are pain in the gall bladder and high and low blood pressure.

Not uncommonly, people may preface the presentation of symptoms with "yesterday I made an anger." A common admonition is "do not make an anger and you will not get sick." While people frequently characterize themselves as being "an angry person," anger is not a solitary act. It emerges in all people, "angry people" or not, out of failed social relations, or from a sense of injustice. One "makes an anger" because of a breach of moral values: when children who ought to obey their parents do not; when husbands who ought not to betray their wives do; when husbands get drunk and they ought not; when husbands dissipate their meager funds on drink and other women and the wife is left with no money for her daily expenses; when siblings who ought to share in taking care of their elderly parents leave one with the entire burden; when a man ought to be the supreme authority in the household and is not; when a young man coming out of the factory is attacked by a policeman who steals the two weeks' wages he earned in the factory; or when a man loses a dispute because his opponent bribed the authorities.

Angers are made when tacitly accepted ideologies are violated, as when women, conceding to the prevailing standards of male dominance and female submission, fail to realize the rewards of submission, as when the spouse spurns them. Angers are made when neighbors harass one's children. Joan, who lived on top of a garbage heap in a house constructed of tin and cardboard, attributed her perpetual pains in the head and in the *cerebro* to lack of food and to the anger resulting from conflicts she was having with her neighbor. For Joan, as for many others, inimical social interactions and their moral underpinnings took precedence over miserable physical surroundings and living conditions in provoking her anger.

Angers are "made" and embodied when human beings are caught in the contradictions between the realities of daily existence and prevailing cultural ideologies. In Mexico there is a strong ideology of monogamy and romantic love, while the realities are that men maintain more than one woman. While a woman usually accepts that men are inherently sexual beings and women are not, she makes an anger when she learns that her husband failed to give her money to meet her daily expenses because he cohabits with "another woman." More and more, parents and particularly mothers are confronted by the contradiction that children ought to obey them and yet fail to do so. In the face of such conflicts angers are made and sickness ensues.

Paradoxically, while making an anger can produce a sickness, it can also protect one against witchcraft, yielding a profound contradiction in Mexican ideology that when left unresolved will tend to prolong the sickness that "making the anger" had provoked. There is a commonly held belief that if one has a "strong character," meaning one is "an angry person," one is protected from witchcraft. Thus, while "making an anger" and being "an angry person" can produce sickness, it can also protect one against witchcraft and its dire effects. I will return to this important point shortly.

Nerves

Anger closely converges with nerves. Nerves explain sickness and are an outcome of sickness. The term also refers to a sickness state. Nerves pertains to a state of being that is often associated with anger, as well as to a wide variety of physical symptomatologies and to existential conditions experienced in the entire body. Nerves as a state of being refers to an agitated state, a state of worry, anxiety, and desperation, when "one begins to think and think," when "the entire body trembles and aches," and when one feels that nothing seems to go right. Patients at the hospital, however, do not present nerves as a primary complaint but rather associate it with jabbing pain in the heart, a caesarean, contraceptive pills, abdominal pains, high and low blood pressure, unpleasant dreams, dryness in the mouth, forgetfulness, pain in the *cerebro*, the economic crisis, inability to pay bills, being beaten by one's husband, being away from one's family, and sleeping alone.

Nerves can be inherited from one's parents, but in the words of one patient, "Everybody in Mexico is nervous because of the economic crisis." According to a young girl whose mother participated in the study, her mother developed nerves because of the economic crisis, when people stopped buying her mother's merchandise, candies, hairpins, and tissues. Over 50 percent of the patients in the study reported they developed a state of nerves following the earthquake, when like the earth, people's bodies began to tremble. It must be underscored that while nerves is usually used to explain sickness, many people attribute nerves to the sickness itself. Thus, nerves could be as much a result as a cause of sickness.

The close association between anger and nerves can be gleaned from the following examples. A young woman sought treatment for nerves because she shivered, she had a pain all over her body, and she had "made many angers." She had suffered from nerves and "making angers" since she was five years old, when her father and then older brother "used her to put his 'worm' [colloquial for penis] between her thighs." A woman's twelve-year-old son was murdered; she made an anger and began experiencing nerves. Finally, Mary reported that she was suffocating ("*me ahogo*") and had no way of "*desahogarse*" to "unsuffocate," or unburden herself. When her husband had accused her of having stolen his money, she became angry, and she also visited a family where a young girl had been murdered. In her words, "All that enters into the body as nerves," and in this instance, generalized adversity became transformed into specific symptomatology of pain in the "mouth of the stomach." In these examples, anger, nerves, and sickness comprise simultaneously the etiology and the sickness state.

As I propose elsewhere (Finkler 1989), nerves is embodied adversity that also encompasses sickness itself, and in its concurrence with anger, nerves is an embodiment of moral evaluations and indignations. Physicians reinterpret nerves in terms of physiological dysfunction. They objectify and separate the disorder from the patient's experience in which the disorder is embedded. Thus, a young woman with chest pains, a choking feeling, tiredness, sleeplessness, pain in feet, and forgetfulness attributed her condition to nerves and associated it with the fact that she had just lost her boyfriend. The physician ascribed her condition to faulty synapses of the nervous system.

Along with anger and nerves, *susto*, usually described in the literature as an illness state (O'Nell and Selby 1968, Rubel 1964; 1984; Uzzell 1974), is also significant etiologically. Within the hospital setting it was never presented by patients as an illness state but rather as its attribution. *Susto* is ascribed to a sudden fright that produces jabbing in the heart or chest, fainting, bloating, dry mouth, and high sugar levels, or diabetes, abortions, and a variety of other symptoms. To cite an example, a man's car had broken down and he was attacked. This event produced a bloating of his stomach. When experienced together with anger, as it often is, it can cause "pressure" or other dysfunctions, including a state of nerves. *Susto* in and of itself, when not accompanied by anger or nerves, is morally neutral; it usually is a response to unforeseen frightening events, as, for example, the earthquake. *Susto* took on a special meaning against the background of the earthquake that became etiologically significant. The 1985 earthquake resulted in a "super" *susto*. It became embodied by people who had experienced it directly. As I noted before, a large percentage of the people in the study attributed their sickness and ongoing illness condition to it.

Personal anguish resulting from the earthquake became expressed through the body. Examples abound. A twenty-eight-year-old woman who witnessed the fall of several downtown buildings as she came out of the subway has since been sick. On the first day of the earthquake she had a bone stuck in her throat, and after the second day, she felt her "innards had come out," and she could not walk. She was unsuccessfully treated by many physicians for the condition. A middle-aged woman who resided in the center of the earthquake zone and who sought treatment for chest pain reported, "Since the earthquake every time something shakes in the house I have pain here," pointing to her chest. One of the patients declared that while before the earthquake he felt ill occasionally, since that time, his mouth has been continuously dry, and he has been sick all the time. A man seeking help for kidney pain and constant trembling attributes them to the earthquake. Another woman attributed a diagnosed case of high blood pressure to the earthquake coupled with her having worked hard all her life. In fact, one senior female physician similarly ascribed her own essential high blood pressure to the natural disaster.

While environment, diet, work, and emotional discharges are the predominant etiological beliefs, several others merit noting, including *aire*, heredity, and witchcraft. *Aire*, believed to be produced by tormented spirits possessing the body, and a not uncommon traditional belief in the countryside (Finkler 1985), was rarely implicated in sickness in the study group. Interestingly, only three patients in the entire sample mentioned *aire* in relation to chest pains. *Aire* is rarely drawn upon from the cultural pool of attributions by the subjects in the sample, owing possibly to the fact that tormented spirits usually roam around cemeteries that, unlike in rural villages, are located relatively far from people's dwellings in Mexico City.

Heredity

Heredity is cited as an illness attribution, or more often as a potential explanation for a serious condition. Inasmuch as none of the subjects in the study experienced cancer or cardiovascular disease, inheritance was not a commonly invoked proximate cause. However, people often indicated that they feared their current illness was symptomatic of a serious condition, such as cancer or heart failure. Notions about cancer vary: It is a tumor, it is very painful, one dies from it. One gets cancer because one had many children. Cancer is the most often cited sickness that people fear, and it is regarded by many as inheritable. Along with inheritance, it is also believed that mothers can transmit sickness to their offspring during pregnancy when they "make an anger," when they experience a *susto*, or when their wombs are exhausted. For example, one patient attributed medically diagnosed ovarian cysts to the fact that she was the youngest of fifteen children. By the time she was born she regarded her mother's exhaustion as having affected her health state. In the same way as high and low blood pressure, the folk belief in the inheritability of sickness emerges out of the folk interaction with biomedicine's understanding of inheritable diseases, of which the patient is made conscious through the medical history.

Witchcraft

Inheritance and congenital transmission of sickness are occasionally associated with witchcraft. In fact, witchcraft is not an uncommon explanation for sickness when medical treatment fails. At the initial interview witchcraft was not cited as the cause of any specific symptom or of the illness episode for at least two compelling reasons. First, patients would be leery of attributing their problem to witchcraft within a hospital setting where they know such beliefs were frowned upon. Second, people usually attribute an illness to witchcraft only when all medical treatments have failed (also Finkler 1985). In fact, it is very common for people to conclude that their condition was due to witchcraft *because* biomedicine failed to remove their sickness. In this way there is a symbiotic relationship between biomedical failure to successfully resolve a patient's sickness and the belief in witchcraft (Finkler 1985). In view of the fact that patients had not exhausted their biomedical options when they sought treatment at the hospital, they were not likely to draw upon witchcraft to explain their illness state at the time of the first hospital visit.

It must be emphasized that while beliefs in witchcraft exist in the pool of shared beliefs, not all people arrive at this conclusion, even when medical treatment fails. There is a great deal of ambiguity about witchcraft beliefs. For example, when patients were asked whether witchcraft was done to them, approximately 58 percent claimed they did not believe in it, while the remaining 42 percent were equally divided between answering "yes," witchcraft had been performed on them, and "they didn't know." Many people stated that they did not believe in it themselves, but they ascribed the belief to others or knew people who were victims of witchcraft. Some people stated that they avoided their neighbors and other strangers to avoid the possibility of having witchcraft performed on them.

Belief in witchcraft is problematic in Mexican culture. For many people belief in witchcraft frequently creates unresolvable contradictions. To admit to belief in witchcraft is to admit to being ignorant, because the society at large condemns such beliefs as ignorance and frowns upon them. On the other hand, to deny attributions to witchcraft is to assume culpability for the sickness rather than blame another for one's misfortune. Witchcraft, like anger, reflects social intercourse "gone rotten." As I have emphasized elsewhere (Finkler 1985), while defiance of a witchcraft ideology abates suspicion and fosters a more favorable social environment among friends, neighbors, and especially in-laws, jilted spouses, or girlfriends, it also shifts the responsibility for the sickness to personal acts, such as "making an anger." Additionally, physicians validate assumptions of personal culpability by imputing the patient's sickness either to anger or to some failure of the patient's organism. I hypothesize that when culpability is shifted from others to oneself, it tends to exacerbate the sickness and militate against its speedy resolution. Several patients in the study for whom biomedical treatment failed suspected they had been bewitched, as, for example, Paulino, a fifty-year-old man, who had seen numerous physicians. He believed that he had been bewitched by his previous spouse, whom he had jilted.

While for some witchcraft becomes a satisfying explanation for a sickness that stubbornly refuses to be alleviated medically, it also enmeshes the individual in a conundrum. The individual must resolve the paradox that one possesses either an "angry character" that failed to protect one, or a weak disposition leaving one unable to defend oneself, a trait that men are especially reluctant to acknowledge. I propose that when a person of either sex is enmeshed in these types of contradictions, it impedes the healing process.

To reiterate a point made earlier, attributions are not discrete beliefs; rather, they become woven into culturally coherent statements that give meaning to the sickness event. Malfeasance becomes intertwined with beliefs about the nature of one's character and with beliefs of inheritance, as can be gleaned from the following example. A man attributed his child's sickness to witchcraft on the grounds that the witchcraft was intended for him. But since he was the possessor of a strong character, "he was an angry person," it ricocheted on his wife during her pregnancy; she then passed it on to her child, who developed the sickness that was being unsuccessfully treated by physicians. Admittedly, this reasoning may not be encountered regularly, but it serves to illustrate how traditional etiological beliefs, anger, witchcraft, and inheritance become interwoven to yield a unitary explanation for the individual.

Whereas etiological beliefs assist in making sense of one's illness state, the proposition is advanced that such beliefs also create contradictions sufferers must resolve to facilitate the resolution of their sickness.

To complete the general discussion of culturally shared attributions, it is noteworthy to examine the frequency with which the study sample drew upon them. Men and women resort differentially to the fund of culturally shared attributions, although the difference is not statistically significant. Table 3.1 displays the attributions most commonly cited by men and women in the study.

Table 3.1: Most Common Attributions of Illness by Sex of
Patient (in percent)

Attribution	Males	Females
Environment	8.0	5.3
Diet	12.9	6.3
Work	12.9	12.6
Don't know	22.5	24.0
Emotional	43.7	51.8
Discharges (includes nerves, anger, fright, and overall adversity)		
	100.0	100.0

As shown in Table 3.1, a higher percentage of men than women also attributed illness to environmental causes. This can be explained by the fact that men are usually exposed to pollution and smog because their activities take them outside the house more than women. Twice as many men as women attributed their sickness to diet. Close examination reveals that while more women expressed the belief that they got sick because of eating the wrong foods (for example pork, spicy foods) and inadequate food, men tended to attribute their sickness to eating food sold by street vendors.

Women were more aware of dietary deficiencies because they often have less access to money for food. They usually feed their families, including their husbands, before they themselves eat, whereas men are more mindful of the foods they buy from street vendors. While a higher percentage of men ascribed their sickness to environmental assaults and dietary causes, a higher percentage of women attributed sickness to emotional discharges.

When attributions were ranked along sex lines in terms of how often a particular category was used to explain the symptoms the person was experiencing, emotional discharges ranked first among women, while environment ranked last; among men environment was ranked first and emotional discharges last.

The fact that a higher percentage of women than men attribute their sickness to anger and nerves and rank them first as the cause of illness is not unexpected. Women are more enmeshed in moral contradictions than men, who from the women's perspective perpetrate their anger and nerves. Women, unlike men, must resolve the prevailing ideological paradoxes about monogamy and the realities of male polygyny: Men abandon women, while women rarely abandon men, and women must compete with "the other woman" for scarce resources a man ought to provide his family.

Women must also negotiate relations with their children, the sort of contradictions that provoke profound anger and produce sickness. Children are expected to obey their mothers but often don't. Since the women carry the greater burden of disciplining the children and spend most of their waking time with them, they are more affected by children's disobedience than men. In view of the prevailing cultural etiological understandings that nerves and anger are sickness producing and that women are more often caught up in situations leading to anger and nerves, it is not surprising that women get sick more than men, a phenomenon that I have discussed elsewhere (Finkler 1985a).

In sum, people do not rely on one attribution to explain their symptoms. A concatenation of etiological causes are given that are culturally shared, but some patients also include idiosyncratic elements such as childhood experiences. Consider, for instance, a man with virtilago, who attributed his abdominal pains to nerves that resulted from difficulties he encountered in his business. He ascribed the virtilago condition to having been beaten by his uncles as a child after his father had left the family. A woman ascribed her pains in the *cerebro* and in the "mouth of her stomach" to having been an orphan from an early age. Another woman attributed her ailments to the fact that her husband would not accept her child from a previous liaison.

Examination of the ways in which people in the study present and explain symptoms illuminates the close links between daily life and etiological beliefs. Elucidation of etiological beliefs and typical symptoms sheds light on the ways in which physicians understand and practice biomedicine and reveals the cultural underpinnings of biomedical practice.

Notes

1. According to one physician who worked both at the Salud Hospital and had a private practice of wealthy patients, the poor patients in this hospital minimize their symptoms, whereas his wealthy ones exaggerate them. It would be important to explore the differences in symptomatic presentation across class lines in Latin America.

4

Health Care Delivery in Mexico

In this chapter I survey health care delivery in Mexico, including the variety of options available to people. I also describe Salud Hospital and the health-seeking trajectories of the study sample.

In his typology of health care delivery systems, Kleinman (1978) delineated three sectors: the professional, which involves practitioners with formal training and political legitimation; the folk, which includes a wide variety of traditional healers; and the popular, which refers to home self-care. Biomedicine is the predominant professional health care delivery system in Mexico. The mixed economy of Mexico, combining state-managed and private economic enterprises, is reflected in biomedical health care delivery. Biomedical health care is provided by state institutions and by private physicians. Additionally, there are alternative healing systems including professional and folk. The former includes homeopathy and acupuncture; the latter includes Spiritualist healing, *curanderas*, and a number of others.

Biomedicine in the Public Sector: Institutional Health Care Delivery

The Mexican Social Security Laws guarantee health care to all employed workers. The state has taken charge of its population's health through its three major public institutions. These state institutions each operate networks of extensive, independently administered, primary, secondary, and tertiary hospitals and clinics. The National Institute of Social Services (IMSS) was established for workers in 1943. With the expansion of the Mexican bureaucracy the Institute for Social Security for State Workers (ISSSTE) was founded in 1960 (Cleaves 1987). Subsequently, other government enterprises, including the National Oil Co. (PEMEX), the Railroad Workers, the Electrical Workers, and the Society of Marines, launched health services for their workers (Lopez Acuña 1980).[1] All these institutions are financed jointly by the federal government, employers, and employees. People who lose their jobs forfeit medical benefits provided by these institutions.

About half of Mexico's population is covered by these government health care programs (Soberon Acevedo and Narro 1984). The remaining population of unemployed workers, peasants, self-employed merchants, and shopkeepers have access to health services provided by the Department of Health (SS), which manages a network of hospitals and health care centers in rural and urban areas. These, like Salud Hospital, furnish primary, secondary, or tertiary services. Salud Hospital, where the study was carried out, is one such hospital. Health care provided by the Department of Health is open to all citizens, including foreigners. Only token fees are charged.[2] Unlike the IMSS/ISSSTE systems, the Health Ministry institutions fail to provide free medication. Salud Hospital maintains a pharmacy that sells medications at very low cost but its supplies are usually inadequate. Patients seeking treatment in Health Ministry hospitals must purchase drugs from private pharmacies. The cost of medications was difficult to assess because of price disparities among pharmacies and daily variation owing to the inflationary economy. Generally speaking, the price of medications ranged from as little as 500 to 1,000 pesos for Maalox to about 6,000 to 7,000 pesos, depending on the manufacturer, for antidiarrheal medication, the most common medication dispensed to patients.

While Salud Hospital itself enjoys a national reputation for supplying excellent health care, by and large the Ministry of Health facilities are considered poorer than those operated by the IMSS and ISSSTE systems. Physicians employed by the latter are also paid higher salaries than those working for the Ministry of Health.

The Mexican government allocates a small part of its national budget to health care relative to the rest of Latin American nations (Alvarez 1987; Horn 1983; Peña-Mohr 1987; Lopez Acuña 1980). One recent report disclosed that during the past six years, medical expenditures have been reduced from 2.6 percent to 1.7 percent of the gross national product (Alvarez 1987), with 70 percent of the budget earmarked for curative rather then preventive medicine. Most important, within the context of our focus on Salud Hospital, 49 percent of the national health budget was earmarked for the Social Security Service as compared with only 16.5 percent for the Ministry of Health (Baez 1988) to maintain its network of services.

The relatively poor funding is reflected in the impoverished conditions under which the physicians carry out their activities in Salud Hospital. Not only are quarters congested and poorly lit, but physicians must share stethoscopes, blood pressure monitors, and other basic medical tools. Not surprisingly, the differential budget allocations within the public medical sector reflect the Mexican government's commitment to the development of capitalist industrialized institutions, many of which are multinational corporations. By guaranteeing free health care to the working population, the government subsidizes the industrial-capitalistic model of development by providing health care to the employed through the Social Security systems at three times the level given to the Health Ministry servicing the population of unemployed. By providing health care to factory workers and the state bureaucracy, the Mexican state safeguards a healthy labor force for the capitalist, industrialized sector of society. The Ministry of Health facilities such as Salud Hospital furnish a last resort for the urban unemployed, the petty merchants and street vendors, unemployed women with children, and peasants, after private physicians' treatment has failed.

As we saw, the earthquake and the economic crisis added new financial burdens to the public sector health care due to the collapse of or damage to several of the major public hospitals.[3] After the earthquake physicians were displaced from their posts and subemployed, and patients shifted to existing hospitals (Alvarez Cordero 1986). Due to the economic crisis, persons who usually relied upon private physicians turned to the Health Ministry hospitals, including those from the middle class and self-employed merchants who uncustomarily sought treatment in Salud Hospital.

Biomedicine in the Private Sector

The elite and the poor are most likely to avail themselves of private physicians. Physicians usually function in a two-tiered economy of public and private enterprise. Doctors employed by state institutions also have private practices. While their institutional salaries are equal, in the private sector their fees vary commensurate with their specialization and the economic means of the clientele they service.

There are private hospitals servicing the elites and a plethora of private physicians in the Federal District whose fees may be exorbitant.[4] The private medical sector includes not only renowned physicians who occupy posts in government institutions such as Salud Hospital, but also doctors who could not gain entry into state-controlled institutions. Physicians holding posts in the public health care institutions often remarked that unaffiliated physicians robbed their patients by charging them high fees and prescribing expensive medications.

While there is a limited system of peer watch in the public hospitals, private physicians are judged through the lay referral system (Freidson 1962), and their professional performance varies considerably. From the point of view of patients who lack access to the Social Security system, private physicians have the advantage that they can be found in many neighborhoods and they can attend to patients with dispatch by avoiding the bureaucratic maze of public sector medicine.

Salud Hospital

Salud Hospital was built at the beginning of the twentieth century and is regarded as a pacesetter for its advances in biomedicine. This hospital services patients from the entire country, including Mexico City and its environs. It provides primary and tertiary care for patients, including internal medicine and all its specialties, surgery, obstetrics and gynecology, pediatrics, plastic surgery, preventive medicine, rehabilitative medicine, emergency service, a blood bank, general laboratory tests, Xrays, and laboratory services. The task of the hospital's social work services is to assess the amount each patient is charged for laboratory analysis, Xrays, and other technological services provided by the hospital.

The outpatient clinic in Salud Hospital was inaugurated in 1965 and provides general medicine as well as all medical specialties and other hospital services. However, while the Outpatient department services the majority of patients using the hospital, most of the hospital resources are funnelled into complex technologies and specialty services, including surgery, for which the hospital is especially well known.

The hospital services several hundred patients a day. For a few cents first-time patients obtained an identity card in which their trajectories in the hospital were recorded. After having received their IDs, new patients were directed to a specially designated physician for a "preconsultation." All women were instructed to have Pap smears done and they later presented the results to the attending physician. The preconsultation usually lasted for less than a minute and new patients were routed to the appropriate outpatient medical service based on their presenting symptoms during preconsultation. Patients lined up in front of the preconsultation physician's cubicle and approached him one by one. As they entered he immediately inquired what was wrong with them and then made the referral and recorded it in the patient's ID. I observed over 150 of these preconsultations provided by various physicians on different days. The following are randomly selected transcriptions of the procedure.

Patient (middle-aged woman): My arms hurt.
Doctor: You have pain in the joints?
P: No.
D: Internal medicine.

P (young woman): I have pain in my stomach.
D: Internal medicine.

P (middle-aged woman): I have headaches.
D: What happens to you, are you nervous?
P: Yes. I have gone to a doctor and he gave me palliatives.

D: You are very green.
P: Yes.
D: Neurology.

P (middle-aged woman): My period lasts nine days.
D: You menstruate a lot. Gynecology.

P (young woman): I have a rash and a lot of itching.
D: Dermatology.

P (young male): I have headaches and swollen cheeks.
D: Did you fall?
P: No. I had a fright and I got angry.
D: Neurology.

(A man entered and said nothing at first.)
D: What is wrong with you?
P: I am suffering from nerves. I also have nausea in my intestines.
D: What else is wrong?
P: I feel poisoned by constipation.
D: How many days?
P: Constantly.
D: It's nervous colitis. Internal medicine.

Referrals to specific services depend largely on the physicians' training and specialty. Two patients reporting the same symptoms will be referred to different specialties, depending upon the preconsulting physician they happen to see. Patients whose presenting complaints were headaches may have been referred either to Neurology or to Internal Medicine. Those reporting pain in the kidney were referred to Urology or Internal Medicine, while women reporting pain in their ovaries were usually told to go to Internal Medicine or to Gynecology. Most patients with multisystemic complaints or diffuse symptomatology and patients with abdominal pains, back pains, and chest pains were usually referred to Internal Medicine. If patients reported abdominal pain and the preconsultation physician was a resident in surgery, they were usually referred to Surgery rather than Internal Medicine.

Patients were randomly assigned to physicians in the medical services designated during the preconsultation. Preconsultations and consultations in the outpatient clinic were conducted in dimly lit cubicles, usually separated from one another by an accordion curtain. Each contained one cot used alternately by two physicians and two writing desks each with two chairs. A nurse, whose task was chiefly to weigh, measure, and take patients' blood pressure, worked for at least three physicians. While the hospital provides morning and afternoon service, the bulk of patients were seen in the mornings, chiefly because many people were not informed that consultations were given in the afternoons. Afternoons were usually quiet, the pharmaceutical salesmen had left, and the relatively few doctors working the late shift attended to patients at a less frenzied pace. Typically physicians in either shift saw between three and five new patients a day and attended to five to fifteen returning patients. Patients were turned away if there were more new patients on a given day than could be covered within the physicians' quotas.

Nonbiomedical Treatment Options

Homeopathy enjoys an extensive following in Mexico, even among some biophysicians, and it is the chief professional competitor with biomedicine. This prominence has a latent effect on the structural positions of physicians in Mexico, if not on biomedical hegemony, and for this reason it merits brief consideration.

Homeopathy was brought to Mexico in 1850 and quickly became a significant health care option. In 1895 the National School of Homeopathy was established and it is currently being supported by the Ministry of Health. Students in the homeopathic school follow the same curriculum as medical students, except that they are taught pharmacopoeia, which forms the basis of homeopathic therapy, rather than pharmacology. In keeping with homeopathic physicians' professional training, they have a right to work in government medical institutions. However, biophysicians who control the public hospitals impede the appointment of homeopathic doctors, restricting their practice to the private sector.

Writing in 1888, the medical historian Flores y Troncoso (1982) observed that according to homeopathy, sickness was produced by a loss of balance of the two fluids comprising the human organism, electric and magnetic. It was founded on the Hippocratic notion that sickness was best treated by medicines which provoke disease in healthy people. If a particular medicine could produce a sickness, it could also cure it. According to homeopathic practitioners and other sources (Mendiola Quezada 1972), homeopathy assumes that no two individuals' organs function exactly the same way, and that since each illness episode is unique to the person, the treatment must also be unique. The capsules prescribed by homeopaths presumably contain specific compounds tailored to each patient. It could be said that while biomedicine is based on notions of nosological entities shared by a majority of people, homeopathy emphasizes the individuality of the person's condition and individualized treatment.

One of the physicians in the hospital associated with this study also practiced homeopathic medicine. According to him, it is necessary to question patients about their moods, the sensation they are feeling, and if they had experienced any frights in order to arrive at a homeopathic diagnosis. The patient's mental state uncovered through questioning, combined with the presenting symptoms, is the basis of homeopathic clinical judgment. In this physician's words, "for the homeopathy, fever and rashes are not very significant, temperament tied to the nervous system is."

The validity of homeopathic medicine as a therapeutic regime has been doubted from its inception. Flores y Troncoso wondered whether homeopaths were "priests of science or only merchants that traffic in the pains of humanity" (1982:259). However, Flores y Troncoso claimed that while homeopathy belonged to the history of art, it ought not to be totally discarded, for "homeopathy cures illusions of sickness with an illusion of remedies," easing self-limiting and nervous illnesses derived from the "influence of the imagination" (1982:647).[5]

Various patients in the study sample have been treated by homeopathic physicians, who may charge as much as 17,000 pesos a consultation (about $10), more than fees normally charged by biophysicians. Patients usually fail to differentiate between homeopaths and biophysicians, except to note that homeopaths give little capsules while physicians give medications. The homeopathic capsules are regarded by most people as being less harmful than pharmaceutical drugs and as having the same but only a slower effect on the condition.

The popularity of homeopathy in Mexico is not surprising considering its affinity to Mexican folk etiological understandings of the role of emotional discharges in sickness. Their medications, presumably tailored to individual patients, are compatible with a patient's conceptions of his or her sickness being unique. Despite epistemological dissimilarities, both biomedicine and homeopathy advance a common fundamental principle: Sickness is cured by the ingestion of pills, a perception widely shared by patients.

Acupuncture has gained popularity and there are courses in acupuncture given by visitors from China. Physicians are permitted to practice it. While there are no professional chiropractic schools, chiropractic treatments are available in Mexico City, although these are not as popular as homeopathy or acupuncture. There is a plethora of other medical modalities, including naturalists, along with a wide network of health food stores and secular and religious folk practitioners among whom Spiritualist healers are the fastest-growing group (Finkler 1985). Other types of folk health practitioners include *curanderas* (secular folk healers), bonesetters, traveling vendors, medicine hucksters, herbalists, and specialists, such as those I noted in the previous chapter, who treat "fallen ovaries" and "open *cintura*" (waist).

Mexico has a long history of usage of herbal medication.[6] Herbal remedies are favored by all classes in Mexican society. Some physicians also prescribe herbal teas for nerves and other conditions. One physician indicated that he prescribed a medicinal plant (nopal) rather than standard biomedical treatment for his diabetic father.[7]

Patients' Trajectories Within Health Delivery Options

Fifteen percent of the patients participating in the study were entitled to IMSS or ISSSTE services, but they sought treatment at Salud Hospital because they were dissatisfied with the treatment they had received in these institutions.[8] For the majority of patients the hospital is a last resort, used after seeking treatment either from private physicians or other Health Ministry clinics. Paradoxically, while patients view the hospital as the last bastion for primary care, the hospital authorities claim that the hospital ought to supply secondary and tertiary but not primary care to patients, even in the outpatient clinic.[9]

For the overwhelming majority of patients in the study, their health-seeking trajectory began with a visit to one or more private physicians. Private physicians either lack the technological apparatus that patients often expect or may charge as much as $50 for Xrays and other laboratory analysis, sums patients in the study could not afford. Other reasons patients gave for soliciting therapy in Salud Hospital included their desire to be seen by specialists, their desire for laboratory analysis and Xrays, and the conviction they will not be made to pay for unnecessary treatments and visits in a government hospital. Less common reasons include seeking treatment as a diversion from household chores and the opportunity to talk to new people. Some came to accompany a sick relative and took the opportunity to solicit treatment for themselves as well.

In keeping with my findings from a previous study (Finkler 1981b, 1985), I have found that biomedicine was the first and foremost resort to health care among the majority of people in this group as well. When biomedical treatment failed, then other modalities, homeopathy, acupuncture, and folk healing were sought, or herbal medications administered. Approximately 12 percent of the people in the study group had resorted to alternative treatments, predominantly herbal medications, concurrently with biomedical treatment.

Table 4.1 displays types of health care sought by patients in the study prior to their hospital visit for the condition they came to treat at the hospital.

As is shown in Table 4.1, private physicians were the first entry into the medical stream for those patients who had sought any kind of medical help before coming to the hospital. The findings suggest that for more than half of the people in the study, the hospital was indeed regarded as providing primary care services, a view of the hospital that was not shared by the hospital authorities.

For many people pharmacies, where pharmacological drugs are often dispensed by people with only a primary school education (Finkler 1985; Logan 1988), are a major, if not the only, health care resort.   Only 6 percent

Table 4.1: Type of Treatment Sought by Patients Prior to
Hospital Treatment by Sex of Patient (in percent)

Treatment Type	Females	Males
Private physician	29.2	50.0
Health centers	16.0	3.1
Self-medication		
(patent medicine)	6.4	6.8
Herbal medicines	6.4	1.6
Have not done		
anything	42.0	38.5
	100.0	100.0

of the population relied on pharmaceutical drugs before seeking hospital treatment. Self-administered herbal remedies were widely used prior to biomedical treatment, but often after medical treatment had failed.

The differential trajectories for women and men disclosed in Table 4.1 are noteworthy. More men had sought treatment from private physicians than women. This finding reveals the well-established fact that men usually have more disposable funds than women, including funds to pay for private physicians, but going to private physicians also saves them time away from gainful employment. For patients who "doctor shop," that is, seek treatment from various physicians, as people in the study sample have done, the variety of diagnoses they received for the same condition was perplexing to them. To cite but one of many examples, a patient was told by one physician she was suffering from rheumatism, by another that there was nothing wrong with her, and by a third that she was parasite burdened.   The variety of diagnoses provided by biophysicians contrasts with the parsimonious explanations furnished by Spiritualist healers, partially explaining the attraction of the latter.

In this chapter our focus was on medical care available in Mexico and how patients resorted to it. In a later chapter we see the trajectories followed by individual patients before they came to the hospital. Now we turn to the history of medical practice in Mexico in general and biomedicine in particular, the predominant medical modality.

Notes

1. For an additional listing of several other government institutions see Lopez Acuña 1980.

2. For example, in Salud Hospital general admission to the hospital in 1986 was 40 pesos (about 3 U.S. cents) and in 1988 it was raised to 100, equivalent to about the same amount. Cost of laboratory analysis ranged from 55 to 130 pesos in 1986 and was raised to 100 to 200 pesos in 1987, while Xrays ranged from 200 to 300 pesos in 1986 and in 1987 were raised from 400 to 1,300 pesos. These peso amounts varied depending on the value of the dollar on a particular day but usually were equivalent to no more than 5 to 30 U.S cents. Xray materials were sometimes unavailable during the study period, in which case patients were required to purchase the negatives in the private sector that could cost as much as 10,000 pesos or $7 to $10. Electrocardiograms cost between 175 and 400 pesos in 1986 and 300 and 500 pesos in 1987, while the cost of an ultrasound ranged from 375 to 775 pesos in 1986 and 600 to 1200 in 1987 (all less than a dollar irrespective of the exchange rate for the particular day). While all fees are minimal, they are assessed for each patient by a hospital social worker using a three-point scale that is applied on the basis of how the patient appeared to the social worker: very poor, mildly poor, or affluent.

3. One of the largest social security hospitals collapsed during the 1985 earthquake, as did several of the ISSSTE and Health Ministry institutions.

4. Visits to a specialist may range from 15,000 to 35,000 pesos ($10 to $20) and 5,000 to 15,0000 pesos ($4 to $10) for a visit to a general practitionera.

5. Homeopathy has many detractors in contemporary times, including physicians and committed positivists. In fact, in 1988 a series of articles was published in a major newspaper and argued that homeopathy was not a science and had no validity (Fernandez de Castro 1988, 1988a, 1988b).

6. The extensive Sonora market in Mexico City sells only medicinal plants and the vendors are not adverse to advising clients how and when to administer them.

7. Nopal, the leaf of the prickly pear, is widely considered a good remedy for diabetes.

8. According to these patients, physicians in such institutions do not pay attention to them, never examine them, or ask them any questions; they only listen to the symptoms and prescribe medications. Physicians who work or have worked in these institutions indicated that the patient load is much higher than in the Salud Hospital.

9. In fact, some consideration had been given by the hospital administrators to eliminating the outpatient service precisely because the hospital considers itself a tertiary care institution providing, to its distress, primary care. After I completed the research there was a brief interval when patients were turned away and referred back to local health care clinics. Only those considered to have serious impairments were attended there. However,

the outpatient clinic physicians strenuously objected to turning patients away, and the new policy was quickly abandoned.

PART TWO

Biomedical Practice in Mexico

5

History of Medicine in Mexico

In this chapter my concern is with the development of contemporary biomedicine in Mexico, recruitment into the profession, and with physicians' social position in Mexican society that also reverberates on biomedicine's impact on people in Mexico. I begin with a brief overview of medical beliefs and practices prior to the European conquest. While arguably there is continuity from the past to the present, the historical panorama illuminates the ways in which medicine is embedded in broader historical and social processes, especially in the relation between the conquered and the conquerors, as well as between Mexico and other nations. Mexican medicine has witnessed considerable sociopolitical and sociocultural changes, corresponding to the major historical epochs of the society.

The Preconquest Period

There is an extraordinary rich literature on the great civilizations of Preconquest Mexico and on its medical beliefs and practices.[1] The Spanish kept meticulous records about the people they had conquered in 1521. According to Aztec beliefs, sickness was caused by punishment from the gods, by spirit intrusions, by bewitchment (Somolinos d'Ardois 1978), and by natural causes. They treated the resultant pathological lesions and patients' symptomatic complaints with a wide variety of techniques, including surgery for abscesses, wounds, and fractures, trepanation, and dental incrustations using gold and jade (Viesca 1986:126). Arguably the most distinguishing aspect of Preconquest medicine was its extensive pharmacopoeia, displayed in the markets of Tenochtitlan, the Aztec capital and present-day Mexico City, that astounded the conquistadores (Díaz Castillo 1963). Over 3,000 plants may have been used for medicinal purposes by the Indians of Mexico, as well as minerals and animal products (Somolinos d'Ardois 1978). This variety reflected Aztec political domination of the diverse ecologies, rendering a vast assortment of *materia medica*.

The Aztec cultivated botanical gardens the flora of which were associated with the gods, accessible only to the privileged. Among the best known sacred plants was the maguey (*Agave sp.*) from which *pulque*, an intoxicating juice of about 12 percent alcoholic strength, was extracted (Finkler 1974).[2]   It was used in surgery for treating wounds and traumatic lesions (Ortiz de Montellano 1975; Viesca 1986:156).

The highly stratified and specialized Aztec society was mirrored in its medical practice. Two major categories of practitioners included those divinely inspired and closely linked to the priests and artisans, and ordinary commoners, whose accumulated knowledge was transmitted from father to son. The divinely empowered physicians gained their knowledge by serving as apprentices in special academies (*calmecac*). They employed prayers and sacred medicines cultivated in botanical gardens. They were primarily religious personages and only secondarily curers whose powers could both heal and harm.

Surgeons and herbalists calling upon knowledge vested in generations of practice formed special types of artisan groups. These artisan-doctors included many specialists, such as sorcerers, diviners, and astrologers. Some even regard them as the forerunners of today's medical specialists (Cardenas de la Peña 1976). They used a variety of naturalistic and magical healing techniques, but chiefly they depended on the usage of medicinal plants. There is an extensive debate concerning the Preconquest versus Spanish origins of contemporary folk medicine and its beliefs (Foster 1953; Ortiz de Montellano 1989). There is little doubt that much of the *materia medica* used by the Preconquest populations continues to be widely used in contemporary times by folk practitioners (Finkler 1985) and some biophysicians.

The Colonial Period

The Spanish conquest was a cataclysmic event in the history of the peoples of Mexico (Wolf 1959, 1982), bringing diseases that had hitherto not existed in the New World, including smallpox, measles, and typhus. These epidemics rendered the native healers impotent in the wake of their onslaught (Crosby 1972). While the annihilation of the population by disease was an inexorable epidemiological outcome of the meeting of two populations long separated geographically, the conquerors deliberately and systematically destroyed the indigenous society, language, and culture. Nevertheless, referring to indigenous rituals, Wolf observed that while the Conquest demolished the ideological framework of the Aztecs, it "substituted the Christian economy of Salvation for it. At the same time, this dominant liturgy was joined to local belief and practice by missionaries attempting to anchor it in local understandings and by local practitioners striving to render it expressive of local interests" (1982:148).

With the process of simultaneous destruction of native life and amalgamation of indigenous and Spanish beliefs by native populations on a local level, the conquerors appropriated native medical knowledge and practices selectively, rendering Spanish medicine in Mexico distinct from its practice in Spain. Whereas the early Spanish physicians who arrived in the New World rejected indigenous medical knowledge, by the sixteenth century Spanish physicians had merged Aztec expertise in the usage of botanical plants with the Hippocratic-Galenic medicine that was practiced in Spain. Hence, medical practice in Mexico became distinct from that in Spain not only because of its relative isolation from the mother country, but because of its incorporation of the indigenous pharmacopoeia. As more and more Spanish physicians came to Mexico, they became instilled with indigenous lore that led to a fusion between Spanish and Preconquest medicine (Somolinos d'Ardois 1979:162).

Medical historians point out that medical practice begins to parallel the structural transformations that took place in Colonial society. Broadly sketched, Colonial society quickly became differentiated into three major social strata: the Spanish conquerors and their offspring, the Criollos; the Mestizos, the overwhelming majority of the Mexican contemporary population representing a genetic and cultural mixture of Spanish and indigenous peoples; and the Indian populations that during the Colonial period remained separate from the other two groups.

Corresponding to the three general groupings of Colonial society, there were three types of medicines practiced at the time: indigenous, Mestizo, and the Spanish medicine of the universities (Aguirre Beltran 1982). Indigenous healers, usually branded as sorcerers by the Catholic Church and the Spanish conquerors, like their predecessors relied on revelation and mystical experience and their extensive knowledge of the indigenous flora and fauna that comprised their *materia medica* (Aguirre Beltran 1982). The Mestizo *curanderos* merged indigenous medical practice with Spanish folk knowledge to create Mexican folk medicine, also incorporating indigenous *materia medica* and astrology as well as Judeo-Arabic practices, Catholic saints, Christian prayers, and fortune-telling derived from medieval medicine. The Mestizo *curanderos* thus had an expanded repertoire of medical practice drawing upon both indigenous and Spanish folk traditions (Aguirre Beltran 1982).

At the top of the hierarchy stood Spanish medicine and its practitioners. The *medicos universitarios*, physicians of the universities, were the Spanish and Criollos, the officially trained physicians who were, according to Somolinos d'Ardois (1979), greatly influenced by Arabs, Jews, Hippocrates, and Galen.[3]

The first university with a faculty of medicine was established in Mexico in 1551. During the Colonial period the Lady of Succor and the priests enjoyed the prestige that flows from healing, and all strata of Mexican society demanded the medicinal drugs produced from animal, mineral, and vegetable matter of both new and old world origins.

The Spanish established hospitals in Mexico as early as 1524 to deal with the devastating epidemics following the Conquest. Despite the establishment of hospitals and the development of universities and schools of medicine, according to Flores y Troncoso "the medical sciences (referring to medicine, surgery, and obstetrics), were all in a lamentable state of backwardness and so it was in the Colonial period in Mexico" (1982:481).[4] Scholasticism prevailed in medicine. Excepting anatomy, Hippocrates and Galen were taught in Latin and no dissections were performed (Chávez 1987). Medical education followed the European pattern of the period, but additionally in Mexico there was a faculty of astrology and botanicals (Chávez 1987:56). News from Europe traveled slowly, particularly new developments in medicine. Those that were not Spanish in origin hardly reached Mexico. Consequently, the decadence that overtook Spanish medical practice also prevailed in Mexico (Chávez 1987:68). Given the low prestige of physicians coupled with their low salaries, the least able students entered the profession at the time.

The history of Mexican medicine sheds light on the complex nature of relations between the rulers and the ruled. Even this synoptic view of medical history in Mexico brings into relief the interaction between the conquerors and the conquered. Normally, we look at how native populations assimilate the ideologies and practices of the superordinate society. Less attention has been given to how the subordinate culture influences the superordinate one, as exemplified by Spanish absorption of indigenous medical knowledge, a recognition by the conquerors of the medical mastery of the vanquished.

It is noteworthy that knowledge and beliefs about medicinal plants were incorporated into Spanish medicine, rather than suppressed, as other native cultural practices had been, and this fact may partially explain the contemporary cultural commitment to herbal remedies by all Mexicans. The Colonial period following the Conquest brought about great discontinuities in Mexican society and culture, including medical practices. The threads of continuity in medical activities were maintained in the daily actions of the people with the Spanish conquistadores and their inheritors blending the local culture with their own, especially the *materia medica*. As we move to the period of independence, we encounter the supreme irony: Alien medical beliefs and practices became heralded, and indigenous knowledge became denigrated.

Independence

Following independence, usage of medicinal plants was brought into question. In fact, with Mexico's independence from Spain in 1810 the thread in medical practice was severed and a new era in Mexican medicine began. Perusal of Mexican medical history following independence reveals how Mexican physicians eagerly embraced the new ideas in medicine that were being promulgated in Europe, especially France. The intellectual extrication from Spain was facilitated by the reform laws during the Liberal Reform period, dominated by Benito Juarez (1855-1862 and 1867-1872). It led to numerous social transformations, including the separation of church and state (Casio Villegas 1956; Finkler 1983). Thus hospitals were disengaged from the church (Barragan Mercado 1968).

Positivism became a dominant theme in Mexican society in general and in the medicine of this time. Mexican scholars and physicians developed ties with the scientific and intellectual establishment of Western Europe, particularly France. French positivism gained further intellectual and political footholds in Mexico during Maximilian's (1864-1867) brief rule, boosted by notions of a shared Latin heritage. Biomedical practice during the nineteenth century reflected the new era's domination by positivism, which became further heightened in the latter part of the nineteenth century with the dictatorship of Porfirio Díaz (1876-1910).

The period following independence laid the foundation for contemporary biomedical practice. All scholars of Mexican medical history mark October 23, 1833,[5] as the day of inception of biomedicine in Mexico. On this date Valentin Gomez Farias instituted the Establecimiento de Ciencias Médicas, the direct antecedent of the Faculty of Medicine at the National Autonomous University (UNAM). The Establecimiento de Ciencias Medicas ushered in the French model of scientific medicine (Chávez 1987; Martínez Cortes 1987; Palau 1979). As the name itself suggests, medicine was declared a scientific discipline. Galen's and Hippocrates' teachings were overthrown, sweeping in the theories of Marie Francois Xavier Bichat, considered by many as the founder of modern medicine. Using cadavers, Bichat had demonstrated that disease was not found in organs but in their tissues (Martínez Cortes 1987; Laín Entralgo 1982; Reiser 1978; Shryock 1979). He advanced the theory that in the absence of investigations of organs and tissues, the study of patients' symptomatology would fail to yield a coherent understanding of disease (Laín Entralgo 1982; Reiser 1978).

New disease paradigms emanated from Claude Bernard, whose goal was to develop a "medicine without the sick" (Martínez Cortes 1987:77). Surgeons, not Galenic doctors, receptive to the new ideas of the time were called to teach in the new academy. French texts replaced the classical medieval ones, and Mexican physicians studied in France with Rene Laennec. Laennec, the inventor of the stethoscope, revolutionized medical practice in Europe by objectifying the patients' sickness. Whereas previously signs and symptoms were the same order of phenomena (King 1982), with the invention of new medical instruments such as the stethoscope (Martínez Cortes 1987; Reiser 1978), new distinctions were introduced between objective and subjective measures. The physician's observations became signs, objective measures of disease unrelated to a patient's consciousness. These became differentiated from subjective experience, and symptoms presented by the patient were no longer considered reliable indicators of sickness (King 1982).

Unlike in the past, when physicians had gained an understanding of a disease from patients' reports (Jewson 1976), the new clinical medicine required the physician to know how to interpret symptoms as signs and detect pathology gleaned by using the stethoscope or by auscultation and percussion (Martínez Cortes 1987:83). Other medical technologies were introduced in Mexico at this time, including hypodermic needles, anesthesia, and antiseptic measures in surgery.

A new era of medical education was introduced that included anatomy, physiology, hygiene, obstetrics, surgery, pharmacology, clinical medicine, and legal medicine. The new medical stars were the surgeons (Chávez 1987), reversing the practitioners' Colonial relationship. Concomitant with the fluorescence of European medicine, traditional medicine, based upon medicinal plants, continued to thrive. The new constitution of 1857 guaranteed absolute freedom to all to practice any kind of medicine, including use of Prehispanic medicines (Flores y Troncoso 1982). Flores y Troncoso, himself a physician, did not discount traditional medicine, which, according to him, could be the scientific medicine of the future. Interestingly, Flores y Troncoso bemoaned the fact that popular medicine was not incorporated into medical practices and that physicians had confidence only in practices imported from foreign countries. He observed that while physicians employed chloroform, imported from England in 1856, for obstetric purposes, ether, hypodermic needles, hypnosis in small operations (1982:653), and potassium bromide as an antispasmodic measure, *pulque*, used in ancient and Colonial Mexico as a medicinal remedy, was relegated to a table beverage of the poor to maintain their energy for hard work. It ceased to be used by physicians.

Flores y Troncoso astutely commented that "although produced in the country [Mexico] like so many other of our products, we receive them after they had been taken to foreign countries (1982:654). He continued: "We accept what is good that is not ours, or that which had been exported before, and then returned to us at a higher price and we reject what is produced here" (1982:681). Flores y Troncoso brings into light the irony that under Spanish domination native *materia medica* was incorporated into Spanish medicine, whereas during independence, it was renounced. His lament regarding the degenerated use of indigenous pharmacopoeia is echoed by contemporary physicians who decry Mexico's dependence on foreign multinational pharmaceutical companies, and on North American texts such as Cecil and Harrison.[6]

Contemporary Biomedicine

The North American influence on Mexican biomedicine was a post-World War II phenomenon. Following independence and until that time, biomedicine in Mexico looked toward the developments in French medicine. Following World War II the French influence waned, and the North American medical model dominated Mexican biomedical practice.

The Mexican Revolution of 1910 ushered in more than a decade of chaos. During this period Mexican society was considerably restructured. The oppressive dictatorship of Porfirio Díaz was brought down, agrarian reform (Finkler 1978; 1980) was promulgated, and workers were guaranteed new rights. Medical advances came to a halt at least until the 1920s. Along with the political and social revolution against the regime, there was also a rebellion against positivism, a hallmark of the Porfirio Díaz regime, and consequently against medical institutions that prided themselves on practicing scientific medicine (Gortari 1980). In the 1920s when the country began to return to stability, new reforms were implemented at the Faculty of Medicine, which at the time was dominated by the French school of medicine.

The new influences on North American medicine began with the Flexner Report of 1910, which firmly anchored medicine in the biological sciences and introduced sweeping reforms in medical education;[7] the North American influence on contemporary Mexican biomedicine came in full force in 1943 (Flores Carbajal 1988; Frenk 1978; Fuente et al. 1984).[8]

Medicine, as it is practiced at present with all its specialties, came into its prime in Mexico in 1943 and it was promoted by the national institutions. That year the Ministry of Health and Assistance came into existence, as did the Social Security system (IMSS), which was rooted in Article 123 of the 1929 Mexican Constitution (Lozoya 1984). Various other public institutions followed, including research institutes. New hospitals were built promoting tertiary care and medical specialization (Soberón 1984). The basic sciences were incorporated into medical education, and postgraduate and continuing education was introduced (Soberón 1984). Laguna observed, "Our concepts of the basic sciences followed from models developed in Western industrialized societies and have facilitated in large measure the implementation of curative medicine that revolves around medical specialization, growth of complex and expensive technology, and the concern of the doctors and institutions have focussed on difficult and complicated medical problems, on rare medical problems of an organic nature" (1984:67). According to Laguna, medical practice in Mexico has been transformed in the last forty years from empirical practices and "imprecise and blind norms to a professional process within scientific norms, though based on observation and analysis" (Laguna 1984:70). In short, according to this and other physicians and scholars of biomedicine (Fuente et al. 1984), the medical profession has pursued a scientific course, and its major efforts have been dedicated to the basic sciences in medicine.

During the 1940s the majority of young physicians went to study in the United States; in Mexico biomedicine paralleled medical developments there along with its specialization and its organization of hospitals and teaching institutions (Ortiz Monasterio 1984; Mendiola Gomez 1979).[9]

Medical education "has followed the international tendencies of specialization, basically influenced by the North American school" (Ortiz Monasterio 1984:80). Specialties were defined around the model of the "Boards" in 1965. In 1946 an inexpensive Spanish edition of Cecil was made available to medical students, facilitating the transmission of American biomedicine.[10]

Mexican physicians take great pride in the fact that with the creation of specialties and vigorous research activities (Chávez Rivera 1984), medicine in Mexico stands on an equal footing with biomedicine practiced in industrially developed countries. Chávez Rivera was concerned that the specializations have created elitism, but he argued that elitism is a product of the intellect, "the indispensable instrument in the advancement of scientific knowledge" (1984:267). In his view, the quality of medical treatment is linked to the progress of Mexico.

The Mexican medical model, like the American, is based on Cartesian dualism, which separates the body and mind and holds a mechanistic concept of the human body (Engel 1977; Osherson and Amara Singham 1981). While Mexican medicine is patterned on the North American model (physicians often can be heard telling a sick person that "the machine has broken down"), Mexican medicine has a distinctive Mexican cast and it must be understood within the local socioeconomic and sociocultural contexts. For this reason biomedical practice must not be compared with practices in other sociocultural settings, as, for example, the United States, as we are wont to do.

Psychiatry

I pause briefly on psychiatry in Mexico, which unlike biomedicine has not had the same impact there as in the United States. While psychiatry in the orthodox Freudian tradition has its adherents in Mexico, especially among elites who can afford it.[11] Eric Fromm and his school have had the most influence in Mexico. Irrespective of the theoretical orientation, however, psychiatry is relegated to a secondary role. In Salud Hospital with all its specialties and advanced technology, the psychiatric service occupies a very small office with two cubicles.

Psychiatry has not taken root in Mexico for many reasons. According to one psychiatrist and some physicians in the hospital, the popular view is that psychiatry is only for the "crazies" (*los locos*), and patients eschew referrals to psychiatry. Indeed, I witnessed very few patient referrals to psychiatry. Patients with "emotional problems" were often referred to neurology rather than psychiatry. In fact, the two patients in the sample who were referred to psychiatry were offended and angry with the physician because they did not consider themselves "crazy." Referrals to neurology reflect the European influence on Mexican medicine, where the lines between psychiatry and neurology were not clearly drawn and where concepts of the somatic basis of mental illness were pursued (Shryock 1974).

Psychiatry failed to gain a firm foothold in Mexico because of its prevailing notion of the autonomous individual rather than the autonomous family of which the individual forms a part. The notion of the autonomous individual goes against dominant cultural understandings in all sectors of Mexican society, where, as I noted before, the family and not the individual is the fundamental unit of society.

Importantly too, early Freudian notions regarding a relationship between sexual deficits and emotional disturbances, voiced by some Mexican psychiatrists, flow counter to traditional cultural etiological notions of emotions that emanate from social interaction and the life world.

Recruitment into the Profession and Medical Education

The biomedical model of disease and its treatment is transmitted to its practitioners through the education of physicians. Recruitment into the profession also bears on our understanding of physicians' status in Mexico and on medical education. Medicine is taught in government-supported universities, foremost of which is the UNAM in Mexico City. Other state-supported universities in Mexico City, arguably less prestigious than the UNAM, include the Politecnicum and the Metropolitan University. Individual states also have government-sponsored medical schools. There are at least two prestigious and costly private universities in Mexico City that, like the National University, inculcate a strict biomedical model and teach biomedicine as a scientific discipline.[12]

Recruitment into the School of Medicine at UNAM since the 1970s was governed by a policy of overall democratization of education, and admission was for all practical purposes without restriction to all graduates from the UNAM preparatory school. During the peak recruitment into the profession in the 1970s there were 5,000 medical students attending the Faculty of Medicine. In the 1970s, accompanying the oil boom, a political decision was made to open twenty-five new medical schools in the country, and there was a 130 percent increase in admissions since 1970 (Frenk 1978). There was a sevenfold increase in medical students between 1970 and 1983 (Soberón and Narro 1984). According to one educator the open admission policy resulted in declining educational standards because, in his words, "you cannot fail everybody."

The curriculum consists chiefly of the basic sciences with little exposure to clinical practice. According to Frenk (1978) and Flores Carbajal (1988), 90 percent of the curriculum entails biological sciences and only 10 percent of medical education is dedicated to social medicine and psychology. During the Lazaro Cardenas regime (1935-1939), rural medicine was introduced in Mexico through the Social Service program out of the president's commitment to the rural population who suffered a grave shortage of physicians (Flores Carbajal 1988). The Politecnicum's School of Medicine was originally established to service the health needs of the rural population with a strong emphasis on social medicine and anthropology. Subsequently, however, the UNAM curriculum was copied, and currently biomedicine is taught in its orthodox form there (Flores Carbajal 1988). In most universities, in fact, medical education since World War II became totally influenced by North America, focusing on biology with "conceptions of fragmented human beings, that emphasize studies and treatment of systems and organs separated from the social and psychological causes of disease" (Flores Carbajal 1988:6). This historian of medical education in Mexico decried the emphasis on technology and the absence of a humanistic perspective: Both tend to ignore social and psychological factors in disease.

The major exposure physicians receive to clinical practice and the medical needs of the Mexican people is through the Social Service program, which requires medical students to practice medicine for a year in the countryside. With few exceptions, all physicians must spend a year in a rural town or village, and for those who come from relatively comfortable homes in Mexico City it may be their first exposure to rural realities of poverty and lack of modern amenities. In the words of one physician, social service was "a watershed in my life."

Medical education and Mexico's emulation of the North American biomedical model along Flexner's prototype[13] have been criticized by some Mexican physicians and scholars of Mexican medicine on at least two counts. First, there is the often heard criticism of biomedicine's biological reductionism and dualism: It fragments the human body and addresses the disease rather than the patient (Martínez Cortes 1987). This criticism is widespread in the United States as well (Engel 1977; Hahn and Kleinman 1983; Kleinman 1988; Powels 1973). It has been amply discussed and its arguments are well known; I referred to it earlier and I will not dwell on it here. The substance of these criticisms, biomedicine's organic orientation, concomitant with the ways it is taught and practiced, has created various struggles for Mexican physicians, which I will discuss in the next chapter.

Second, the assertion is made that biomedicine in Mexico fails to address health issues rooted in public health problems associated with poverty, inequality, and capitalism (Horn 1983), a criticism that has also been lodged against the medical establishment in North America (Navarro 1976, 1986; Waitzkin 1983).

I pause to examine the critique of biomedicine voiced by Mexicans pertaining to its failure to address the needs of the nation. Mexican critics of biomedicine assert that because "the Flexner report has been the most powerful influence on medical education in Mexico" and "medical investigations are based upon United States models, they have little relevance for the realities of Mexico" (Frenk 1978:21). It is said that students learn about diseases, diagnostic procedures, and complex technological therapeutics but not about primary care. Mexican students learn little about predominant pathologies in the Mexican population. The books they use, such as Cecil or Harrison, fail to reflect Mexican realities. These texts speak little to infectious pathologies, parasitosis, or about the complex relationship between ecology and infectious disease (Frenk 1978). Scant attention is paid to mechanisms of transmission, which Frenk argued persuasively are rooted in social causes (also Evans et al. 1981). According to Frenk, medical schools use manuals in microbiology that discuss microorganisms not seen in Mexico. They discuss Mediterranean fever, North Asian fever, and Montana fever, but fewer than four pages focus on salmonellas that produce gastroenteritis, one of the most common diseases in Mexico. Frenk noted that "the inadequacies of the health needs of the Mexican population that characterize the programs and the texts used in the schools of medicine are a reflection of the positivist education that has been copied from foreign programs." This creates "contradictions for Mexican physicians who assimilate the most recent technical and scientific advances from other countries, while the national pattern of disease continues to be similar to that of the last century" (Frenk 1978:24).

Echoing Frenk's criticism, one physician participating in the study observed that instead of practicing good traditional medicine (i.e., clinical medicine), they practice bad first-world medicine; they are not taught solid clinical practice, for example, how to interrogate a patient. Moreover, physicians lack preparation to use the technology of the first world, which is not readily accessible to them.

Related to this line of criticism, physicians deplore the emphasis on specialization in Mexico (Cleaves 1987) when the country desperately needs primary care physicians rather then cardiologists and other specialists, especially in rural areas. In the words of another physician, "In Mexico there is a hierarchy in the medical profession and the specialists hold the most important positions and esteem. It is like a military service with only generals and colonels." To the lament of the generalists, it is the specialists who enjoy the greatest prestige and the large practices because not all medical school graduates are admitted into residencies in government institutions.[14]

Physicians' Social Status

The distinction physicians make between specialists and generalists leads me to dwell briefly on physicians' social and economic position in Mexican society, because it also bears on their role as healers. Biomedicine has established its hegemony in Mexico and dominates health care delivery there. In the words of one patient, "Biomedicine is like the ruling party, the PRI [Institutionalized Revolutionary Party]." There is a pervasive conviction in the power of biomedicine to cure all ills. People have phenomenal faith in the curative powers of biomedicine--so much so that, when it fails them, they are frequently led to believe that they have become bewitched (Finkler 1985). The reasoning is as follows: If biomedicine could not cure an ill, then it must have been due to malfeasance, for if the disturbance was not produced by witchcraft, then biomedicine could cure it.

But while biomedicine's validity is not doubted as a curing system, its practitioners' prestige and power is not commensurate with the system itself (Cleaves 1987). Physicians hold power over patients through the diagnosis and causal explanations they provide. In Wolf's words, "The ability to bestow meanings--to 'name' things, acts,...and ideas--is a source of power" (Wolf 1982:388). Yet, as physicians, they lack the power and prestige that one would expect to emanate from biomedicine's authority as a healing system. While patients have great expectations of biomedical technology and pharmaceutical drugs, in the minds of patients, physicians are viewed as part of an undifferentiated mass of healers with whom one may disagree, say, about a diagnosis.

Doctors are conscious of a time when physicians enjoyed great prestige. In the words of one young physician, in the 1950s doctors were "persons of respect and money, but since the 1970s [when he graduated from medical school], a doctor is the same as anybody else." In the words of another physician who occupies a relatively high post in the medical bureaucracy, "By and large today physicians are like any other workers, especially those that are not specialists." In fact, the physicians working in the outpatient clinic are often regarded as exiles to the "Siberia of the hospital." They occupy low status within the profession because they are internists, taken to mean generalists, and some are not markedly removed from their patients' standard of living or style of life.

The medical profession has not achieved the prestige and power in Mexico as it has, say, in the United States (Freidson 1970) for several important reasons, reasons that also illuminate broader sociopolitical processes of the nation-state in which biomedicine is embedded. First, as part of the government bureaucracy, physicians are subordinate to the state apparatus that controls the institutions in which they are employed. Physicians' power is derived from the bureaucracy in which they serve. The bureaucratic mantle undermines their prestige and power, which might otherwise emanate from the knowledge physicians possess as doctors. Instead, their authority flows from their position in the bureaucracy, which is controlled by the state and the institutions with which they are affiliated: IMSS, ISSSTE, or the SS.

Second, and related to the first, while the government health institutions are controlled by the state, they are autonomous entities allocated separate budgets (Cleaves 1987). The separation of the government medical institutions fragments the medical profession. It places physicians in competition with one another, reflected in differing salary scales for physicians in the various institutions. The profession's divisiveness precludes the development of a corporate consciousness and limits its organizational potential. In the words of one physician whose views also reflect those of his colleagues, "Doctors are completely disunited." These factors--bureaucratic state control, and competition among institutions--fragment the medical profession, deflate its power as a profession, and minimize physicians' identification with their profession.

Third, the state's formal support of homeopathy as an alternative healing system to biomedicine aids in reducing the medical profession's power as the sole legitimate health care delivery system, while concurrently reinforcing its own control over the medical profession. Concomitantly, from Preconquest and Colonial times medicinal plants have been widely used across class lines and given legitimacy by the conquerors. Physicians themselves support alternative therapies, including traditional herbal medicines. The readily available, legitimate alternative sources of health care militate against complete dominance of the medical profession as the exclusive health provider in Mexico.

Fourth, the power and prestige of physicians have been further diminished more recently by recruitment policies determined by the state designed to democratize admission. Whereas once physicians were recruited from among the elite, they now originate from many social classes. In the words of one physician discussing unrestricted admission to the medical schools, "Doctors started coming out like sheep."[15] Not unexpectedly, the rapid expansion of medical schools in the 1970s resulted in a surplus of unemployed doctors. The glut of physicians enhanced further the state's ability to exert its power over the profession by making employed physicians thankful for the jobs they held.

Last, it ought not to be overlooked that the broader dependency relationship between Mexico and the United States also bears on physicians' power in Mexico. The authority of physicians is diminished by its dependence on the professional legitimation of the North American medical establishment. As bemoaned by one prominent physician, recognition within the medical profession is given when one's work is first published in the *Journal of the American Medical Association.*

It is noteworthy that many physicians are caught in a bind. While their prestige emanates from an affiliation with one of the government institutions, a good portion of their income comes from their private practice. To maintain themselves at a moderately comfortable standard of living, most physicians in Salud Hospital hold at least two jobs in governmental institutions (Cleaves 1987) and also maintain a private practice. In fact, one physician noted that one day's earnings in his private practice were equivalent to two weeks' salary in the hospital. On the other hand, the fact that he had a post in the hospital enabled him to attract patients to his private practice.[16]

A doctor's economic power is further eroded with the lack of state restrictions on the sale of almost all medications. Patients have ready access to drugs in which they have great faith without the need for prescriptions. Any employee in a pharmacy readily prescribes medication (Finkler 1985), as do neighbors, friends, and relatives. Moreover, individuals themselves may resort to their past experience with a particular drug, which they can easily purchase at any time.

I have given some consideration to Mexican physicians' circumscribed power and prestige because they relate to the manner in which biomedicine is practiced in Mexico. The limited influence individual physicians have on their patients opens the way to view the physician not as the ultimate authority about a diagnosis but as one among many different medical practitioners. It may be one of several factors that lead patients to question and often refute a physician's diagnosis, but agreement with the physician is an important ingredient in affecting the patient's perception of recovery, as we will see in Chapter 10.

The control exerted by state policies leading to fragmentation of the profession may restrict a doctor's development of allegiance to the profession. Physicians' limited identification with the profession influences how biomedicine is practiced, allowing for more idiosyncratic diagnoses and treatment. The diversity in diagnosis of the same symptoms given by different physicians results in patients' confusion about the nature of the sickness, a confusion that may also influence the healing process and lead patients to seek alternative healing regimens. Additionally, such lack of conscious allegiance illuminates in part the fact that many physicians conserve their cultural beliefs about the virtues of alternative healing modalities.

Notes

1. Chávez 1987; Flores y Troncoso 1982 [orig.1886]; Foster 1953; López Austin 1980; López Austin and Viesca 1984; Martínez Cortes 1965; Somolinos d'Ardois 1978, 1979; Viesca 1986.

2. For a discussion of how the plant and the beverage are used in contemporary times, see Finkler 1974.

3. The first physicians who came to Mexico may have been converted Jews, including the great Protomedico Francisco Hernandez.

4. All Spanish sources were translated by the author.

5. In keeping with the Mexican practice to celebrate each profession by a special day, October 23 was designated as "Doctor's Day."

6. The foremost texts in internal medicine used in American medical education that were made the Mexican physicians' "bibles."

7. For the influence of the Flexner Report on American medicine, see Berliner 1975; Starr 1982.

8. Fuente et al. is comprised by a series of articles that deal with biomedicine in Mexico since 1943.

9. At present forty-three specialties are taught in thirty-one hospitals of the Ministry of Health, forty-three hospitals of the Social Security system, and twenty-six of the hospitals of the Federal Health Insurance plan. Also, for an exhaustive list of all the centers of investigation of basic biomedical sciences, see Soberón 1984.

10. One physician was quick to point out that there was not one Mexican contributor in the latest edition of Cecil.

11. The practicing psychiatrist at the hospital indicated that while his salary is like most at the hospital, he charges 50,000 pesos a session, which at the time equaled more than a month's minimum wage.

12. The Metropolitan University has the reputation of training physicians for primary care, and graduates of this university are said to have less prestige and less access to the medical institutional structures that are generally controlled by UNAM graduates.

13. The Flexner model of medical education was introduced to the Faculty of Medicine by its director, Raul Furnir, in 1954-1955 and it laid emphasis on technological rather than clinical practice. See Frenk 1978.

14. In 1987-1988 there were 1,400 positions in the public institutions for specialists and 57,000 candidates who took the examination for admission.

15. Indeed, in 1987 there was a successful student strike, and one of the major issues of the strike was a desire by the university rector to institute more restrictive admissions policies to the university as a whole, including the Faculty of Medicine.

16. In 1986 physicians working in the outpatient clinic were paid approximately $100 a month for 80 hours of work. Subsequently, their salaries

were raised to about $400 a month, more commensurate with salaries paid to IMSS doctors, but their official hours were raised to 160 hours a month.

6

Biomedical Beliefs and Practices

General Considerations

In the last chapter we saw that the American biomedical model was transplanted to Mexico. We must therefore ask, in what ways does a system of knowledge spawned in one society become translated in another? What are the invariant and variant aspects of biomedicine?

To address this question requires us to give some consideration to the core universal characteristics of biomedicine. Contemporary biomedicine is based upon a norm of generalized knowledge and experience (Pellegrino and Thomasa 1981; Gorovitz and MacIntyre 1976) about disease entities and their course. It is practiced within a dyadic encounter between an individual experiencing distress expressed in bodily symptoms and a physician trained in a university to minister to the patient's physical symptoms. To alleviate the patient's malady requires the physician to make a diagnosis, informed by etiological understandings of the patient's symptoms (Feinstein 1973), medical history taking, exploration of symptoms, and signs derived from a physical examination, using various diagnostic tests and technological apparatus. Clinical judgment is based upon a process of exclusion of hypotheses as new information comes to light. A diagnosis, therefore, is provisional (King 1982) and entails a degree of uncertainty, despite the fact that physicians are trained for certainty (Atkins 1975). Biomedical knowledge entails a scientific and systematized understanding of physical pathologies based upon a duality of body and mind. Once the disease entity is established it is usually treated pharmacologically with medications produced in pharmaceutical laboratories.

I hypothesized that biomedicine in Mexico will reflect its purported international character. Decidedly, on first glance biomedical practice in Mexico is not very different from its counterparts the world over. It is easily recognizable by its technological accoutrements (e.g., stethoscopes, sphygmomanometers, scales, Xray machines), and its practitioners by their white coats. More important, however, the nomenclature used by biomedical practitioners forms part of an international vocabulary of disease entities, and the medications they prescribe go by similar names, suggesting the internationalization of pharmacological treatments. Biomedicine and the pharmaceutical companies that manufacture its medicines have produced ostensibly an international culture.

But despite these similarities, biomedicine is differentially practiced in Europe (Marsh et al. 1976), in Germany, (Maretzki 1989), and in Japan (Lock 1980). My observations of and discussions with seventeen physicians and close collaboration with eight reveal that in Mexico certain domains of biomedicine are culturally molded, some are idiosyncratically constructed by their practitioners, while others retain international configurations.

The structure of the medical consultation, a general understanding of the organic basis of disease, and diagnostic nosologies form part of the international aspects of biomedical practice, but emphasis on clinical practice reflects Mexico's historical affiliation with France. Etiological explanations and consideration of typical symptoms resonate on cultural beliefs, while diagnosis and treatment are influenced by idiosyncratic and international understandings. Diagnoses are derived from clinical reasoning as well as from physicians' stereotypic personal and cultural understandings of pathology (Gaines 1982).

Mexican physicians must confront conflicts stemming from their cultural comprehensions and the international biomedical model which they are taught and to which they accommodate differentially. In this chapter I describe in general terms biomedical practice in Mexico, and I propose a model of invariant and variant facets of biomedicine that sheds light on those aspects of a system of knowledge that remain constant across cultures and those that are subject to individual and cultural interpretation. In the next chapter, I shall draw some comparisons among the various physicians that illustrate the variability in biomedical practice.

The hallmark of biomedical activity is the diagnostic process, identifying disease entities using universal nosological classifications, and treatment. Much has been written about the diagnostic process, whether it is an art (Cassell 1976; Munson 1981) or a science (Reiser and Rosen 1984; Feinstein 1973). Theoretically, diagnostic reasoning flows from etiological understanding of the disease symptoms (Feinstein 1967; King 1982). When an organism is invaded by noxious pathogens, the etiology is easily established. It is only when there is no obvious invasion of the body by pathogens, when the diseases are of a congenital or degenerative origin, or when the disease entities lack unique etiologies that causality becomes unclear (Engelhard 1975:132; McKeown 1979). Nevertheless, according to the biomedical model disease is rooted in physical pathology and organic dysfunction. Psychoanalysis has influenced the development of psychosomatic conceptions of disease as governed by unconscious psychological processes (Armstrong 1977, 1982; Figlio 1982), particularly when a specific cause cannot be detected.

Since the Flexner Report, which as we have seen had served as a model for Mexican medicine, biomedicine has been cloaked in a scientific mantle and nourished by physics, chemistry, and biology (Berliner 1975; King 1982; Starr 1982). Ideally, the diagnostic process ought to follow scientific procedures of hypothesis testing as well as interpretation of patients' symptoms in an artful fashion. Diagnosis is usually based on a patient's subjective presentation of symptoms and doctors' objective assessments of signs measured by a variety of techniques, including physical examination, auscultation, percussion, medical history taking, and an array of technological assessments (Reiser 1978).

Clinical reasoning entails a constant reevaluation of the initial diagnosis of the patient's condition, a ruling out of some hunches, and refining or changing the diagnosis as new information is gleaned about the patient from diagnostic tests, signs, and symptoms. Clinical judgment involves the weighing of alternative possibilities and "reasoning back to causes" (King 1982:300). Uncertainty exists about almost all diagnoses. They are subject to revision as new information about the patient unfolds (King 1982). King, for example, distinguished between good and bad medical practice: Good medical practice calls for reflection, evaluation of alternatives, the making of a deliberate choice, and not administering therapy automatically in response to a set of symptoms (King 1982:301).

Excepting surgery, biomedical treatment techniques rely heavily, if not exclusively, upon pharmacological remedies to eradicate noxious pathogens or, more commonly, alleviate symptoms, if only temporarily. Generally speaking, most medications act to alleviate the symptoms rather than eliminate their causes (Thomas 1977; Pellegrino 1979). Increasingly, however, the symbolic aspects of biomedical treatments are being recognized (Comaroff 1982), including the power of the placebo that rests in the medications, the diagnosis, and the diagnostic apparatus (Brody and Waters 1980; Sox 1981; Spiro 1986).

As I noted previously, contemporary biomedicine has been criticized for its reductionism and dualism, the objectification of the patient, and isolation from his or her social and cultural environment. The reliance on technology and the quest for objective--that is, scientific--measures of disease through the development of complex diagnostic technology has led to an obliteration of the patient as a whole being removed from his suffering (Kleinman 1988) and to the reduction of the human being to a mechanical body.[1]

The current emphasis on technology in American biomedical practice is being viewed with some alarm by practitioners.[2] Mexican day-to-day primary care practice has not become dependent on technology as yet, but it has produced dilemmas for its practitioners.

Biomedicine in Mexico

While recognizing that biomedicine practiced in Mexico has its roots in developments in North America, Mexican physicians speak of Mexican medicine, by which they mean clinical medicine and which they contrast with North American technological medicine.

Emphasis on clinical rather than technological medicine in Mexico is associated with its historical antecedents and ideological affinity to France and with structural constraints rooted in national economic and political priorities. Structurally, biomedical practice forms part of a bureaucratic state system that has placed its priorities on tertiary care. Indeed, Mexico possesses the complex modern medical technology of any economically developed country (Piahaud 1979), but Salud Hospital outpatient service lacks even the basic diagnostic tools.

There exists, however, an ideological commitment to clinical medicine rather than technological medical activities, which engages Mexican physicians in a struggle that is perhaps not unique to Mexico (Armstrong 1977, 1982; King 1987) between emphasis on clinical and technological medicine. This struggle stems as much from economic constraints as from an ideological disposition to interpret sickness in traditional terms. Concurrently, as physicians trained in the biomedical model, they reinterpret sickness in a biomedical idiom. If we consider the core of medical practice--etiology, diagnosis, and treatment (Elstein 1978; Feinstein 1973, 1983; King 1982)--the etiology of sickness is chiefly understood in the traditional Mexican way. Physicians make diagnoses using biomedical nosological categories shaped by an individual physician's training and interest. Treatment varies with a particular physician's background but consists primarily, if not exclusively, of pharmacological monitoring of the body's physiological processes with some attention paid to diet.

Etiological Beliefs

By and large, Mexican physicians tend to be drawn into latent conflicts between their intuitive cultural understandings and their medical training, which they resolve by reducing cultural holistic notions of sickness to organic dysfunctions and mind/body duality. They invoke etiological explanations that are closely linked to cultural notions. These explanations tend to be reductionist, in much the same way as biomedicine is. This reductionism contrasts with the patients, whose explanations are fluid and who incorporate a variety of emotive and existential suppositions to make sense of their sickness. Patients may include anger, nerves, fright, daughter running away from home, the earthquake, and any other experiences that become embodied and expressed symptomatologically.

Physicians combine biomedical with traditional folk understandings to explain sickness. In the majority of cases, the physicians' etiological explanations correspond with traditional folk understandings relating to emotional discharges such as anger, nerves, and fright; to a lesser extent, to environmental and social causes; and to diet. I hasten to add that most physicians show little concern for underlying causality and only limited interest in proximate causes incorporated by the diagnosis. To cite an example, a patient with headaches was diagnosed as having scoliosis and flat feet, to which the physician attributed the patient's headaches. When I questioned the physician about the underlying cause of scoliosis, the physician was stopped short and hard-pressed to explain its etiology, which after some thought he attributed to poor sitting position and bad posture.

My findings suggest that physicians' etiological beliefs about underlying, if not proximate, causes are heavily laden with traditional etiological beliefs that become reinterpreted in medical terms. With the one exception of a physician who adhered to an orthodox biomedical model of physiological dysfunction, most provided an interpretation of underlying, and in some instances proximate, causes of a given set of symptoms, akin to the cultural etiological explanations discussed in Chapter 3. These include climatic insults and dietary deficiencies, but mainly disease is attributed to nerves, angers, or social causes. These are not uncommonly perceived stereotypically as patients having "problems at home" related to poverty resulting from their "ignorance and lack of education." Emotive experiences such as nerves tend to be translated into organic terms; for many, the result is a problem of the nervous system, which for some is also associated with the spinal column.

More specifically, diet and climatic changes are part of the etiological folk baggage for both physicians and patients. Many physicians associate poor diet with the overall poor health state of the population they treat. Often they attribute specific gastrointestinal dysfunctions to the spicy Mexican diet and to the eating of pork, which is considered an irritant to the stomach.

Tonsillitis, or a general pain in the throat, is almost always attributed by physicians and patients to inclement weather or to getting wet. Two physicians combine folk and environmental explanations by including air pollution in the city as an important factor influencing respiratory and tonsillitis problems.

There is great ambiguity among physicians with regard to the etiological role of nerves. Some physicians retain their cultural understanding of nerves as a state of being, while others consider nerves as a psychological disturbance. For some, nerves is a physiological dysfunction of the nervous system, for others it is an emotionally uncontrolled state, and for still others it is attributed to social causes. Irrespective of their interpretation of nerves, all physicians, with one exception, usually asked patients during the physical examination or history taking whether they were nervous. They usually medicalize it in terms of a physiological condition not uncommonly associated with a disorder of the spine, requiring intervention by neurologists or even orthopedists.

According to one physician, 90 percent of patients suffer from nerves, which he regards as a neurological problem. For example, a patient reported to this physician that she was very nervous; the physician explained that she was suffering from rheumatism in the spinal column, and the spinal column, being in the center of the nervous system, produced her nervous state. This physician imposed on patients the notion that they are nervous or have "made an anger," even in the face of the patient's denial. For example, he asked a patient with abdominal pain whether she was nervous. When she said no, he nevertheless insisted that nerves was the root of her problem. In the case of Nomi, who suffered from a serious kidney impairment, this physician attributed her disturbance to nerves.

Yet another physician regarded nerves as a condition of the nervous system that is lodged in the head and spinal column and affects all other bodily functions. When a young male patient complained of chest pain, the physician attributed the symptoms to a disturbance of the nerves that entered the heart, so she diagnosed his condition as polineuritis. For a third physician, nerves as manifested by pain in the *cerebro* and gastritis has an economic origin that affects rich and poor alike, whether "one worries about one's stocks or about having enough food to eat."

It is noteworthy that with few exceptions, physicians frequently diagnose patients with problems of the spine. Their emphasis on the spinal column may reflect a reinterpretation of nerves as a dysfunction of the nervous system that is lodged in the spine and that causes a nerve sickness.

Three physicians regarded nerves as rooted in emotional or psychological states of anxiety rather than in the nervous system. They attributed numerous symptoms to nerves, including intestinal problems and abdominal pains. When a woman patient reported that she had experienced a fright because she had witnessed a shooting the day before and she was terrified, the physician responded with, "You are very nervous." In this case the physician's ontological view of nerves disassociated the woman's condition from her experience of terror. Still others dismiss a variety of symptoms, including chest pain, with the statement, "It is only nerves." One young physician responded to a patient's statement, "I am very nervous," with "Yes, but what other disturbances do you have," giving short shrift to the patient's declaration. One physician attributed nerves in women to menopause, not an uncommon attribution for a variety of symptoms experienced by women over forty years of age.

Reflecting the population at large, some physicians regard "making an anger" as a result of being nervous, others view nerves and anger as synonymous, and still others separate experiences of anger from nerves. But no matter how physicians perceive the two dispositions, almost all physicians routinely ask patients as part of the medical history taking whether they have "made an anger" recently, irrespective of the nature of the symptoms the patients present. In their view emotional upsets and anger cause numerous symptoms. In one case the physician diagnosed a patient as suffering from colitis, irritable colon, and neurosis, attributing the woman's condition to anger and emotional upsets resulting from her grave conflicts with her husband. According to one physician, when a patient reports symptoms in every bodily organ, it suggests to the physician that they are due to an anger. Anger can thus explain generalized as well as specific symptoms, including, of course, high and low blood pressure.

All physicians relate patients' symptomatology to adverse life circumstances, which some physicians regard as determined by one's character at birth and social circumstances. Others regard the symptomatology as intrinsic to economic conditions in Mexico. Predictably, different physicians dealt with and interpreted the symptoms in various ways. One physician attributed almost all sickness presented by patients in the hospital to wife-beating and economic problems. He distinguished between subjective sickness that he regarded as "conversions" and objective sickness such as appendicitis, a condition that could be measured. This physician argued that the medicalization of life's problems, with physicians prescribing medications for harsh life circumstances, simply aggravated the people's economic situation because they were confronted with the new and additional expenses of medications.

Other physicians, who ascribed patients' symptoms to life's problems, regarded these patients as a nuisance, especially when the patients were women. For example, one physician noted that when a woman turned up with new symptoms every time she came to see him, it was most assuredly "a case of somatization caused by her husband's lack of attention to her." He usually had not found anything seriously wrong with patients of this type.

Even physicians who regarded sickness as rooted in social causes still had a relatively stereotypic and reductionist understanding of it: Stereotypic because they judged the population they treated as an undifferentiated mass of "the poor," and reductionist because they diminished causality to poverty alone. Most physicians fail to *fine-tune* each patient's suffering and its causes within the context of the patient's life. In short, by attributing sickness only to people's poverty, physicians fail to discern patients' presenting symptoms as expressions of embodied adverse existence moored both in society and in phenomenology, a point I will explore in Chapter 11. By medicalizing life's problems and emotional discharges, which are essentially moral and existential statements, physicians promote a demand for medication and the resulting growth of the pharmaceutical industry (Brudon 1987; Gereffi 1983; Villanueva and Quintana 1982).

Additionally, medication becomes a major expectation of treatment and attribution for recovery. By medicalizing and reinterpreting lived experience and emotional states--for example, nerves as a problem of the nervous system or deviated spinal column--physicians remove the patient from his or her pain and its attendant cultural denotations and envelop the patient and themselves in a drama, which is the medical consultation, a point I shall explore in Chapter 8.

In much the same way as physicians' attributions retain a traditional cast, so too do their responses to patients' presentation of typical symptoms, such as pain in the *cerebro*, pain in the lungs, pain in the kidneys, and high and low blood pressure. Generally speaking, most physicians intuitively recognize the metaphoric content of the self-diagnosis of high and low blood pressure and treat it medically. Physicians understand the cultural meanings of these symptoms; for example, when patients speak of feeling crestfallen, dizzy, or lazy, physicians spontaneously respond by checking the patient's blood pressure. By doing so, they are dealing with profound sadness and suffering in a biomedical and physical way and concurrently impose on a folk level a corporeal grasp of existential experience.

Almost all physicians, when asked about high and low blood pressure, equated low blood pressure with dejection and being crestfallen (*decaimiento*), described in the words of one physician as "the sky falls down on you." The experience of both reflects vicissitudes in the patient's experience. Rather than denying the existence of this condition, however, they reinterpret it in physiological terms. In the words of one physician, "pressure must be measured," and it is then treated medically. One physician entered it into the medical record as neurasthenia and treated it as a nervous disorder.

The proposition is advanced that the phenomenon of patients' experiencing high and low blood pressure reflects a structuration process (Giddens 1979) between macrophenomena, biomedical practice, and micro-events shaped by cultural understandings (Harre 1981; Knorr-Cetina 1981). To patients "low pressure" clearly symbolizes adverse emotional and lived experience that produces a sense of despair; "high blood pressure" denotes a state of agitation and anger. High and low blood pressure is, in the words of one woman, when "things have gotten out of control." Physicians medicalize these meanings by interpreting them in the biomedical terms of blood pressure and treating them; in turn, patients come to physicians to seek treatment for an existential condition that they identify as high and low blood pressure. The majority of physicians, like patients, attribute "pressure" to nerves or anger, especially when it goes up. One physician blended emotional, existential, and physiological explanations to explain the cultural concept of high and low blood pressure by linking it to nerves. According to him, pressure was unstable and went up and down as a consequence of nerves. The nervous system fails to regulate the pressure mechanism. In this view emotional instability and suffering lead to discharges of catecholamines affecting the nervous system, thus resulting in labile, "unstable" pressure.

Interestingly, when a patient reported "pressure," as one of his or her symptoms, physicians asked if the condition had been experienced by a family member; they then recorded it in the medical history without associating it with the symbolic meaning that they intuitively knew as members of Mexican culture. In fact, one physician in her late fifties diagnosed herself as having high and low blood pressure. When she measured her blood pressure it was 110/70. She remarked to me that she was suffering from low pressure that she attributed to her anemic condition and cardiac lesions, and which went "up and down" due to nerves, fright, and anger. One physician attributed a woman's high and low blood pressure to "making an anger" and sadness because her brother was murdered, both coupled with the woman's suffering from a potassium deficiency. In this instance he blended his folk understandings with a biomedical explanation of the condition. Physicians attribute high and low blood pressure to emotive states, but also to menopause, change in climate, renal problems, cardiac impairment, nervousness, and frights (*susto*, or anxiety).

Physicians usually deal with typical symptoms within the context of the patient's presentation. It is only when a patient presented a self-diagnosis of high and low pressure, even when his or her pressure reading was 110/70, that the physician corroborated it and treated it pharmacologically. One physician, who adhered to an orthodox organic explanation of disease, categorically denied that high and low blood pressure was a valid medical category and he never treated it. He regarded it as a "nondisease" (Robbins et al. 1982) and claimed it was "an expression of mood vicissitudes."[3]

Some physicians adhere to idiosyncratic etiological explanations not shared by others. There is a trend among various physicians to attribute maladies not directly related to parasites to the spinal column and flat feet. While the spinal column is associated with the nervous system, it is also a sui generis explanation for at least one physician. Here the etiological explanation may be totally idiosyncratic rather than cultural and is in line with his stated failed aspiration to do a specialty in orthopedics.

Another physician's attributions concomitant with diagnoses reflected her personal view of male sexuality and morality, as when she ascribed a male patient's kidney infection, another's chest pains, and a third's abdominal pains to what she assessed to be their excessive sexual activities. She usually diagnosed unmarried male patients as homosexuals. In the case of a hairdresser, she explained that when men have anal intercourse, "It goes way up to their spine, and upsets the entire nervous system," leading to sickness of all kinds.

Physicians' idiosyncratic causal explanations are not readily accepted by patients. A patient with chest pains denied that his ailment was related to his diagnosed scoliosis and flat feet. Given that determining underlying, if not proximate, causality is not inherent to the diagnostic process but dependent upon clinical experience of symptomatology, a physician's etiological understandings are susceptible to cultural and individual malleability.

The Diagnostic Process

Despite the importance of medical history taking for getting at an accurate diagnosis of a patient's condition (Hampton et al. 1975; King 1987), Mexican physicians struggle with reliance on the North American emphasis on technology versus reliance on patients' presentation of symptoms and medical history. Ironically, industrially advanced societies have begun to question dependence on technology[4] and are reexamining its use (Feinstein 1983), while in Mexico the issue is its absence rather than its overuse.

Mexican doctors are conflicted between what they regard as two different types of medicine: clinical and technological. When Mexico modeled its biomedical practices and beliefs on North American forms, it produced conflicts for practitioners for at least two reasons. First, historically, Mexico continues to have strong intellectual ties to France and admiration for its culture. This French heritage, rightly or wrongly, is viewed as relying on clinical rather than technological medicine associated with North American practice. In fact, French culture is regarded as a variant of Latin culture, and physicians take pride in Latins being the best clinicians. Second, lack of economic resources places constraints on accessibility to medical technology. While Mexico possesses all the modern medical technological accoutrements in its private and large public hospitals, on a day-to-day level the public hospital physician lacks even the simplest medical tools. Physicians experience conflicts with regard to the use of technological supports, which they at once admire, but consider expedient in reducing expenses for the hospital and the patient, despite the fact that patients may desire electrocardiograms and Xrays.

One physician observed that he often had male patients in their twenties and early thirties who reported chest pain. He knew that it was much more common for a patient at that age to have muscular discomfort than angina or a myocardial infarction, but he knew there may be exceptions. He reasoned that while on the one hand, myocardial infarctions were encountered more and more in this age range, on the other hand, the medical facilities at the hospital limited him to routinely order an electrocardiogram for every young man who reports chest pain. The physician was, however, troubled by his contradictory experience because these young patients felt better when an electrocardiogram was normal.

Physicians often ordered routine laboratory tests (complete blood profile, fecal culture, and urinalysis) and employed other diagnostic measures to support rather than to formulate a diagnosis. I found that with one exception, physicians ordered routine laboratory tests in 15 to 20 percent of their cases. One physician ordered laboratory tests for a third of his patients. With some small variation, physicians rarely ordered Xrays and other diagnostic technologies such as ultrasounds and electrocardiograms (one physician did in 4 percent of the cases, while two physicians never did so).

Interestingly, if physicians were faced with conflicting evidence between patients' symptomatic presentation and laboratory test results, they usually gave more credence to patients' symptoms. For example, although stool analysis for ova and parasites showed as negative, if the patient presented symptoms which the physician judged to be indicative of amebiasis, the diagnosis and treatment were based upon the patient's symptomatology and not on the test results. The test results were assumed to be incorrect. One physician uniformly diagnosed all patients as having parasites and never ordered fecal stool examinations. Most physicians routinely diagnose parasitosis.

As part of the diagnostic process, physicians take exhaustive medical histories. In keeping with their understanding of the epidemiology of parasitosis in Mexico City, all physicians question patients about stool evacuations to the extent that they instill into patients a consciousness of their bowel movements they had not possessed before. Generally speaking, the exhaustive medical history for diagnostic purposes increases patients' awareness of their bodies, heightening the experience of their symptoms.

The medical history taking varies in emphasis. Some physicians questioned patients about the minutia of their stools, while others asked about bowel movements in general terms. Some physicians also extensively questioned patients about their sexual activities. According to one physician referring to his female patients, Mexican male machismo may be hurtful to women. This line of questioning required patients to reveal the most intimate details of their beings.

Physicians complained that patients did not report all the symptoms necessary to assist them in making an accurate diagnosis. Several patients I interviewed failed to report to the physicians symptoms that they reported to me on the first interview prior to the medical consultation. In some cases it may have been headaches, in others, vaginal discharges or even diarrhea. The latter two signs were frequently taken for granted by patients and became known to a physician only if the patient was questioned about them. With one exception, all the physicians performed a physical examination by auscultation and percussion.

Theoretically at least, physicians make their diagnoses on the basis of patients' presenting symptoms, medical history taking, and a physical examination. But in the final analysis clinical judgments were based upon physicians' stereotypic epidemiological understandings of the patient population, individual physicians' training and experience, and moral values that were often unrelated to patients' symptomatic presentations and medical history, not unlike what has been observed by others in the United States (Gaines 1982). The diagnostic process incorporates habitual reasoning that the patient population seeking treatment in the Salud Hospital outpatient clinic is parasite burdened. Irrespective of the patient's symptoms, he or she was invariably diagnosed with parasitosis by the majority of the physicians. In one extreme case, the physician diagnosed all his patients with parasites, regardless of the symptoms they had presented.

It is common knowledge that parasitic infections are endemic across Mexico, although it is disputed to what degree individuals may be simply carriers as opposed to experiencing parasitic disease, especially amebiasis (Gutierrez 1986, 1987; also personal communication 1987a). A large number of infected individuals are healthy carriers, and some contend that physicians overdiagnose and overmedicate for this disease. According to Gutierrez, "The fundamental problem consists in a tendency of erroneously diagnosing amebiasis in cases of diarrhea and dysentery due to the difficulty in practicing laboratory examinations" (Gutierrez 1986:375; also 1987, 1987a). Physicians in the study disputed such findings and claimed that patients' symptomatology clearly warranted a diagnosis of parasites, with amebiasis and tricosephalus being the primary pathogens.

Diagnostic validity was usually established when a patient reported on a return visit that he or she was feeling better as a result of the drug the physician prescribed. Paradoxically, using symptom alleviation through medication to corroborate the correctness of a diagnosis removes the authority of physicians, but also reassures them of the precision of their diagnosis. When a patient, after having taken the prescribed medication, returned to report that there had been no, or only minor, improvement, the physician revised the diagnosis, not uncommonly to a problem of the spinal column or nerves; or the physician made a referral to a specialist.

Treatment Management

Unlike etiological beliefs that are heavily laden with folk understandings, and unlike diagnoses that vary with physicians' individual training and experience, the medical encounter and treatment, generally speaking, follow the international aspects of biomedicine with its dyadic interaction, referrals to specialists, and reliance on medication. The structural configurations of the physician-patient encounter do not differ among physicians, and they closely resemble the doctor-patient encounter in the United States. The relationship is paternalistic, with an active physician and a passive patient, which is characteristic of the Szasz and Hollander (1956) model of guidance and cooperation. The superordinate-subordinate relationship places the patient in a passive role vis-a-vis the physician. While structurally the encounter does not differ among physicians, individual nonverbal and verbal communicative styles may. This includes whether the physician stands up to shake the patient's hand or remains sitting, oblivious to the incoming patient; or whether the physician interacts with the patient by smiling or acting grumpy.

There is wide variation in physicians' referrals to specialists ranging between 8 and 11 percent of the cases, although one physician never referred patients to specialists. Physicians often tended to rely on their own expertise for diagnosis and treatment rather than referrals, which patients often expected. Physicians were sometimes critical of those who used the referral system and regarded them as incompetent to treat. The fact that patients have great confidence in specialists but are not referred to them has some influence on the way they perceive the treatment they have received. On the other hand, referrals sometimes place an unnecessary economic burden on patients, especially those who are referred to Orthopedics, where they may be ordered to obtain Xrays and prescribed a special brace they can ill afford.[5]

Medication is a physician's treatment of choice. Only one physician failed to prescribe any medication to as many as eight of thirty-seven patients in the sample he saw. With the exception of one physician who emphasized diet and exercise and who prescribed little medication, most physicians prescribed on the average three medications per patient; the range was between 1.7 and 5.5 medications per patient.

Because physicians commonly diagnose parasitosis, most prescribe an antiparasitic treatment to all patients. Two physicians even prescribed antiparasitic treatment to the entire family and especially the spouse on the grounds that these parasites were transmitted when underwear was washed together, or by sexual intercourse. Given the sociocultural importance of the family, it is surprising that more physicians do not make this type of recommendation, but biomedicine's individualistic cast normally directs treatment to the individual rather than to the group of which a patient is a part.

In Mexico, as in the United States, there is a popular cultural belief that vitamins have special potent force. Physicians variously prescribe a variety of vitamins and tonics, with one physician prescribing them to every patient and one not to any. At least two physicians recommend popular herbal teas for nerves and fright (e.g., te de tilia [*Tilia occidentalis*]).

Treatment is usually both segmented and piecemeal. The physician assigns a different diagnosis to distinct parts of the body, for example, the kidneys and stomach, and treats each problem separately. When a patient reports several ailments in different parts of the body, the physician may ask the patient which ailment the patient wished to have treated first. Thus, almost all patients are initially treated for parasites and then for the other disorders they report.

Beyond medication, diets are variously prescribed. One physician prescribed the same diet to 24 percent of the cases observed, whereas other physicians prescribed diets between 8 and 12 percent of the time. This suggests that most physicians are cognizant of diet as part of a treatment regimen. The most physiologically oriented physician recommended a diet in 2 percent of the cases only, and this recommendation mainly entailed salt reduction for hypertensives. Only one physician regularly prescribed exercises. Treatment also included recall visits. One physician routinely recalled hypertensive patients, and by doing so, the few hypertensives in the sample maintained a blood pressure at a level that eliminated the symptoms for which they came to seek treatment.[6]

With one exception, physicians preached to patients, imposing their own values and their morality, which patients usually regarded as part of their treatment. The nature of the advice varied with the sex and age of the physician as well as with the patient. Their counsel usually revolved around male-female interaction, interaction with other family members, and the importance of education for children. When patients were later questioned about the attribution for change or recovery from their condition, they noted that they had followed the advice of the physician. People expect advice from elders and people in a position of authority.[7] Some physicians transmitted their moral values to patients. One physician, an especially devout Catholic, preached incessantly to both men and women about the importance of church weddings and not abandoning one's family. This physician sermonized to young men against drinking alcoholic beverages, homosexuality, and promiscuity. According to her, too much sex at a young age leads to a man's impotence at age forty. Male physicians preached to young women about the importance of maintaining their virginity and about their obligation to listen to parents who protect them against losing it.

To the extent that patients follow physicians' advice, and I have some evidence to show that they do, physicians not only treat patients' symptoms but also alter to some degree their perceptions, if not their existence.

A Model of the Cultural Transformation of Biomedicine

At the beginning of this chapter, I posed the question: What are the variant and invariant biomedical domains? I discussed the core components of biomedicine,[8] including diagnosis, etiological explanations, and treatment that are played out in an encounter between a physician and a patient. Using the Mexican case, I propose a model of biomedical practice as it becomes transferred from one society to another. The model suggests that while biomedicine shares a universal nosology of disease entities and employs a universal diagnostics vocabulary, the diseases also become shaped culturally by typical symptoms.

Within a given culture, causal explanations comprise a mixture of universal recognition of disease entities and culturally specific conceptions of sickness. While proximate causes are usually understood in biomedical terms, especially when they are embedded in diagnostic categories, underlying causes of a disease entity are likely to be shaped by cultural denotations. The structural relationships encompassed by the doctor-patient encounter to implement treatment assume universal configurations, entailing a dyadic, asymmetric interaction among the practitioner, the expert with generalized knowledge, and the sufferer, who comes with a particularized experience of pain and disorder.

The diagnostic process is universally based upon symptom exploration, medical history taking, and technological supports. In the final analysis, however, diagnostic reasoning is informed not only by a universal understanding of causality and disease processes but by the individual practitioner's personal experiences and training, which become reinterpreted culturally or idiosyncratically.

Treatment is distinctly pharmacological, but it may also draw upon cultural and individual proclivities that may include diet, traditional medicinal pharmacopeia, and counsel. The medical consultations I present in Chapter 8 bring into full view the model of biomedical practice. Studies of biomedicine cross-culturally will further enable us to elaborate on this representation and will illuminate the sustaining transformations that a system of knowledge undergoes from society to society.

In this chapter we have seen the general trends of biomedical practice as exemplified by physicians in Salud Hospital. In the next chapter consideration is given to the individual variations of biomedical practice that further illuminate the general trends.

Notes

1. There is now a small movement in Mexican medicine to see the patient in his totality much along the biopsychosocial model promoted by Engle (1977).

2. See, for example, Budry 1986; Grady 1988; King 1987; Pinckney and Pinckney 1989.

3. In fact, I presented him with the verbatim symptomatology and blood pressure reading of a patient whom we will meet later (Chapter 8), who was treated by one physician for high and low blood pressure. This physician immediately indicated that there was no disease and that there was nothing wrong with the patient.

4. See "Going Overboard on Medical Tests," *Time*, April, 25, 1988.

5. The regular price for Xrays in the hospital is about $2; however, when the hospital machines are broken and patients must have them done in private laboratories, they may cost as much as $10, an expense that most of the patients cannot afford.

6. It is noteworthy that diagnosed hypertensives who upon follow-up reported full recovery were treated by the one physician who kept these patients on recall, while those hypertensives not on recall failed to report any recovery, suggesting that for hypertensive patients, physicians need to rely on recall visits for them to maintain the medication regimen.

7. When the CMI was administered to patients and the question was asked, "Do you feel you need advice from others?" people uniformly said yes and did not regard this as an indication of emotional weakness.

8. These are shared by all healing systems (Kleinman 1988).

7

Variations in Biomedical Beliefs and Practices

In the last chapter, I described general trends in biomedical practice as exemplified by physicians in an Internal Medicine outpatient clinic at Salud Hospital. It is important, however, to attend to the variations by comparing beliefs and practices of the different physicians. Too often individual diversity is overlooked in favor of uniformity, when in actuality there are obvious distinctions within generalized shared understandings. A comparison of individual physicians' diagnostic and treatment activities reveals the idiosyncratic (also Hahn and Gaines 1985), cultural, and international aspects of biomedicine as elucidated by the model set forth in the last chapter. The variability in beliefs and practice we encounter among physicians in Salud Hospital suggests widespread individual variation in the profession as a whole.

It must be emphasized that the brief descriptions here do not do full justice to the complexity of physicians' understanding of disease and its treatment. In this chapter I broadly sketch and highlight the positions of eight physicians bearing on disease causality, diagnosis, and treatment, as well as alternative healing systems that together with biomedicine form part of the total Mexican medical system. I compare, for example, two physicians who represent two extreme stances toward body/mind dualism. For purposes of anonymity, I refer to all physicians by numbers rather than names.

Description of Individual Physicians

Physician 1, in his early thirties, the son of a lower level government employee, was trained in public health as well as medicine. His etiological explanations reflect his epidemiological training and popular Marxist notions of disease being rooted in adverse social, economic, and ecological conditions related to poor diet and general poverty. He blamed patients for their ignorance, lack of education, and bad habits (as, for example, drunkenness), which he associated with faulty education and poverty. His diagnoses, based upon symptom exploration, medical history, and physical examinations, were always biomedical, even when he recognized that a patient could be having "emotional" difficulties that he attributed in a generalized way to conflicting family relationships rooted in poverty. His diagnoses usually revolved around parasites or emotional problems. The latter he ascribed to stress, which became translated into insults to the nervous system. He treated these conditions with muscle relaxants. In the case of a woman who had marital difficulties which he imputed to her "emotional" problems, he nevertheless diagnosed her condition as "prediabetic" and later as "hypoglycemia." He treated patients with medication and had little confidence in folk therapies. He had the reputation for counseling patients. In one case where his counsel had no effect, he referred the patient to psychiatry. On the other hand, a patient whose only symptom was forgetfulness he referred to neurology.

Physician 2, in his mid-thirties, originated from one of the southern Mexican indigenous speaking communities. He was trained in general medicine and combined traditional folk and biomedical explanations of sickness. He regarded the underlying causes, if not the proximate causes, of sickness episodes to be anger, nerves, or existential conditions, which he reduced to stress. He established a diagnosis on the basis of a patient's presenting symptoms, medical history, and an attentive physical examination. His diagnostic repertoire revolved chiefly around parasitic infections, but he was not committed to any one specific diagnostic category. He treated patients with intractable conditions with medication and referred them to specialists if necessary. For instance, he attributed Esperanza's incessant headaches to nerves and poverty; he treated her with medication and finally referred her to Neurology. He had great faith in alternative healing because his grandmother was a traditional curer in his village. He thus regarded alternative healing, including acupuncture, chiropractic, and homeopathy, as viable treatment options which he himself, however, did not employ. This physician had perhaps the most conflict about his role as a medical practitioner because he felt impotent "to help the poor people to escape their poverty," which he regarded as the real underlying sickness. He was very attentive to popular beliefs related to emotional discharges and asked all patients whether they had "made an anger" before they got sick. This physician was very conscious of the prejudices against the poor and people of his origin. He never fixed responsibility for his patients' sickness on their "ignorance and lack of education."

Physician 3, in his mid-twenties, came from a Mexico City elite family and adhered most closely to what is commonly understood as the scientific biomedical model. His etiological explanations focused on organic dysfunction. His diagnostic repertoire was extensive, but frequently it was a variant of a parasitic infection. The diagnoses were based upon symptom exploration, medical history, and physical exploration of some, if not all, patients. The treatments he prescribed were uniquely pharmaceutical. However, he was the only physician who prescribed no medication whatsoever to about 25 percent of the patients he saw during the study period and prescribed only aspirin to a few others. As we will see in the case of Sharon, he ruled out all possibilities of organic dysfunction before he considered the possibility of an emotional problem, which he differentiated from problems of the nervous system. Nerves, for example, he explained as emotional rather than neurological. In cases that he regarded as "emotional disorder," such as anxiety related to problems of living, he referred to Psychiatry. He considered all types of alternative practitioners, for example, practitioners of homeopathy and acupuncture, as charlatans.

Physician 4, in his mid-forties, came from a small community in southwestern Mexico. He first aspired to become an orthopedist. He uniformly attributed to and diagnosed all patients as having a dysfunctional spinal column, usually scoliosis, flat feet, and amebiasis. Although he took a copious clinical history and carried out meticulous physical examinations, his diagnoses never varied, irrespective of the patients' presenting symptoms. He referred them all to one physician in Orthopedics. In addition to this standard diagnosis, he sometimes included obesity. He regarded nerves and other emotional discharges as problems of the nervous system, which he occasionally referred to Neurology or discounted. While he prescribed pharmaceuticals to his patients because "I am in the hospital," he had great faith in traditional pharmacopoeia. In fact, he treated his father's diabetes with traditional medicinal plants rather than pharmaceutical drugs.

Physician 5, a woman in her mid-thirties who came from an upper-middle-class family, followed closely the standard biomedical model. Her etiological explanations were rooted in organic causes, yet she usually inquired about patients' nervous states, which she regarded as problems of the nervous system. She usually passed over problems that may have been characterized as emotional, and her diagnoses and attributions were always within a biomedical idiom. Her repertoire was relatively restricted. In addition to parasites and muscular contractions, her most favored diagnosis, based upon patient exploration of symptoms, clinical history, and physical examination, was "anginas" or tonsillitis. She disclaimed any knowledge of alternative healing.

Physician 6 was a woman in her early sixties of middle-class origins. For her the underlying cause of all disease was a variant of the nervous system, the center of which is situated in the spinal column. The nervous system became afflicted by fright, nerves, or anger, all of which could be transmitted from parents to children through the blood. Proximate causes would include anemia, alcoholism, high and low blood pressure, or in men's cases excessive sexual activity. Her diagnostic repertoire was extensive and based solely on patient symptomatic presentation. The treatments she provided were purely medical.

Physician 6 prescribed almost twice as many pharmacological drugs as did other physicians, and she often included vitamins or native herbal medicine. In keeping with popular beliefs, she differentiated pharmaceutical drugs from herbal medications on the basis that the former simply worked faster than the latter.

Physician 7, a man in his mid-sixties, had studied and practiced acupuncture, homeopathy, and iridology in addition to biomedicine. In his view biomedicine and homeopathy have the same origins in the teachings of Hippocrates, who, according to Physician 7, promulgated the laws of similarity, or homeopathy, and difference, or allopathy. Physician 7 advocated that medicine must be heterodox because biomedicine could identify diseases but not cure them. This physician adhered to the psychosomatic roots of sickness. According to him, all sickness had its origin in emotional-psychological stress or nerves, which he sometimes separated from the nervous system and sometimes reduced to a disequilibrium of the nervous system. In his words, "All disease was functional, there was nothing wrong with most patients." He relied heavily on the generalized concept of stress to explain the antecedent causes of a variety of diagnoses. He also invoked Chinese concepts of yin and yang to explain conditions that were of parasitic origin. He reduced nerves and anger to disorders of the nervous system, metabolic dysfunction, or stress, which in the final analysis he related to the endocrine system.

His diagnostic inventory was varied, however, and was based chiefly on symptomatic exploration and medical history and supported by physical examination. He was one of the few physicians who failed to find parasitic infections in most patients. The emphasis of his treatment was on exercise and diet. Generally speaking, his treatment course was eclectic, and as he liked to point out, "When biomedical drugs fail, I give homeopathic treatments or acupuncture," in much the same way as patients resort to alternative treatments when biomedicine fails. If he assessed that a patient would benefit more from acupuncture than pharmaceutical drugs, he would provide the acupuncture treatment, as he did for two of the subjects of the study. In addition to prescribing acupuncture treatments or homeopathic medicines, he would prescribe gingerroot for pain in the abdominal region, as well as traditional teas that were used for nerves and anger.

Physician 8, in his mid-thirties, originated from a petit bourgeois Mexico City family. He was trained in epidemiology and regarded disease as rooted in the adverse ecological environment of the people. While he was attuned to the role of poverty in sickness, he was sensitive to the existential conditions of his patients, that is, to conflicts that may have produced an illness episode, such as being an adolescent, difficulties at work, and conflicts with parents or spouses. He adhered to an organic model of disease, and like Physician 3, he explained proximate and antecedent causes in terms of physiological dysfunctions and nerves. His diagnoses were based on symptomatic exploration, clinical history, careful physical examination, and on the characteristics of the neighborhood in which the patient resided. If the patient lived, say, in Neza, he automatically deduced that the patient was suffering from parasitic infections. Indeed, amebiasis was his most frequent diagnostic category. When other diagnostic categories and treatments failed to alleviate the patient's disorder, he diagnosed obesity or scoliosis and referred the patient to Orthopedics. Physician 8 treated all patients with pharmaceutical drugs and took an agnostic position with regard to traditional therapies, which he believed do neither harm nor good.

These brief depictions call attention to the diverse backgrounds and stances of the various physicians. Physicians 3 and 5 followed most closely the standard biomedical model taught in the universities. Physicians 1 and 8, both with degrees in epidemiology, attended to public health conditions most. Not surprisingly, Physician 2, who originated from a poor community, was the most attuned to patients' economic plight and never disparaged the behaviors of the poor.

Individual Variations in Physicians' Practice

My findings suggest that diagnoses are usually influenced more by the physicians' personal inclinations and experience and less by patients' presenting complaints. Given that patients referred to the outpatient clinic of Internal Medicine were randomly selected for the study and also assigned to the physicians at random, I anticipated that the nature of diagnoses, treatment, and the number of diagnoses would be randomly distributed. My hypothesis was only partially borne out. While physicians shared various diagnostic categories, certain diagnoses were made exclusively by some physicians. On the other hand, the number of diagnoses per patient was evenly distributed among the various physicians.[1]

Analysis of the diagnoses given me reveals that while there were some shared by all physicians, others were made exclusively by only one physician. This suggests that some physicians at the hospital employ a larger diagnostic repertoire than others in their day-to-day practice. There were ninety-eight diagnostic categories used by the physicians for all patients in the study. All physicians diagnosed amebiasis, colitis, obesity, hypertension, urinary tract infection, anemia, and arthritis. On the other hand, only two physicians found patients to have neuritis and polyneuritis. These diagnoses usually were given to patients who reported typical symptoms, such as jabbing pain in the chest and heart or pain in the "lungs." Some of the physicians incorporated diagnoses not included by any other doctor, such as depressive psychosis, hypothyroidism, myomas, varices, duodinitis, spondylitis, hyperlordosis, fallen bladder, and spastic colon.[2]

Table 7.1 displays the number of patients seen by each of the eight physicians, the combined total number of diagnoses for patients seen by each physician, and the average number of diagnoses per physician.

Table 7.1: Number of Patients and Diagnoses by Physician

Physician Number:	1	2	3	4	5	6	7	8
Patients per doctor	13	11	37	32	12	40	14	24
Total number of diagnoses for all patients	31	24	84	135	25	158	32	65
Average number of diagnoses per patient	2.3	2.1	2.2	4.3	2.1	3.8	2.4	2.8

Table 7.2: Diagnoses by Individual Physician (in percent)

Physicians	1	2	3	4	5	6	7	8
Infections or parasites	35.5	41.7	44.0	54.0	48.0	57.6	25.0	44.6
Metabolic or systemic disorders	19.4	12.5	14.3	10.4	8.0	5.0	9.4	9.2
Degenerative traumatic or sequela	16.1	12.5	3.57	23.0	28.0	10.1	18.8	12.3
Psychological	9.7	12.5	12.0	0.7	4.0	1.3	15.6	10.8
Pregnancy	-	-	1.2	-	-	-	-	-
Specific etiology	19.4	20.8	20.2	11.1	8.0	24.7	28.1	21.5
Healthy	-	-	3.6	-	-	-	-	-
No diagnosis	-	-	1.2	0.7	4.0	1.3	3.1	1.5

The majority of physicians diagnosed a mean of slightly over two conditions per patient, suggesting little variation among physicians with respect to the number of diagnoses they made per patient. Interestingly, Physician 4, with the highest mean number of diagnoses, never examined any patient physically. She based her diagnoses exclusively on clinical history and patient presentation of symptoms.

To elucidate the diagnostic categories, the infections or parasites category comprises several subcategories, including digestive, genitourinary, and respiratory disorders. The metabolic or systemic group incorporates diabetes mellitus, arterial hypertension, obesity, and anemia. Degenerative, traumatic, or sequela comprise chiefly diagnoses of scoliosis, deviated spine, and a few cases of arthritis. Specific etiology is perhaps the most complex category. It includes a large variety of diagnoses that, according to the physician who constructed the classification, could not be placed in any other categories because their etiology could not easily be established or because the diagnoses did not fit any known medical classification, as in the case of "discharges." This group includes a single diagnosis, such as gallstones, ulcers, hemorrhoids, nervous colitis, or nervous gastritis, which could not be placed in the subcategory of digestive track dysfunctions because the etiology was unknown. Ovarian cysts and inflammations, hernia, dysmenorrhea, and nephritis all failed to fit into the genitourinary subcategory of infections and parasites because they were not of infectious origin. Other diagnoses included in the general category of specific etiology are discharges, and conditions of the nervous system of unknown origin.

While we see a degree of uniformity in the types of diagnoses made by all physicians, the variation in the frequencies of diagnostic categories is intriguing in view of the random selection of patients to physicians. Physicians tended to display a predilection for certain types of diagnoses, which may or may not reflect the patient's presenting symptoms.

Not unexpectedly, the highest percentage of diagnoses for all physicians is found in the infections or parasites category. In light of all the physicians' shared expectation that the patient population experiences amebiasis and parasites, this finding is not surprising. Interestingly, however, Physician 7 whose eclectic practice includes homeopathic treatments and acupuncture, has the lowest percentage of diagnosis in the infections or parasites category (25 percent) as compared with the other doctors, whose averages in the infection or parasites category range between 35 and 57 percent. Physician 7, however, has the highest percentage of diagnoses in the specific etiologies group, which in his case refers chiefly to nervous colitis, nervous gastritis, and endocrine imbalance.

Interestingly, too, Physician 5 made 12 percent of the diagnoses in the respiratory category as compared to 1 to 5 percent for the other doctors, reflecting her predilection for a tonsillitis (that is, anginas) diagnosis. Physician 5 had the highest percentage of diagnoses in the degenerative category, with seven out of the twelve patients diagnosed as having arthritis and muscle contractions. Physician 4 found all of his thirty-one patients to have scoliosis and flat feet coupled with infections, including parasitosis.

Physician 8 also showed a tendency to diagnose scoliosis. In fact, eight of the twenty-three patients he saw were thus diagnosed. Only three of the eight physicians, including Physician 7, whose diagnoses in the degenerative and traumatic category refer to muscular and arthritic conditions, failed to diagnose any of their patients as having scoliosis. To reiterate a point made earlier, I postulate that the prevalence of diagnoses focusing on the spine may have roots in its association with the nervous system, a biomedical translation of a cultural category.

Turning to the psychological category, Physician 7 had the highest percentage of diagnoses in this group. For him, nerves was the major cause of sickness, which he regarded sometimes as an emotional problem, while at other times as a disorder of the nervous system analogous to neurasthenia. Predictably, Physician 4 and Physician 6 show the lowest percentage of diagnoses classified in the psychological category. Physician 4 either ignored or reduced emotional problems to "it's only nerves" and rarely addressed issues relating to nerves or other emotional discharges per se. Physician 6, with minor exceptions, tended to reduce symptoms that traditionally are considered of psychosomatic origin, including chest pain, to a diagnosis of polyneuritis or a condition of the nervous system.

As might have been expected from a random selection, the majority of the physicians have similar percentages of diagnoses clustered in the "specific etiology" category. Exceptions are Physicians 4 and 5. Physician 4 utilized the most narrow diagnostic repertoire. His diagnoses were largely confined to scoliosis and parasitic infections. Physician 5 tended to focus on tonsillitis and muscular degeneration.

To highlight the comparison among physicians, one patient who was treated by two participating physicians for the same symptoms illuminates the diverse ways biomedicine is practiced. Jose's case affords us a glimpse of how two physicians deal with the same patient and the same symptoms. He was the only subject who was treated by two different physicians during the study. He was initially seen by Physician 5, who left the outpatient service. When Jose returned for treatment of the same symptoms four months later, he was assigned to Physician 8.

Jose

Jose, twenty-nine years old, reported that he took the opportunity to request a consultation for himself when he came to accompany his wife to the Obstetrics and Gynecology clinic for prenatal care. He explained that he had experienced pain in the *cintura*, or lower back, for seven to eight months. Initially, he attributed the impairment to excessive work and later to a chill. He believed his condition was serious and he feared eventually his body would be paralyzed. He described his pain thus: "I feel heat and as if constricted by a corset." It started when he lifted a heavy stone onto a truck five years earlier, but the intense pain began eight months before he came to the hospital. Before the visit to the hospital, Jose had been treated by his father-in-law, a bonesetter, who gave him a massage and put a plaster on his back. This relieved his pain temporarily.

He was seen by Physician 5, who carefully wrote down all his symptoms and a clinical history without looking at Jose, who sat reading a comic book when he was not responding to the interrogation. Jose recounted that he was having pain in the *cintura* that it was affecting his "lungs" or *pulmon* (meaning "back"), that he had this pain for seven months, and that he thought he twisted something inside because he had lifted a heavy object. The physician asked about the object he had lifted, whether he could move at the onset of the pain, and whether it was very painful. He reported that yes, he could move, but movement was excruciatingly painful, and as a result he couldn't breathe. She inquired if he had had an Xray, which he had not, and whether he felt better with the bonesetter's treatment. She explored with him the point of origin in his body from which the pain emanated and whether he could bend down. He said he could but only with pain. She explored his symptoms, took a medical history, and asked about diabetics in the family, whether his parents were alive and healthy, and whether anyone in the family had tuberculosis. He responded that his parents were well and had not had any of the diseases she had asked about. She inquired about his personal habits and instructed him to smoke less. She asked about his occupation, and she gave him a referral to Orthopedics, where they would do further studies. She diagnosed the pain as due to a muscle contraction, but she wanted to rule out any lesions in the spinal column. She told him that until his back was Xrayed in orthopedics, she would give him a muscle relaxant for when he was in great pain. She instructed him to return after he was seen in Orthopedics.

After Jose left she explained to me that she had given him an analgesic for the pain and that in all probability he had a deviated disc. She added that he may also have had a spastic colon, since his pain made him tense and anxious. Once she had the results from the orthopedic studies, she would then attend to his colitis and parasites, but at the time her main concern was with his back. It is worthy of note that Jose never complained about abdominal dysfunctions, and he even told her in response to her questioning that he did not have any problems with moving his bowels. When I asked whether there was any problem with his spine, she indicated that the clinical evidence did not suggest a deviated spinal column.

Upon his return to the hospital, Jose was assigned to Physician 8. He again reported the same symptoms, now of about a year's duration. The students who usually surrounded the physician during consultations took the clinical history. Jose reported that he had had the same pain continuously for four months. When the doctor asked him about his visit to Orthopedics, Jose began explaining the difficulties he and his wife were having with their youngest child, who was born with a heart murmur, but he was not given the opportunity to finish the narration. Jose did not report to the doctor, as he did to me, that he could not get the Xray done and that he was very dissatisfied with the visit to the orthopedist. He said only that he had been prescribed a muscle relaxant (Naxodol) but that he never had an Xray taken. In response to the physician's questions, he indicated that he was no longer taking the medication. The physician gave him a physical examination and asked him to stand up normally with his heels together. He immediately diagnosed the condition as lumbago, related to the scoliosis and an "unstable spinal column." He ordered an Xray and prescribed a muscle relaxant (Robaxisal) and a recall visit in a week.

The doctor recorded the diagnosis as "lumbar scoliosis with right side convexity." He noted, "Based upon physical exploration patient was experiencing pain in the lumbar region of the spine that augmented with intense effort and diminished with rest with a tendency to incapacitation." The doctor indicated that a large percentage of the population suffered from lateral curvatures of the spine because of incorrect sitting and standing. According to the doctor, the condition was treatable with muscle relaxants, which he had prescribed, as well as with corsets, massages, and hot-water pads. In addition to the prescription he ordered Xrays.

The patient did not keep the scheduled appointment, but returned unexpectedly to see the physician three weeks later with Xrays taken in the hospital on negatives purchased in a private laboratory because the hospital had none. Jose reported that he continued to have the pain, though it was relieved somewhat with the analgesic (Robaxisal) prescribed by the physician. The physician suggested to the patient that he was feeling better, as we see from the verbatim exchange after the doctor asked the patient about the effects of the medication.

Doctor: You do feel better now?
Patient: Well...
D (in a tone both declarative and interrogatory): You don't have any pain, you are taking the medication?
P: Well, yes.

The physician looked at the Xray, confirmed his initial diagnosis of scoliosis, and noted the asymmetry of Jose's legs. He referred the patient to Orthopedics again.

This comparison between the two physicians reveals the diverse clinical diagnoses made of the same syndrome, reflecting individual preferences for specific types of diagnoses that were largely independent of the patient's pains. Physician 5 focused on muscular contractions. Physician 8 diagnosed the condition as scoliosis, a diagnosis he frequently made, especially when he had ruled out any other possibilities. Physician 5 totally excluded the possibility of scoliosis and diagnosed, as she usually did, muscle contractions and colitis. Physician 8 made the scoliosis diagnosis following his physical examination, which was confirmed for him by his reading of the Xray, and made no reference to parasites.

It is instructive to compare how two physicians who represent the opposite ends of the mind-body duality treat individual patients. Physician 3, while recognizing the nonsomatic aspects of a patient's symptoms, addressed sickness in terms of pathophysiological disorders that he treated solely with medication. He was totally committed to an organic model of sickness. Physician 7 adhered to a psychosomatic model. He claimed that the overwhelming majority of patients' maladies were attributable to psychological problems and nerves, which he diagnosed using biomedical nosologies. He depended greatly on naturalistic treatments, with special emphasis on diet. His biomedical treatments were informed by a combination of theories related to diet and Chinese and homeopathic medicine.

The two physicians' medical postures respecting etiology, diagnosis, and treatment underscore the inherent dualism in biomedicine that also reverberates on the patient's diagnosis and treatment. A dualistic interpretation of any kind, when diagnoses are made solely on psychosomatic or organic grounds, be they emotional discharges or physiological dysfunctions, affects adversely the course and outcome of the treatment. The cases of Sharon and Nomi bring into relief both the dilemma created by medical reductionism either in terms of the body or the mind and the variations in biomedical practice respecting the diagnostic process. One physician relied on technologies used by different specialists to support his diagnoses, while the other relied on clinical symptomatology. The two patients, like all patients, would have been better served if their sicknesses had been understood as lived experience manifested in a single body and mind and treated in a multidimensional way.

Sharon

Sharon was treated by Physician 3 and seen seven times. She was eighteen years old, weighed 91 pounds, measured 4'8", and had a perpetual shy smile on her face. She had come to Mexico City a year earlier from north central Mexico to work as a live-in maid to a young professional couple without children. She came to the hospital accompanied by an older cousin (her mother's sister's daughter). The cousin was permitted by the physician to attend the consultation, which lasted seventeen minutes, and she did much of the speaking for the meek Sharon, despite the fact that the doctor addressed his inquiries to the patient and not to the cousin. In fact, the cousin was the first to speak during the encounter, reporting that the girl had been suffering from headaches, back pain, and sleeplessness and that she imagined things and had nightmares.

(Uncustomarily, Physician 3 addressed this patient in the familiar "tu," as befits an older person addressing a younger one.)

Doctor: What do you imagine?
Patient: Snakes on the roof, ugly animals, and bad people.
D: Since when?
P: It's been a while.
Cousin: It's been a while. (The cousin then explained that she did not want Sharon to watch television because Sharon then imagined things of terror.)
D: Is that what you imagine, the same as on TV?
P: No.
D: You are frightened? (He said in a declarative and an interrogatory tone.)

(Sharon replied that she was and the cousin declared she didn't want Sharon to watch television because then she had bad dreams and screamed.)

(The doctor declared that it was normal but...)

D: What is not normal is that you have headaches. Did you go to school?
P: Yes, till the fifth grade.
D: Did you have headaches when you went to school?
P: No.
D: Never?

(He continued to explore the reasons for her headaches in relation to her habit of watching television.)

D: Are you in pain without television?
P: Very little. When I have the light turned off and I watch television, they say I have pain. Yes. (That is, other people tell her that is the problem.)
D: No, not what people say you feel. Do you have headaches with the television?
P: It hurts a bit.

(The doctor explored her ability to read small letters by showing her a calendar.)

D: Can you see letters?
P: Yes, but no.
D: You don't read them well, you don't distinguish the letters?
P: Yes, but ...
D: Let's see, read this. (She looked at the calendar.)
Cousin: You know what, I think she is very nervous, very very nervous.
D: Yes, but here you can be calm with us. Can you read these letters on a calendar?
P: Well...
D: What is the last word?
P: What?

D: Yes, you see it well, you can distinguish the letters?

P: Yes. The letters [say] "March."

D: So you can read. What does it say here?

P: August.

D:When you use your eyes does your head hurt more?

P: No, oh yes, a little more.

D: When you are looking at something does it hurt more?

P: No.

D: Let's see, cover one eye. What does it say?

(Sharon was able to read all the words to which the doctor pointed.)

D: So you can see pretty well. In any event, we will send you to have your eyes examined. Maybe you need glasses and that is why you have headaches.

(The cousin declared that Sharon started getting the headaches when she arrived in Mexico City and she began watching television. She was seen by many physicians who gave her medicine and sent her for analysis, but Sharon failed to improve.)

Cousin: And she has pain in her back.

D: But you are lazy always, true?

P: No, yes, on Saturdays and Sundays, yes, I sleep.

Cousin: If she is not doing anything she falls asleep right away.

D: And appetite, how is it?

P: Sometimes I have a little.

Cousin: Sometimes she comes out with rashes on her body and a doctor gave her a cream but it didn't help. She itches a lot, and the rashes open and pimples come out.

D: You have them now?

P: No, sometimes when I wash the stove.

D: With detergent?

P: Yes.

D: Why don't you get gloves?

Cousin: She itches.

P: And sometimes my whole body stings.

D: Anybody in your family have diabetes? Do you know what it is? It's when the sugar level rises.

P: No.

D: Any other sickness, "pressure"?

P: Yes, pressure, one of my aunts.

D: What does she have?

Cousin: A mother's sister has pressure, she does not have diabetes, nothing.

D: Nobody else?

Cousin: No, she has low pressure, but no diabetes.

D: What diseases have you had?

P: I had anemia and I am allergic when I wash with soap.

D: Anemic. Any other illness that you can remember, operations?

P: No.

D: Nothing like that?

Cousin: Yes, she had fever of the stomach, or something like that.

D: When did you begin menstruating?

P: Fourteen.

D: How often?

P: Every month.

D: How many days do you bleed?

P: What?

D: How long does your period last?

P: Sometimes four, seven days, like that?

D: Have you had sexual relations?

P: No.

D: I think that there is nothing wrong with her, but in any event I will send her to Ophthalmology so they can give her a checkup and I will order a blood exam to see if she is anemic.

Cousin: I say yes, she is always like this. I don't know what she has. I took her to another doctor but she continues to have headaches that don't stop, and she cannot sleep.

D: She is nervous.

Cousin: And then the TV. I don't like to watch it, because in the house where she works she watches and my aunt thinks it's because of that.

D: Your mother is here in Mexico?

P: No.

D: Where is she?

P: (Names the state.)

D: What is happening is that you want to go back to your mother, isn't that so?

P: No.

Cousin: Doctor, is her height okay? We regard her as very short. Her sister is much taller.

D: Your sister, how tall is she? Taller than your mother?

P: Yes, they are taller, and my brothers as well. One of my mother's sisters is my height.

D: It's normal. Do you know who was Napoleon? He was shorter than you, do you know?

P: No.

D: You don't know. You don't remember from school he was shorter than you? But you may still grow within the next two years.

Cousin: I don't believe it.

D: You will still grow about two inches. What else do you want? We will also order a fecal stool test, a blood test, and refer you to an ophthalmologist, and give you an appointment in two weeks.

Cousin: Yes, I think so.

(The doctor explained the date and time, and where she needed to go to have exams done.)

Cousin: Thank you.

D: It's pure nerves, the nightmares, don't pay attention to them.

After the consultation, the doctor informed me that he believed there was nothing wrong with Sharon, that her eyesight was the reason for the headaches, and that she was most certainly malnourished and anemic. It also seemed to him that the problem was her nerves. He diagnosed her condition as malnutrition, parasites, and nerves. He did not prescribe any medication.

She returned for her scheduled appointment, which like all subsequent appointments, lasted about five minutes. The results of Sharon's laboratory analysis were entered in the medical record, and they revealed that she had parasites (ucinaria) of a kind uncommon in Mexico City but found in the region from which she originated and that cause anemia. The doctor claimed that this particular species thrived in humid soils, and entered the body through the skin. Sharon, however, claimed during the interview that she had not gone barefoot. According to the doctor, the tests showed that Sharon was not anemic yet, however.

The cousin, who again accompanied Sharon, reported that they had gone to the ophthalmologist and that the doctor there told Sharon that she had a cataract from birth. This physician claimed that was not her problem and led her to understand that she misunderstood the ophthalmologist's explanation. He revised the diagnosis on the basis of the test results and explained that Sharon's problem was parasites. He prescribed antiparasitic medication and indicated to her that she should not be concerned by temporary side effects of the medication such as dizziness.

Sharon returned for her scheduled appointment a week later. She reported that she took the medication. She was asked whether she was feeling better (the doctor both inquired and declared), to which she replied "yes"; and whether she now didn't have the headaches anymore, to which she responded with "a little."

Doctor: Now you have less headaches, now you don't feel lazy? (question/statement)

Patient: (Sharon laughed.) Sometimes, I still feel lazy.

D: Less than before?

P: Yes.

(The doctor inquired whether she was sleeping better. She answered that she still could not sleep, and when he asked for the reason, she responded, "I don't know. I feel nervous.")

D: Say, my God, at eighteen you begin to be nervous. You are very young to be nervous at eighteen. What do you think about when you cannot sleep?

P: Nothing.

Sharon was weighed during this visit and her weight had not changed. This time the doctor prescribed another antiparasitic medication and explained to her how to take it and alerted her not to be frightened by the medication's possible side effects, including dizziness and coffee-colored urine. His diagnosis was slight anemia caused by parasites.

Sharon kept her next scheduled appointment but this time she came by herself. The doctor inquired whether she took the medication and how she was feeling. She replied that she did take the medicine but continued to have headaches. When he asked her about the pain in her back, she indicated that she still had the same pains, and she also had pains in her stomach. (At the initial interview she reported to us that she had pains in the "mouth of the stomach," but she had not mentioned this to the physician until this visit.) He declared that she had ucinarias.

Sharon reported she had a headache only once that week, but that she had had stomach pains the night before. The doctor then referred her to Neurology so that "they could assess why she was having headaches." He asked her if she could tell in advance the onset of the headache. She said, "No, it just starts like that. Sometimes I feel it slow and sometimes very ugly." After referring her to Neurology he gave her a return appointment for two weeks later.

During the next visit the doctor reviewed the medical record, which suggested that it was not an ophthalmological problem; the parasites had already been treated, and it was not a neurological problem, for the neurologist referred Sharon to Ear, Nose and Throat (ENT) for Xrays. The neurologist suspected that it may be sinusitis, so he ordered an Xray of her head. When Physician 3 asked if she had catarrhs, she responded that she did not. He asked whether she had green mucus coming out of her nose and although she said no, he concluded that her problem was chronic sinusitis because of the referral to ENT. He felt relieved that finally there was a concrete diagnosis. While gratified that a diagnosis had been made, Physician 3 was also puzzled because it was unusual for headaches to be the only symptom of sinusitis. But now he could understand why her headaches would be more intense in Mexico City than in her native state: It was drier in Mexico City, leading to increased inflammation. When I pointed out to the doctor that the climate in her native state was as dry as Mexico City's, he indicated that the polluted air in Mexico City aggravated the problem.

Physician 3 gave her yet another appointment for a week later, which she kept. Results from the Xrays ordered by the ENT specialist were not available. The medical record indicated that Sharon had an inflammation of the nasal membranes. The doctor told her not to worry, and she left convinced that her problem was sinusitis.

She returned a week later, reporting that the ENT specialist had prescribed an antibacterial drug and a decongestant (Bactrim and Gotinal) for her sinus infection. She was told that if there was no improvement, she would require an operation of the cornets. Sharon reported she was feeling a little better and that her headaches were less frequent. The doctor again gave her an appointment for two weeks later and instructed her to follow the treatments she was getting from the specialists. Physician 3 noted that Sharon's enlarged cornets were producing the headaches.

She returned a month later and reported that the medications prescribed by the ENT specialist produced stomach pains and dizziness, and therefore her employer had told her not to take them. The headaches were less severe, but her insomnia was worse and she had not slept for two days. She reported that the ENT physician thought she still needed an operation. In the meantime he prescribed Cafergot (an antimigraine medication) but it made her feel sick. Physician 3 doubted that Sharon suffered from migraines and believed that the medication she was taking ought not to have made her feel sick. He told her that she was very nervous but that nothing was wrong with her. At this time, Physician 3 concluded that her only problem was the parasitic infection, which should have been cured with the treatment he had prescribed. He gave her no further appointments but told her she could return to see him at any time.

Sharon was seen by Physician 3, by an ophthalmologist, by a neurologists and by an ENT specialist. Physician 3 finally concluded that there was nothing medically wrong with Sharon, except that she was suffering from emotional problems and anxiety. He reasoned that it may not even have been sinusitis because Sharon's disturbances changed every time.

I have presented Sharon's trajectory in great detail because her case is instructive for various reasons, but within the context of our present discussion, it suggests that while we could not exclude Sharon's parasitic infection, more information about her life was needed to capture the reasons for her headaches, back pain, and insomnia. While the doctor intuitively recognized on Sharon's initial visit that she might not have any "organic" dysfunctions, the paradigms that animated Physician 3's clinical judgments led him to regard and treat Sharon as a solitary corporeal body.

On follow-up at home, Sharon revealed that she understood the doctor's diagnosis that she had "worms" caused by her having walked barefoot, because he gave her medication for it, but she believed that her problem was not "worms": Her sickness was the headaches that she had been experiencing ever since she arrived in Mexico City. She liked Physician 3 because she was relieved to hear that she was not suffering from anemia or allergies, as a private physician had told her, and therefore her problem was not that serious. She was confused by the ophthalmologist, who she thought told her she had a cataract (which did not appear in the medical record) but that she did not need glasses. She excluded any possibility of an operation, because her employer and her mother were against it. She was frightened by all the visits to the doctor. It was true that she was nervous, particularly when she was among strangers or when she was alone. She was, in fact, alone in the house all day while her employers were at work.

Of all the medications prescribed for her, the only one that made her feel better was an over-the-counter medicine, whose name she did not know, that a young woman friend gave her. This friend had recently left the city. Sharon reported she was feeling very alone and that she had nobody to talk to, especially now that her closest friend had left her, coinciding with the time that her headaches intensified. Her only exchange with her employers was about what she would cook for the day. Sometimes, she was locked in her room and she felt as if she were going to choke.

Sharon was indeed isolated from her family; her closest relative in Mexico City was her overpowering cousin. She had lost her closest friend. While the physician noted that Sharon missed her family, he failed to connect her symptoms with her isolation. Had the physician explored Sharon's symptoms within the context of Sharon's life, it is quite possible that he could have also understood that her sickness was embodied isolation and solitude, which are against the norms of Mexican society. An eighteen-year-old woman, alone, unmarried, and away from her natal family is in Mexican society likely to feel extreme deprivation rather than, for example, independence, as in American society.

Sharon's case depicts the characteristic way in which Physician 3 usually dealt with patients: on an organic level. In his own opinion, he was uncomfortable with patients who may have had what he identified as "psychiatric problems."

Nomi

Nomi was treated by Physician 7, whose clinical judgments are informed by a psychosomatic approach to sickness. Nomi's case, in fact, illustrates the dangers of the converse of physiological reductionism, when medical diagnoses are based on etiological understandings that sickness is rooted solely in "mental" causes.

Nomi, thirty-six years old with a sixth-grade education, was married for twenty years and had seven children. She came to solicit treatment for left-sided abdominal pain. She had sought treatment from many physicians. The first consultation with Physician 7 lasted fifty minutes, during which time he explored her symptoms, examined her physically, and prescribed treatment. The doctor dedicated a good part of the time to explaining his prescribed diet. The transcript of the verbal exchanges between the physician and patient is typical of this physician's interactions with patients.

(In the physicians' customary way, the patient was addressed in the formal you ["usted"].)

Doctor: Good afternoon.

Patient: Good afternoon.

D: How can we serve you?

P: Well my stomach hurts, doctor.

D: All of your stomach?

P:(She pointed to the area of the pain, which was all around the middle and left side of the abdominal and lumbar region.)

P: I cannot eat. Everything makes me sick. My pain is very intense.

D: Have you lost weight?

P: How much do I weigh now?

D: 66.700 kilograms (146 pounds).

P: I weighed 74 kilogram (162 pounds).

D: So you did lose weight. How long have you had these disturbances?

P: Well, it's been a long time.

D: Please tell me in months or years, but accurately, how long have you had this pain?

P: I have had this pain for fifteen years. That's a lot, doctor.

D: Quite. Very well. And what treatment have you received for this?

P: None, doctor. I sought treatment in many places. I went to the health centers, and recently to a private physician when I got very sick.

D: Yes.

P: I have pain and temperature.

D: Let's see. Have you brought all your prescriptions?

P: Here is the prescription; these are the analyses.

D: Now, we will see. Let's go backwards. What else do you want to tell me, so that I can try to cure you?

P: The kidneys.

D: Pain in the kidney, since when?

P: I don't have pain in the kidneys, doctor.

D: Then?

P: Only that they disturb me when I do my chores in the house. I get tired and they hurt--a little, like a tiredness befalls me. No more.

D: Then, disturbance of a kind of tiredness.

P: And when I urinate, and I try to urinate into a bottle, there is a lot of sediment, dirt. I had an examination of the kidneys, and yes, yes, I have an infection of the kidneys. It's when...

D: And since when have you had the pain in the kidneys?

P: The tiredness, the kidneys--about a year and half.

D: Eighteen months in developing.

P: Yes.

D: Anything else, Mrs., that you want to tell me? Now it is your turn to talk because afterwards it will be my turn to talk.

P: I have had diarrhea for many years.

D: What else?

P: This is the most important.

D: This is what you want to tell me?

P: Yes, doctor.

D: Now I will ask you some questions. The pain you have had for a year and a half, sometimes it is colic? You don't know what is colic?

P: Yes, like, as if my intestines were in knots. Yes, sometimes, but not always.

D: Pain is occasionally colic?

P: Yes.

D: After you eat or even when you don't eat, how do you feel? Bloated?

P: That, yes.

D (wrote and stated): Meteorism. The bloating becomes accentuated after eating?

P: Yes doctor, and every morning when I wake up I feel as if my stomach had been kicked; it's very painful. I want to go to the bathroom and I cannot until I walk a bit and start functioning.

D: Good, and aside from this, do you have grumblings?

P: Yes.

D: Do you expel gases from below?

P: No.

D: You want to but cannot expel them.

P: I would want, but no, and then I take a teaspoon of magnesia and I start having gases.

D: Smells bad?

P: Yes, very bad.

D (repeated and wrote): Gases, through rectum, diarrhea.

P: I have to go three times a day to the bathroom.

D: Always?

P: Sometimes twice, but diarrhea...

D: Diarrhea with mucus?

P: No.

D: You have always been that way? Are you constipated sometimes?

P: Yes, I was constipated; that was a long time ago, about three years ago, and when I moved my bowels I bled and I couldn't go. I wanted to go and forced myself. I was so constipated, it was terrible.

D: And since three years ago until now it's been diarrhea?

P: Diarrhea, and I have been happier this way because it doesn't hurt when I have diarrhea.

D: Since three years ago?

P: I have been able to control it for two or three days, fifteen days and then again.

D: Diarrhea without mucus, without blood. But you do have mucus.

P: When I have the pain and I make a little, then it is pure mucus, and when I don't have pain it is pure diarrhea.

D: Is there no blood?

P: Blood? No, doctor.

D: This sensation when you want to move your bowels and then tenesmus?

P: What is that?

D: That is called rectal tenesmus.

P: That, and I feel that.

D: Sometimes as if you had a wound.

P: Yes, pain. I return from the bathroom and I hug myself.

D: And that is as if you had something nailed to the back?

P: Yes, that is it.

D: Hemorrhoids. What else?

P: Yes, since I got married I had them. My husband gave me that. No, not true: I feel it is from the heat when I sit down. (The latter is a common cultural belief about the etiology of hemorrhoids.)

D: No, no. It is because of the constipation and because of the colitis.

P: Now I understand.

D: How long have you been married? Don't blame your husband.

P: No, I have been married twenty years. It will be twenty years the sixteenth of this month.

D: Very well. Anything else?

P: Doctor, when I have [sexual] relations I am in pain.

D: Always, always has been that way?

P: Almost always, yes. Because one doctor said that it is necessary to love him, to love a lot one's husband, and since I don't love him that much, oh it hurts me!

D: But now, yes, you love him? Or no?

P: A little bit.

D: Then it doesn't hurt you anymore.

P: It hurts now more.

D: God's punishment. (Doctor laughed.)

P: Oh I cannot stand it.

D: Now let us see, let us see.

P: And always when I have a Pap smear I have an infection.

D: And since when have you been having Pap smears done?

P: Oh, since about ten years ago.

D: How often?

P: Sometimes I have it done twice a year; sometimes I forget until I feel sick and then I go again, but I don't have it done often.

D: If you have it done every six months, it's enough.

P: One cleaning woman told me that my intestines were like yoghurt.

D: Tell the woman that she doesn't know and to be quiet. Don't alarm yourself. Very well, then, you have a Pap smear done every six months and it shows an inflammation. Discharge with color.

P: Yes.

D: Yellow?

P: No.

D: White like *baba de nopal*. (*Baba de nopal* refers to the white sap from prickly pear cacti.)

P: I will explain to you one thing; sometimes like now, yes, I have it [the discharge], but sometimes it is dry and I place a few ovules, I don't know what you call them.

D: Since when do you have the discharge?

P: Now.

D: No, not now, since when?

P: Since when? It stops and then I have it again.

D: The first time.

P: Oh my God, doctor!

(The doctor questioned Nomi about her birthplace and how long she had lived in Mexico City. She reported she was brought to the capital at the age of three and returned to his questioning about the vaginal discharge.)

D: Now, since when do you have the discharge?

P: I have, my God, well it's been a long time, like seventeen years

D: Sometimes it itches.

P: Yes.

D: Smells bad?

P: No.

D: It doesn't leave the clothing starchy?

P: Yes.

D: It irritates, it scratches?

P: Yes, a lot.

D: What else? (Wrote in the medical record and repeated): Pain during sexual relations, disturbance of a kind of tiredness in the lumbar region, eighteen months in developing during physical activity. What else? Do you have varices?

P: Yes.

D: Since when?

P: I am in pain when I menstruate since about three years ago.

D: And how are they [the varices] now?

P: I don't know, one has to see; and when I menstruate I am in pain, and I am in pain from sitting.

D: But they [the varices] don't jump out [blow up]?

P: No, no. They are always the same, very ugly. That is because I have not taken care of them.

D: Something else, problems on urination?

P: No. Sometimes yes, but not now.

D: Good. Have there been people in your family with diabetes?

P: My mother. (This actually refers to her grandmother, who had raised her and whom she called mother because her mother abandoned her and her brother when she was a child. The doctor recorded "mother" in the medical record.)

(The doctor continued questioning Nomi about her family's medical history, especially regarding anyone in the family having had cancer and "lungs," which in the physician's parlance refers to tuberculosis, and the patient responded no. The medical history included questions about her menstrual cycle and about the number of pregnancies.)

D: How many children have you had?

P: Seven, and one abortion.

D: Then there were eight pregnancies?

P: Eight pregnancies and seven children.

D: Natural births?

P: Yes, doctor.

D: Abortion spontaneous?

P: How is that? What does that mean?

D: By itself.

(At this point Nomi returned to an important theme in her life respecting her relationship with her husband that the doctor ignored.)

P: But, you know what, doctor? I bleed when I have sexual relations five days before my period. My husband removes blood; when I have relations after menstruation, it hurts me, it itches me, it's ugly ["feo" also meaning terrible], and he is stubborn and does not want to wait and I tell him to get out from there and he sticks.

D: What a man, what a man. (Doctor laughs.) Lets move to this: What operations have you had?

P: Tubal ligation, or how you say it?

D: Salpingectomy.

P: That's it.

D: When have you had it done?

P: Four years ago. What year would that be?

D: About 1982.

P: 1982.

D: Any other operation?

P: No.

D: Any serious operations that you have had?

P: Serious. Never serious, only this one.

(Nomi was instructed to lie down on the cot for her physical examination.)

D: Yes. For fifteen years. It is chronic colitis. We will control it, but it was poorly treated, poorly treated, not well treated, you will see. If you follow the instructions I give you, the diet, the diet above all, in less than one month you will have controlled it [the disturbances]. The abdomen looks pointed. True? From the pregnancies, from the umbilical scars. Surgical scar from the salpingectomy looks normal.

(The doctor proceeded with the exploration.) Inflammation through palpation. With deep palpation we find painful colic, hyperaesthesia. Good, now we move to percussion. Look, it sounds that there is a tympanic sound. This sound should normally exist only here on the left side. That is the gastric chamber. Here it is normal air. The stomach chamber normally gets to this point, but given where you have it, it suggests an increase in air in the abdominal region and together with hyperaesthesis confirms that it is colic. The physical exploration confirmed for us the diagnostic impression as true, the diagnosis that we have made on the basis of the interrogation. Would you like to turn over please with your head down.

P: You are not going to beat me hard? Because it is very painful there, doctor.

D: You tell me, if it hurts.

P: No.

D: Thus in the exploration of the colon, we find hyperaesthesis on the spinal hypophysis of the third, fourth, and fifth lumbar. Do you want to get cured lady?

P: Yes.

(At this juncture, Physician 7 told Nomi what he usually tells all patients.)

D: If you want to get cured, I will give you an adequate treatment. But not only will I cure your sickness; this does not depend on the physician, but on the patient. It depends on how precisely you follow the diet, take the medicine, and you yourself will notice the difference. The treatment will be for three to four months, and before the month is out you will feel better. For the first time you will feel happy.

P: Oh, I wish.

(He examined the test results Nomi brought which she had done in various private laboratories.)

D: Hematology. A bit anemic. (It showed 11.43 grams of hemoglobin, 37 hematocrit.) The results from urine culture are illegible; blood chemistry is within the normal limits, the general urinalysis shows hematuria. Thus we find hematuria.[3] It indicates bacteria but does not indicate which. The results of the general urinalysis have no date. They didn't do a study of the fecal stool materials?

P: What is that?

D: Excrement?

P: The yellow one. (pointing to a piece of paper)

D: Good. On 11 October [three months before the present consultation] you had a series of three coproparascopicos done which show amebas histolytica. And what did it serve that they found amebas histolytica? Now, as to the treatment, the one before the one you had, the prescriptions.

P: No, I don't have them.

(A brief discussion followed about Nomi's previous treatments which, as the doctor mentioned earlier, were in his judgment inadequate. These included Kantrex [antibiotic], Froxona [antidiarrheal], and Synalar cream [antimicrobial cream] for the itching.)

D: Then you were prescribed Pentrexyl [an antibiotic] injections every twelve hours, two antiamebian medications [Libertrim for colic, Libertrim antispasmotic], Neo Melubrina, an analgesic. True.

P: And he told me to come another time because I wasn't getting well with these [medications].

D: Not soon, not ever

P: No, I am not going....

D: I have come to the following conclusion, that you have a chronic colitis, hemorrhoids, unspecific vaginitis, and lumbar spondylitis. Because you have been taking a lot of medication within the past months, laboratory tests are not recommended at this time. If you buy the medicine that I prescribe for you and don't follow the diet, you are not going to get well. If you follow the diet, and don't take the medicine, you will probably get better, so that you will see that most important is the diet rather than the medicine. And I forgot to ask you, I am sure, that yes, do you eat spicy food, salsa?

P: Not anymore.

D: Now, look here. You ate all through your childhood everything. Now for the rest of your existence it is necessary to follow a diet, then also you will take Maalox Plus liquid and I will refer you to Gynecology and please have another Pap smear done. Exercise. I will give you some exercise for the back. You carry heavy things?

P: Yes.

D: Stop carrying heavy things and do the exercises. Your pain in the kidneys is due to carrying heavy things. If you continue to carry heavy things you will continue to have the pain.

P: Why did I come? Better not to have come if I continue to carry heavy things. Why come to the doctor if I don't take care?

D: If you don't eliminate what causes it [the problem], it will not disappear.

P: The doctor cannot be a magician.

D: We are doctors. We don't make miracles. So that there will be very little medicine, you have already spent enough on medicines, true? The Maalox, how would you like it? In tablets or liquid?

P: In tablets. Suspension is awful.

D: Chew tablets at six, ten, fourteen hours. Do you know when is fourteen hours?

P: Yes, two o'clock.

D: Eighteen hours.

P: Yes. Four o'clock is eighteen hours.

(The doctor instructed Nomi to take the Maalox tables at specific hours for ninety days.)

P: And then when I stop taking them, I will feel bad.

D: Why will you feel bad?

P: Because I will get into the habit of taking them.

D: These are not habit forming.

P: No.

D: On the day it is not necessary to take them, you will stop taking them.

P: Let's see if I have recovered when I come back.

D: All depends on you, woman.

P: What will be the diet?

D: This will be the only medicine. The diet, we have to agree that you will follow it. I don't want to impose it on you.

P: No.

(Physician 7 gave Nomi, as he did all his other patients, instructions regarding the specific times of the day she must eat and drink the foods he indicated in the diet, including two liters of camomile tea a day with sugar.)

D: In the he morning you should have a fruit, a fruit cocktail called "macedonia."

P: Cocktail.

D: But must be cooked. All must be cooked.

P: Yes, I will take a jumenx. (This is a canned fruit juice.)

D: Chemical--no.

P: Nothing.

D: Natural, natural, cooked fruit.

P: Where am I going to hide this, because my children will eat it.

D: The secret is that all is cooked. No, you cannot eat anything raw. If you eat these things raw they will harm you.

P: Carrot juice, no?

D: Everything must be cooked. Cooked fruit, including papaya, you can cook.

P: Apples?

D: Apples, pears, above all. You have diarrhea. Apple and pears, but puree. It has cellulose and natural fiber and immobilizes the intestine and removes the diarrhea.

P: Yes, doctor, I feel truly that, yes. I don't want beans and tortillas.

(As the doctor prescribed the diet and gave Nomi instructions on how to cook the creamed vegetable soups and prepare the fish that he ordered her to eat, Nomi observed that she did not have an appetite for any foods, and besides she was very concerned that the diet would give her a big stomach.)

D: Look, now. If I will give you holy water, the holy water will give you a big stomach because of the inflammation you have in the intestine. But if you follow the diet that I am prescribing, right away, after a month you will feel much better.

P: You will give me holy water? Yes, I need it.

D: What better is there than holy water?

P: Why? It still is nothing but water.

D: No, but holy water removes even bad spirits.

P: That is not true.

(Nomi anticipated difficulties with taking the cooked soups and fish to work with her every day.)

D: When you go out selling, then you must take everything with you.

P: Walking?

D: What do you sell?

P: Cinnamon sticks and garlic, and I walk selling and I have been doing it for a long time, because, my husband, what he gives me...

D: Good, you walk.

P: I walk, walk, walk, walk...

D: Good. Then at the hour that you must eat your meal excuse yourself and eat.

P: I will sit down on a bench.

D: Wherever you want.

P: There.

D: And eat at two o'clock.

P: Well, I will do it.

D: Health or work.

P: Yes, it's okay.

D: Then to work and not eat well, you will not be able to work and you will get ulcerative colitis.

P: Yes, I already have one.

D: No.

P: How do you know?

D: According to what you told me. With ulcerative colitis you expel pieces of intestine.

P: Oh, no!

D: There is a big difference. True?

P: Yes.

(The interview terminated with the doctor giving Nomi a return appointment for a month later on the one day of the week when she was not selling in the market.)

D: Good. Then in a month. Think there is nothing easier than this treatment. You have been sick for fifteen years, and if you want to avoid being sick...

P: I won't even attend to my children. Thank you, I am going.

I asked the doctor if he thought her condition was grave and he indicated it was not. Her disturbances were related to her bad eating habits, especially the spicy foods that she had eaten all her life, and to her general emotional state. She has had parasites for fifteen years, but the medicine he prescribed (Maalox Plus) would protect the mucus of the colon.

Nomi saw Physician 7 twice more. First, when she returned a month later for her scheduled appointment, he saw her for seven minutes. She reported that she was feeling very well. In fact, she even told the physician that he was like a magician. But a few days before she had eaten a tortilla and she started having pains, pointing to the left side of her abdomen and lumbar region. She stopped following the diet and ate her favorite enchiladas, because "they are so cheap, fish is so expensive." When she indicated that vegetables were very expensive, he responded, "Better to spend on vegetables than on medicine." She was eating well and, pointing to her stomach, indicated it was getting smaller. He asked if she had done her exercises and she said he didn't tell her to do them. He insisted he had. He instructed her to lie down on the cot to show her how to do sit-ups.

She disclosed that she recently began helping her husband selling in the market and with this change she could not spend time washing and cooking the vegetables and she ate only fish. She reported that because she was eating so much fish, her husband did not want to come near her or sleep with her because he claimed she smelled of fish. In response, the doctor advised her to use lemon after every meal to eliminate the smell. She reported that her headaches were gone (she had not reported having headaches before) because she ate more than once a day.

The doctor insisted that she must do sit-up exercises and tuck in her buttocks and stomach three times a day before each meal to eliminate the pain in the lumbar region. She asked, "How can I do that in the market?" He agreed with her when she said she would attract many onlookers. She informed him that she had pain, pointing again to the left side of the abdomen, but the doctor insisted that these exercises would strengthen her muscles and the pain would disappear. When she worried she could injure the scar she had on her body, he reassured her that the tissues were very strong and grown in. He asked her about the Pap smear she was given when she first came to the hospital but she had not picked up the results.[4]

The doctor insisted that on the next visit she bring him the results of the Pap test. She repeated that she was having pain in the kidneys, and the doctor told her that the exercise would eliminate it. She then pointed out to the doctor, "But I work very hard carrying and lifting and running." He insisted that the pain was due to lack of exercise. She asked, "Isn't it the same to do exercise and pick up heavy sacks?" She went on: "I urinate like atole [which suggests the color of white sap] and I expel from the urine pieces like pineapple. The urine is totally discolored like whipped cream." The doctor informed her that he would order an analysis later on, but at this time she had to do exercise by increasing her movements every three days until she made thirty movements a day. She responded with "I will be like Miss Universe."

He instructed her to continue with the Maalox Plus and again reminded her to bring the results of the Pap smear. When she inquired why he needed it, he replied that after seeing the results he would refer her to Gynecology. The consultation ended with the doctor reminding Nomi to pick up the Pap smear results, and Nomi claiming that her "stomach will twist from the hunger pangs."

She returned six weeks later for a scheduled appointment that lasted fifteen minutes. Nomi was clearly uncomfortable during this interview. During this consultation, the doctor reviewed the case and repeated the diagnosis he made during her first visit. This time she brought the results from the Pap smear indicating that she was perfectly well. Nomi, however, wanted to know why she was having a burning sensation during sexual intercourse. The physician suggested that this sensation was something else and he informed her that he would refer her to Gynecology to deal with her chronic vaginal inflammation.

He inquired about her pain in the *cintura* and she again stressed that her pain was not in the *cintura* (in the lumbar region), but in the left side, which the doctor related again to her tiredness. He stated, "But now it does not hurt." She feebly agreed with him but noted that her stomach was still bloated. He questioned her about having constipation; when she responded that she was suffering from diarrhea, not constipation, he responded, "But not anymore." She stated that she was not following the diet, and the doctor warned her that if she stopped her diet, it would cost her more. She told him that the diet was too difficult and too expensive to follow, nor could she do the exercises either. "You told me to do exercises three times a day, and I run and run, then the dishes, the daily chores, the children; isn't that exercise?" He reminded her that she had been feeling better and to continue with the Maalox Plus. "You cannot program yourself only to work you have to live, rest, and take care of yourself and your body." Nomi answered, "My husband says that 'to rest is only in the cemetery.'" The doctor retorted with "It is impossible that the machine work all the time; exercise is the eternal rest."

The doctor gave her an appointment for the following month and she inquired whether she could come to see him before if she were not feeling well. He asserted again that she would recover with the Maalox Plus, the diet, and the exercise, and it would be cheaper than any other kind of treatment. This was the last time Nomi came to see the physician.

This consultation, like the previous one with Sharon, gives us a glimpse of how a clinical judgment is made. Within the context of our current discussion, it is noteworthy that unlike Physician 3, and in keeping with his usual reliance on clinical observations rather than on technological interventions, Physician 7 used physical exploration coupled with the patient's presenting symptoms to support his diagnosis. He was the only physician in the study who used diet and exercise as a treatment modality.

While informed by concepts derived from Chinese and homeopathic medicine that places great emphasis on balance and harmony, especially psychological harmony, this physician's diagnoses and interrogation style are unquestionably biomedical. We can also clearly see how he imposed a time dimension on Nomi's condition with which she had difficulty dealing. Yet he disregarded Nomi's symptoms and he overlooked her very serious kidney dysfunction. Had the physician made an effort to learn about the context of Nomi's sickness and had he heard when she spoke about her poverty, relating how she worked all the time to eke out a less than minimum subsistence, he would also have realized that it was impossible for her to follow a costly diet requiring a great deal of leisure time at home to prepare. With a bit of more probing, he would also have learned that her sickness, of which the kidney dysfunction was the major problem, was embedded in her abysmal relations with her husband, who beat her from the first day of her marriage because she did not bleed on their wedding night. Nomi's comments during the consultations give us a glimpse of her relations with her husband, to which the physician lent a deaf ear, even admonishing her not to blame her husband when she mentioned that she was having pain during sexual intercourse.

Nomi's reference to pain in the left side of her back and the kidneys was reinterpreted by this physician as *cintura* and understood by him in cultural terms by associating kidney pain with lower back pain. In this case, however, the patient's focus on the kidneys referred to her urinary dysfunctions which she clearly spelled out when she described the texture of her urine.

The cases of Sharon and Nomi reveal not only the diverse ways biomedicine is practiced in Mexico, but also the different etiological assumptions upon which clinical judgments are made. We also see that a reductionist approach, be it organic or psychosomatic, if not informed by the patient's existential circumstances and life's lesions, fails to diagnose or treat the patient's condition. For Nomi, the outcome was quite disastrous. I will describe Nomi's case in much greater detail in Chapter 11, where we will learn more about the life of this extraordinary woman and the ethical dilemmas her case raised for me as a participant observer. As we shall see, the three visits to the hospital were only a prelude to her endless search for treatment of her kidneys.

The medical encounters we have just witnessed also direct our attention to the inherent drama of the consultation, a point to which we turn in the next chapter

Notes

1. As gleaned from my findings, using diagnoses given me by the physicians, as well as classification of them by one physician. I gathered all the diagnoses given me by the attending physicians for the patients in the study. I requested one physician to classify the individual diagnoses into broader diagnostic categories. Using *Principles of Internal Medicine* by Harrison, the physician classified the diagnosis around disease etiology. Of the seventeen physicians whose patients were followed in this study, only physicians who saw ten or more patients in the study sample were included in this analysis. These eight physicians saw a total of 183 patients.

2. According to the physician who did the classification, 10 percent of the 98 diagnoses did not correspond to any known diagnostic biomedical category, as, for example, "unstable column." According to this physician "unstable column" is not an accepted diagnosis within medical nosology.

3. A positive test is a clue to etiology in a patient with acute renal failure.

4. These results are given only in the mornings, while Nomi's appointments were in the afternoons. To get the results she would either have to spend the entire day in the hospital or make two separate trips with each trip taking three hours.

8

The Medical Consultation

In the last chapter we gained a glimpse of the doctor-patient interview, illustrating the diversity in biomedical activities and shedding light on the problematics created by the duality in biomedical practice. The doctor-patient encounter has been of interest to scholars of medical practice for numerous other reasons, however. The medical consultation provides a stage for a multidimensional view of biomedicine in action and how diagnoses are made and treatment courses devised by different physicians; concurrently, it introduces us to the people it serves as the physicians see them and who will form the focus of our attention in the third part of the book.

The clinical interview is regarded as standing at the juncture of micro- and macroanalysis (Cicourel 1981). It is one arena where tacit cultural understandings become molded by macroconceptions in the medical domain and where the lived world shapes broader systems of medical ideas. It is also the core of biomedical practice (Maretzki 1985) or, in the words of Pellegrino and Thomasma, "Clinical interaction is the source of integrity of medicine as a discipline" (1981:64). Most important, the clinical encounter encompassing the doctor-patient relationship is considered by many as the essential component of the healing process; successful diagnosis and treatment depend on it.[1] In Mishler's words, "A complex set of assumptions about the biological specificity of disease etiology and symptoms and about the primary function of physicians as applied bioscientists, has excluded from serious concern how variations in clinical practice and in the conduct of medical interviews affect the course and outcome of patients' illnesses" (1984:10). As I will show in the next chapters, the doctor-patient interaction comprises only one of several elements in the healing process, and only certain aspects of the interaction contribute to patient-perceived outcome. However, as a component of the healing process, the doctor-patient encounter engages the two players in a drama that forms part of the patient's pursuit of recovery.

123

The medical interview is not an ordinary meeting between two strangers. The conditions that bring the protagonists together are *extraordinary*: One is in pain and under duress while the other is expected to eliminate or transform it. By viewing the medical encounter as drama, we observe the inherent tensions and conflicts that are played out in sickness and in the healing process and that also bear on wider social processes.

Guided by Turner's (1974) notion of the "processual" aspects of human interaction as "social drama," Frankenberg (1986) proposed that sickness itself is such a drama. There is no denying that sickness is drama in a human being's life. But as I sat in on over 800 medical consultations, I soon became aware that I was experiencing the unfolding of a drama in the medical consultation itself. I sensed a tension and a gradual *denouement*, as patients uncovered directly and indirectly not only their bodies but also layers of the core of their lives. Yet, paradoxically, we learn from the medical consultation relatively little about patients' lives that underlies the motives for their being on this stage at this particular time. Herein lies a major element of what makes the encounter a drama. From its inception the dramaturgical nature of the medical encounter becomes apparent because the physician listens, but does not hear. Balint emphasized that the physician must learn to listen. During the process of listening the physician "will soon find out that there are straightforward direct questions which could bring to light the kind of information for which he is looking" (1964:121). Balint charges the physician to listen in order to get at information a physician believes necessary to make a diagnosis (Armstrong 1984) but not to hear the anguish of the lived experience and the contradictions the patient must negotiate. The physician cannot hear because the paradigm that guides his or her ordered script admits only revelations related to the physical body, to "objective phenomena," and to a stereotypic social map on which the physician situates the patient. All other assertions are taken as incoherent statements and bracketed as "subjective" and irrelevant (Engel 1977). In the case of Mexican physicians, they were unable to incorporate other types of knowledge, the outpourings of patients' suffering and patient's "incoherent" statements about their lives, not because they lack sensitivity to a patient's agony, but because their perceptions of themselves as professional physicians would have been diminished were they not to adhere to the biomedical model. As Cicourel rightly noted, "The physician is not trained to deal with micro-events as socio-cultural, cognitive and emotional manifestations" (1981:71). Maintaining their self-image as competent physicians requires them to ignore the intrinsic meanings of typical symptoms and "incoherent" narratives, the content of which often revealed the core of the pain the patient was experiencing. As members of the culture, physicians share with the patient the recognition of the magnitude of the patient's narratives and some were clearly pained by them. Ultimately, however, the patient provides accounts orchestrated by the physicians because the doctors' medical training and medical script require it.

Following Turner's model of social drama, the players' interests stand in opposition in the medical encounter. Cognitively, at least, the two actors are bound by a common interest: alleviation of the patient's ailments. The encounter as scripted by the biomedical model brings the two players into conflict, however. Moved by a crisis, the patient arrives on the stage to seek advice from an expert who presumably knows more about how bodies work than the patient does. The physician claims to have a monopoly on the knowledge of disease. He is the authority of what went wrong (Parsons 1975; Tuckett et al. 1985). The patient comes laden with personal knowledge encoded by cultural understandings about the workings of *his* or *her* body and the authority of the specific condition. The patient is *certain* of his individualized experience of pain (Scarry 1985), while the physician is often uncertain of the diagnosis (Fox 1980). In the words of one doctor, "I must sometimes invent a diagnosis" that is based upon generalized, normative, and the physician's personal knowledge of disease entities. In the seventeenth and eighteenth centuries, "It was believed that each individual had his own unique pattern of bodily events which the practitioner had to discern in each case" (Jewson 1976:229). In the twentieth century the idiosyncratic patient disappeared to emerge as part of a generalized class of ills. The physician no longer takes his cues from the patient's individualized symptoms, despite eliciting an exhaustive medical history. The patient's unique personal experience of pain has not changed since the eighteenth century. The physician's guiding script has changed, however, as he converts personal suffering to generic, impersonal disease entities; uncertain diagnoses are scripted by a physical biomedical model, or in some instances psychosomatic constructs, and reflect personal understandings.

Physicians also fail to explain the underlying causes of the diagnoses they make. To cite a compelling example, a patient seen by one doctor was diagnosed as having a "fallen womb" attributed by the physician to the fact that the woman had given birth to fifteen children. The patient, however, wanted to know why other women who had as many children did not experience this affliction. The physician, taken aback by the question, had no response for her except to say, "We are not all equal."

The drama is further sustained because there is no chorus to interpret for the patient what the doctor attempts to communicate. Often, patients may not understand the physician's explanation, and ultimately they must make sense of their affliction, an intensely subjective experience by themselves, as in the case of the woman just mentioned who wished to comprehend why she and not her friend suffered from a "fallen womb?"

Another important dimension of the conflict arises from the physician's need to situate the patient's disease in time and anatomical space. The diagnostic process incorporates a temporal and topographical dimension. For the patient, however, his or her sickness transcends time and body topography. Sickness suspends the temporal dimension of existence, so the patient is frequently unable to pinpoint the date of the onset of the sickness. Sickness and the accompanying symptoms fluctuate in time and body space commensurate with the experiences that they signify. The physician is often frustrated by the patient's inability to compartmentalize the symptoms to a particular anatomical region, to conform to the medical history format, or to locate the symptoms in a time frame, as we saw in Nomi's case. Not uncommonly, the patient is forced to guess or invent an approximate date and specify an anatomical location to satisfy the physician's script.

The traditional dyadic model of the doctor-patient relationship excludes the family (Hahn et al. 1988) that is intrinsic to a Mexican's existence. The doctor-patient encounter individualizes the patient and involves only two players in the drama: the solitary, autonomous patient facing the solitary, autonomous physician, who gazes upon the afflicted individual as the sole sufferer. We witnessed Sharon's clinical interview in which the physician endured the cousin. Some physicians, as in Sharon's case, admit other members of the family, but many do not because the medical encounter is individualized.

Not surprisingly, the biomedical encounter as we know it today and as it takes place in Mexico emerges out of modern Western society's individualism, which has become an all-embracing universal principle (Dumont 1971, 1977; Lukes 1973; Shweder and Bourne 1984). This model conceives of the person as an autonomous unit, independent of and isolated from other individuals and the social and cultural contexts. By not incorporating information about the family and the life world in which the patient is embedded, the medical consultation aggravates rather than allays the crisis for the patient and accentuates the drama.

The dramaturgical event requires a resolution of the crisis by mitigating it, and by transforming the patient's life world which leads to restoration to a healthy state. The aura of biomedicine's invincibility raises the patient's expectations. For some, the medical encounter is a drama in one act. The patient is brought back to his or her usual state and no longer experiences his or her body as "strange." For many, the crisis is not resolved for reasons that are largely separate from the encounter itself; the patient must therefore continue in his or her pursuit of recovery and restoration of order to his or her life.

Some have argued that physicians in America transmit political ideologies during the medical consultation (Waitzkin 1979). As we see in these and numerous other consultations, physicians in Mexico transmit their prejudices about the poor, their morality (especially pertaining to male-female relations and marriage), and religious ideologies, and they exercise power through the prohibitions they impose on their patients (e.g., diets, sexual abstinence). Physicians fail, however, to transmit an ideology about the state which they themselves must serve and which renders them powerless as well. We can thus say that in broader societal terms, the medical consultation is a vehicle for the transmission of numerous ideologies whose content will depend upon the structural position of the medical profession in the society in which it is found.

As we see from the medical encounters that follow, the medical consultation reveals to us the drama of the doctor-patient encounter and the ways in which the microlevels and macrolevels of interaction within a medical context intersect; how the medical interview on a microlevel--what physicians and patients say to each other--becomes transformed on a macro-level into notions about how to formulate one's experience of sickness in physical terms; how sickness is transmitted through inheritance; and how treatment requires tests and medications. Concurrently, these beliefs and practices become reinforced by patients' demands for tests and medication to "make them forget" and for treatment for all their ills, or by common beliefs in the inheritability of disease.

I have set the stage for the presentation of the following verbatim transcriptions of medical encounters by the various physicians to reveal the nature of biomedical practice and its nuances as it unfolds during the medical consultation. (Whenever available, the pressure height, and weight of the patients are also added.)

Concurrently, these transcripts disclose aspects of medical practice that I have discussed in the previous chapter, including ideologies physicians transmit to patients and patients' mode of symptom presentation as compared with the way they presented symptoms prior to seeing the physician. Most important, we discern how different physicians deal with the same presenting symptoms and how their clinical reasoning illustrates the diversity in biomedical practice. I selected consultations with patients from the total number of patients seen by each physician, and individuals whom I also followed on a regular basis, to portray the physician's particular style. As we saw in the previous chapter, there is a diversity of medical orientations among the physicians, but each physician is consistent in the manner he or she conducts the consultation. Thus, these interviews are representative of each doctor's consultation style and clinical reasoning. I have presented in the previous chapter consultations with three patients, Jose, Sharon, and Nomi; I now turn to four additional patients out of the 205 in the study sample.

The routine procedures of the medical consultation always began when patients waiting for a consultation were called by a nurse into a small room to be weighed and measured and to have their blood pressure taken. These data were recorded in a folder that was given to the physician. The patient then returned to the waiting room until he or she was called by the nurse to be seen by a doctor. Folders of new patients were randomly distributed to attending physicians. The new patients were usually seen after the patients on recall appointments. The time a patient waited to be seen by the doctor depended upon the number of return appointments he had scheduled for a given day and the number of interruptions by visitors, students, or pharmaceutical salesmen.

All physicians followed a standard procedure. This included having patients report their symptoms, taking and recording a medical history, preparing a set of forms for each laboratory analysis and diagnostic test they ordered, writing out the prescription, and in the event that they made a referral, filling out additional paperwork. For statistical purposes, all patients were asked where they lived and where they came from. With few exceptions physicians did a physical examination.

Many physicians spent a considerable portion of the medical consultation writing and completing forms. Previously, I discussed the role of medical history taking in the transmission of an ideology of sickness as inheritable. Medical history taking has other residual and unmeasurable effects. While a few physicians write meticulous histories, most jot down the salient symptoms reported by the patient. Some physicians first listened to the patient's symptoms and then wrote, in which case they looked directly at the patient as he or she spoke. Others wrote as the patient spoke and hardly ever looked at the patient.

Irrespective of the length of the written record, the physician's act of writing down what patients say makes many patients feel that they are in competent hands. Many patients remarked that what they liked most about the physician was that he or she wrote down what they had said and it formed part of a permanent record.

Another residual effect of medical history taking is the questioning process in and of itself. Various patients indicated that what pleased them most about a physician was that he or she asked a lot of questions. Ironically, a common belief among younger physicians is that the more questions a physician must ask a patient to establish a diagnosis, the less prepared he or she is as a doctor; a good and experienced physician ought to be able to make a diagnosis with minimal questioning of the patient.

During the morning shift most consultations were interrupted by pharmaceutical salesmen. During the afternoon shift there were hardly any interferences, but as far as I could assess, patients were not disturbed by these interruptions. Nor were they bothered by the number of people present during a consultation. Four to five students were usually present during consultations given by at least three of the physicians during the morning shift, and most had other occasional visitors. When I queried patients about how they viewed the presence of people other than the physician during the interview, all patients gave a very similar response: It showed that many people were interested in them because they were there. Normally, for the purpose of the physical examination, patients were asked to partially undress from the top half of their bodies, which the nurse covered up with a sheet.

The similarities in consultation mask, of course, the difference in the actual content of the questioning and the physicians' general demeanor and stance toward the patient. Two physicians gave great weight to the doctor-patient relationship. According to Physician 7, since most sickness was psychosomatic, the doctor-patient relationship was crucial to curing the patient's ills. Most physicians received patients with courtesy at all times. Physician 6 could sometimes be quite gruff and treated people in the manner of a stern mother.

Arthur

Arthur's case is significant because it illuminates the unfolding drama of a consultation even when the physician combines a folk and biomedical orientation as we see Physician 6 do. Her diagnosis is firmly anchored in biomedical nomenclature and her etiological explanation places great stress on heredity factors, yet she accepted and treated typical symptoms, as was the case with Arthur. Physician 6 treated the patient's self-diagnosed typical symptoms of high and low blood pressure and "created" a disease in orthodox biomedical terms (Helman 1985) where there might not have been one.

During the first interview Physician 6 clearly suggested symptoms to the patient that he was not experiencing, especially those related to urination. The typical symptom of high and low blood pressure was medicalized into several syndromes and treated with massive medications. In this case the patient's condition was medicalized both by the physician and the patient. The physician showed no concern for the patient's life situation, although Arthur speculated that perhaps his sickness was related to his work. This interview clearly illustrates how sexual morality is transmitted in a clinical encounter, as when the doctor condemned multiple partners, yet concurrently expressed widely shared beliefs about male sexuality when she commented to Arthur about the inevitability of his father seeking another woman when his mother was sick.

Arthur reported in the first interview that he came to seek treatment for high and low blood pressure. He presented a slip of paper showing that his pressure had been measured on consecutive days. He feared that he would die from a heart attack. His major symptoms were headaches, dizziness, feeling faint, and feeling numb.

Arthur (pressure 130/80, 144 pounds, 5'6") was twenty-eight years old, and married with one child. He came unaccompanied to the hospital.

The consultation lasted forty-five minutes, but much of the time the doctor addressed the nurse who was also present. It was not uncommon for Physician 6 to begin a consultation by telling patients and any other bystanders about her problems. In this instance she reported on her difficulties in getting her paycheck and the anger it was provoking in her. Physician 6 usually listened to the patient's presenting symptoms and then wrote a few brief remarks in the medical record. She addressed the patient in the formal "you."

Doctor: Let's start. How long have you been sick and why did you come for a consultation? What is your problem?

Patient: I started having the disturbances around May [five months earlier].

D: Starting in May of this year, what did you feel?

P: "Pressure." I have been checking my pressure with the doctor in the college where I study and I brought the record of the changes in my pressure. Sometimes it goes up and sometimes it goes down.

D: From May 1986 till the present you have had an alteration in arterial pressure. It goes up and goes down. It relaxes. Do you sweat?

P: It goes up and down in the morning, when it is very high and very low.

D: And how did you get it?

P: Well...

D: Do you study? Work? Or what do you do?

P: I work and I study.

D: What kind of work do you do and what are you studying?

P: I work in an auditor's office.

D: Auditor.

P: And I am studying public accounting.

D: Are there people in your family--father, mother, grandfather--that have high blood pressure?

P: I don't know.

D: Your mother, what did she die of?

P: Heart.

D: What heart problem did she have?

P: I don't know. I was one and a half years old.

D: Did anyone have angina pectoris [*angina de pecho*], heart arrest, or, what was the problem? You should ask your father what problem she had.

P: I think she had a heart operation.

D: She had a heart operation. Probably she had a traumatic problem, maybe the valvular, due to rheumatism, rheumatic cardiopathy. You were two and a half?

P: A year and a half.

D: A year and a half, correct. And your father is alive? What health problems does he have?

P: He has cirrhosis.

D: Alcoholic. He drinks a lot.

P: Yes.

D: Did your father remarry?

P: No.

D: That was bad. Does he have other children?

P: No. But yes, he had two wives at the same time when he was married to my mother. He didn't marry but he had another woman with whom he had three children.

D: When your mother was alive, he had another woman?

P: Yes.

D: How daring the Mexican [using a diminutive], eh?

P: Yes, from Guanajuato.

D: Of course, the song says life is not worth anything. (She laughed.) Good, he was young; he was a man; he needed to have something; he needed an attraction, incentive in life. Probably your mother was suffering from advanced clinical problems. He needed a woman closer to him. We are not getting into your father's personal life, of course.

P: Of course.

D: You live with two brothers?

P: No, there was a time when I lived with him [his brother]. We are three brothers.

D: Males?

P: Yes.

D: The brothers are here, correct? Did your grandparents die of a serious disease?

P: No.

D: You are now twenty-five years old. (He was twenty-eight years old at the time) What serious ailments have you had?

P: Nothing. Only pressure now. Of my brothers, I am the least sick.

D: Have you had frequent diarrhea problems?

P: No.

D: Have you expelled worms [earthworms (*lombriz*)] or oxyuris?

P: Oxyuris, no. Earthworms, yes.

D: At what age? Eight, nine, more or less?

P: Around that age. I don't remember how old I was.

D: How many earthworms did you expel. How many could there have been? Did you see, Did you expel ascaris?

P: About three, more or less.

D: From that time on you didn't expel any more? Did you get any treatment?

P: Yes.

D: When you were young, since puberty, have you had some problems?

P: No.

D: Your sexual life began normally at puberty?

P: Yes.

D: You are not to exaggerate. You don't run around too much? All this we need to know to see what is the cause of your arterial pressure being dislocated.

P: Yes, before I was married I had another girl with whom I had sexual relations.

D: Good. Did you have children with her?

P: No.

D: Yes, but did "we" have a normal life or a very exaggerated one?

P: No, normal.

D: You were married or lived in free union? You were actually married?

P: I married only once.

D: Yes, the first time you lived in free union.

P: No, she was my fiancee, and I had sexual relations with her.

D: (angrily) Already as fiances, you lived in free union. Here we call things as they are. Your fiancee at the beginning, but once you had relations with her she was not your fiancee, it was another thing. It is called free union, and we will leave it at that.

P: Yes.

D: How long did you live with her?

P: Two years.

D: Now, as to your marriage, how long have you been married?

P: Three years.

D: Do you have children?

P: One, three years old.

D: Male?

P: Yes.

D: You smoke, drink?

P: Sometimes.

D: Sometimes what?

P: Smoke, drink.

D: Smoker, alcoholic, positive. Sometimes, what times is that?

P: Well, every three months, every four months.

D: Didn't smoke three months to date, okay. (laughingly) When you go to a fiesta you drink two or three Cubas [Coca Cola and brandy] and you become happy and you drink with your friends, and after ten or twenty Cubas you toast, you drink pure vinegar, and then you play the guitar.

P: I am very reserved, I am very reserved. I am not like one of those.

D: Exaggerated, what I want to know is the truth you see. (She laughed)

(As with all patients, she questioned him in great detail about his bowel movements and nature of the fecal material.)

D: How often do you get sick in the stomach?

P: Very rarely.

D: Once or twice a year.

P: No, about four or five times.

D: Four to five times diarrhea a year, okay, that is chronic colitis. And already had ascaris, already had parasites. Cannot discard that this is a person with an abnormal colon and intestine, a person with parasites, because parasites are cyclical. When diarrhea cycles begin, could have some little animals, could have tricocefelos, oxyuris, and there is then a normal time when they are asleep, some food that exacerbates the problem and produces diarrhea. Did you take some antidiarrheal medication? You have chronic parasitosis, right? Urination. Have you ever urinated with mucus or blood, no? Never. When you have colic, diarrhea, you have colic?

P: Yes.

D: Do you have pain in the rectum? Your rectum becomes irritated when you have diarrhea?

P: No.

D: Never?

P: No.

D: Nor recently, nothing? When? You drink alcohol, you have pain in the rectum? Try to remember.

P: Well, when I drink, yes.

D: You see, another clinical datum, that you have chronic colitis, rectal tenesmus with alcohol. Now, as to urination, how often do you urinate a day?

P: Twice a day.

D: Do you drink a lot of water?

P: I drink a lot of water when I stop. All day I sit, then when I stop I urinate more often.

D: You urinate in accordance with the quantity of water you drink, but normally you urinate twice a day. When you urinate liquid, your urine is very concentrated, very hot. You feel burning, pain on urination?

P: No.

D: Nothing like that? You have never had pain?

P: Yes, when I urinate.

D: When you urinate, it is very concentrated?

P: Yes.

D: What color? Clear, yellow, very white, very dark?

P: Very yellow.

D: All depends what will happen when you do your analysis, so that we know what the origin of the problem with your pressure is. With the analysis we will see whether it is a renal problem. You feel pain, you feel sudden burning on urination.

P: Yes.

D: You consume too much salt? A little, normal?

P: Normal.

D: You eat salty foods? I like very salty meals.

P: Regular.

D: Your meals are salty, you like salty foods?

P: Yes.

D: You will stop eating salt completely. During one month you will not take any salt to correct the pressure. We will have analysis done (The doctor prepared the forms.)

D: You have never had a venereal disease, gonorrhea, syphilis. Have you had asthma, something else, some other thing. Urticaria (hives)?

P: No.

D: Nothing like that? Anginas [tonsillitis] frequently, catarrhs, pain in the ears?

P: Pain in the ears? No.

D: Frequent anginas?

P: Anginas.

D: How often during the year?

P: Four times a year.

D: Did you receive a treatment to alleviate it, a palliative or real treatment for anginas?

P: I had a treatment for anginas.

D: When? you must be very alert with the anginas because your mother already had rheumatic fever and then mothers transmit it and you get it. We must do a pharyngeal exudate to see the problem because the mother had rheumatic fever, and you can get this problem as well. That was the time when she had a midwife. It's a problem if you deliver at home. And yes, we need a blood chemistry analysis, a urine analysis. Now, since May, what medicines have you had for this ["pressure"]? It is very important, so we can treat the arterial pressure that goes up.

P: Well, nothing--only these were given to me. (He showed a piece of paper indicating Effortil, a drug for hypotension.)

D: Give me the paper where you have written down Effortil. This means that you have had more low pressure than high pressure. Effortil is to raise the pressure only. To stabilize pressure, pharyngeal exudate and electro-cardiogram.

P: Can you give me a moment to go to the bathroom?

D: Yes, of course. But ask where it is. I don't know where it is.

P: Upstairs.

(In the meantime the doctor examined the paper he brought on which his pressure was recorded on a daily and weekly basis six times. First time, 140/90; second day, 120/80; two days later, 120/70; three days later 120/90; a day later, 100/60; and two days later, 110/60.) As she read the piece of paper she reasoned out loud, "Let's see what I will consider an essential arterial pressure, because he does not have many clinical data. But listening to him, there is a problem. He has had parasites. He has a renal problem, because there is pain and burning on urination and his urine is very concentrated. And in addition he has chronic tonsillitis. Let us find out whether the tonsillitis is related to the kidneys, and that will explain the pressure, because it is high; we will give him an appointment for about two weeks."

In addition to the analysis, she ordered an ultrasound of the kidneys "to see how the kidneys are."

Arthur returned to the cubicle and the doctor urged him to have the tests done quickly in case he was suffering from kidney stones, although she doubted it. She also suggested that he tell the laboratory service that it was an emergency in order that he be attended to promptly.

Lastly, she gave him several indications.

D: When you get up in the morning at six o'clock, take your pressure and pulse. Buy a thermometer, and take your temperature daily and also your arterial pressure daily.

P: I will have it done at night in school.

D: We need that you take the pressure in the morning. Can't you take it in the morning?

P: Yes.

D: You will take it in the morning and in the evening, to see what variation there is. If you shiver, what you must do to raise the pressure is eat normally. But eat no pork, or pork rinds, sausage with chile, nothing like that. Otherwise you can eat anything you like, but without a drop of salt, no salt, to see how your kidneys function. Food will taste insipid, but you are in treatment. We will prescribe Neurofor, 50,000 mcg. These are vitamin B [vitamin B12] and they are intramuscular injections. The first bottle must be injected daily, three centimeters deep, the other bottles every third day--and you must follow a diet without eating salt. It's very important to have the studies done and begin your treatment right away. Do you sleep well?

P: No, I suffer from insomnia.

D: With this Neurofor, you will get well. You will take three bottles. It is like you said, the insomnia, the days that you have high and low blood pressure vary. That is why you don't sleep well. (She also prescribed a vitamin- mineral complex, to be taken three times a day after each meal.)

D: You will be called at the front desk.

After this interview she explained to me that her final diagnosis was alteration in arterial pressure--"it goes up and down"--but it is obvious that it went down more than up. She needed to discover the etiology of the problem. The clinical data did not suggest that he was suffering from essential arterial hypertension, because of its fluctuation up and down. She wanted to establish if indeed he had parasites and chronic tonsillitis that could harm the kidneys and cause the pressure fluctuation.

Physician 6 noted to me that the patient had a problem of inheritance of cirrhosis to deal with that possibly could cause the rise and fall in pressure, but she didn't know if the father had cirrhosis before or after Arthur was born and and whether this problem was due to his father's drinking. Finally, she concluded that he had a renal disorder and a disturbance of the liver because he was the son of a chronic alcoholic. She remarked that Arthur's mother had suffered from cardiac pathology, another hereditary factor to be considered. Her clinical reasoning incorporated the fact that Arthur had been married twice: The first marriage was a free union, and in a free union "sexual life is not normal" because the woman could have been with men other than the patient, thus acquiring an infection and contaminating him. She ordered urinalysis to assess if Arthur's kidneys were functioning normally or if he had cirrhosis due to alcoholism. In the medical record the diagnosis was entered as "arterial hypertension."

Arthur returned to see Physician 6 twice more. On the first return visit two weeks later, Arthur's pressure was 130/80. He reported that he continued to feel sick, and this time he mentioned that he was experiencing headaches (front and back) and chest pain. The results of all the laboratory analyses were negative, and his cardiogram was normal. However, based upon the test results the doctor concluded that Arthur was susceptible to staphylococcus aureus and streptococcus. Based upon this presumed susceptibility to staphylococcus aureus, she concluded that he had a renal infection.

Consider the drama that had unfolded during these encounters. Arthur's concern was the fluctuation in pressure, while the doctor wished to know whether he indeed never had gonorrhea "or any such thing." When he responded "no," she questioned him further about his sexual activities before his marriage and led him to admit that he was a flirt then. On the basis of this admission she concluded that he was suffering from renal dysfunction and venereal disease and that this disease was causing the high and low pressure. Additionally, he suffered "intercostal polineuritis of the thorax."

Arthur kept his second scheduled appointment three weeks later. The doctor took his pressure herself, which was 130/90. He reported that he no longer had any pain on urination. He said he felt better, but he was having headaches; perhaps he felt sick because of his work. He took all the medications, except one she had prescribed that was no longer available in the pharmacy.

In response to her questions, Arthur indicated that he was allergic to penicillin and other antibacterial agents, which led her to think that there may be no way of curing him. But when Arthur asked if the infection could be eliminated, the doctor responded. "Of course we can, son. You will take a lot of medication. Here there is nothing that is not possible. In medicine everything can be cured if you are in a condition to be cured. You are a young fellow and if you follow the treatment you will get well, if you exclude salts from your diet, and that is why you have arterial hypertension, and not only is it high but it is also low." At this time she added several new diagnoses: renal infection (nephritis), that is, "the kidney is in disequilibrium," causing the low pressure; massive infection of the colon; salmonellosis; typhoid; and tonsillitis. She prescribed a series of medications including sassix (?), a diuretic to lower the pressure, duroditenil (?) capsules, and diodicenil (?) (antiparasitics) every eight hours as well as Pantomicina 80 mgs (antibiotic) intramuscular injections and Uro Binotal (antibiotic for urinary infections), one with every meal three times a day for eight days, for "your renal infection." She also prescribed Neurofor (injections every third day for polineuritis), dipoprin (?), Uropol (antiseptic for urinary tract infections), and Ponstan (an analgesic) for his pains in the chest, arms, and kidneys. In addition she indicated a traditional fruit drink (*agua de Jamaica*), one glass every hour, "but not when it is cold." She prohibited him from eating foods with salt, a special hardship for Arthur, and urged him to eat vegetables and fruits except watermelon. She prescribed some juices, hot baths, and "never walk on cold floors." She gave him another appointment for two months later, which he did not keep.

During the first interview the doctor clearly suggested symptoms to the patient that he was not experiencing, especially those related to urination. The typical symptom of high/low blood pressure was medicalized into several syndromes and treated with massive medications.

Arthur did not anticipate such diagnoses, although he too interpreted the symptoms in medical terms. Despite the fact that at one point Physician 6 considered the possibility that Arthur's condition was related to his lived experience, especially his work, her final diagnosis was related to her personal views of male sexuality rather than to the results of the laboratory analysis or even presenting symptoms.

In the final analysis, the diagnosis revolved around Arthur's sexuality translated into biomedical nosology--venereal disease--and urinary tract infection (nephritis). The treatment was purely pharmacological. Biomedicine usually holds the individual responsible for his or her disorder. In this instance, we learn that Arthur was responsible for his condition--his alleged promiscuity. From the physician's personal script we glean the doctor's interpretation of Arthur's family medical history: an alcoholic father and a mother who died from rheumatic heart disease, conditions Arthur undoubtedly inherited. But we fail to learn anything about the patient's lived world that could illuminate Arthur's experience of high and low blood pressure.

Medical consultations, like all dramas, provide us with insights into ideologies, in this case, about heredity and about male sexuality. The drama is, however, not resolved with pharmaceutical drugs that physicians prescribe and patients desire, when they come to seek treatment for lived experience that they too medicalize.

Serge

Serge, like Arthur, complained of high and low blood pressure. But he received a very different diagnosis and treatment from Physician 4, who usually diagnosed patients with diverse presenting symptoms in the same way, namely parasites and skeletal disorders (specifically "scoliosis and flat feet"). Physician 4's clinical judgment, exhibits the idiosyncratic nature of the diagnostic process. His script rarely deviated from the standard consultation and treatment procedures we see him follow with Serge.

Serge (pressure 120/80, weight not taken, 6'5"), twenty years old, with preparatory school education, arrived at the hospital dressed in a very heavy sweater despite the fact that it was a singularly warm day. In the first interview Serge reported that he came to seek treatment because he was feeling "very desperate," his pressure went up and down, and he was experiencing an internal pain, tiredness, depression, dizziness, and nausea. Sometimes he heard ringing in his ears and he wondered whether it might not be psychological. He could not explain the reasons for his condition except that perhaps he took too many vitamins and did too much exercise.

Physician 4 briefly listened to the patient's complaints and then took notes as he questioned the patient about his medical history. During the consultation there was a movement of visitors in and out of the cubicle, in addition to the students and the pharmaceutical salesmen. The doctor addressed Serge in the informal you (*tu*) during the interview, which lasted twenty-eight minutes including interruptions.

Doctor: My name is...And how can we serve you?
Patient: Well, I came to see... I came to see if you could help me.
D: Serge, what is your surname? (The name is usually written out on the folder the doctor gets.)
P: Serge...
D: You are very big, good.
P: I have been sick in my stomach approximately six months. I have a lot of gas, and I have been having pain in "lungs" [that is, back] for the past three months. Since that time, my circulation changed and also I have pain in the waist [*cintura*] down to my kidneys and then I feel exhausted.
D: And what else?
P: I have pain.
D: Astemia, tiredness.
P: Yes, tired and I have headaches.
D: Migraine [*cefalea*]. What else?

P: Sometimes my pressure goes up and sometimes it goes down, and I have gone to see other doctors and I have been told that maybe I have parasites, but I have not had any analysis done.

D: Epigastric pain. You have this pain in the "mouth of your stomach?" Is it a burning sensation, or how?

P: No, it only hurts. I feel an emptiness.

D: Emptiness, what else?

P: Sometimes my pressure goes down.

D: Good, you think the pressure goes down.

P: Yes, it happens that sometimes I feel very weak and my pressure has been taken and it is low. Yesterday I played football soccer and I felt very weak and they took my pressure and it was high.

D: Do you have heartburn?

P: Now? Not any more but there was a time...

D: Bitter?

P: No.

D: When you bend down, do you have water coming up, as if when one eats salsa, there is a pain in the "mouth of the stomach" that comes up like belching?

P: No.

D: But you belch?

P: No.

D: What other disturbances do you have? Gases in the belly?

P: Yes, I tell you I went to have tests done.

D: Leave the tests and what you were told. I want to know what happens to you, not what your mother told you. I don't believe your mother. And if you tell me that your analysis came out bad, they are bad. The disturbances continue, true?

P: Yes.

D: You say there is a lot of gas in your stomach, and through the bottom you expel gas. Normal, or a lot?

P: Yes, a lot.

D: And do you have itching in the rectum?

P: Sometimes.

D: Very well, do you salivate at night and wake up with saliva?

P: Rarely.

D: Dry cough in the afternoons?

P: No.

D: You move your bowels in small balls, big ones like a rabbit?

P: No, that is, it has no form.

D: Sometimes very thin and a lot.

P: Always very thin and it has been very loose, loose, loose.

D: With mucus?

P: I didn't notice.

D: Sticky, yes?

P: Yes, and different colors.

D: Are the stools very greasy?

P: No.

D: Sudsy?

P: Yes.

D: Very well. Do you have many nightmares.

P: Yes, well, not nightmares, but I dream a lot and it bothers me. That is, for example, sometimes I have been at the point of losing reality. I feel very depressed.

D: You are an angry person?

P: On occasions, yes.

D: Do you forget things?

P: Yes, recently I have been forgetting things.

D: Very well. You urinate normally? There is no burning, jabbing pain?

P: No, normal. But sometimes I have difficulty.

D: What do you mean about the urine? Do you have difficulties, or what?

P: I make, but I cannot make.

D: You want to make more? You remain with the desire to make more?

P: No.

D: Burning, jabs?

P: No.

D: Has your urine ever looked like Coca Cola?

P: No.

D: Blood?

P: No.

D: Your father, your mother, have they had heart problems, lungs, diabetes?

P: No.

D: Very well. Do you live with animals, parrots, dogs, cats?

P: Yes, I have a dog, but I don't live with him. I don't live in the house where the dog is.

D: Sometimes, yes.

P: Yes, on occasions.

D: What others than the dog? Parrots, geese?

P: No.

D: You have been vaccinated?

P: I had one for rabies.

D: Have you been operated for something?

P: Not long ago I was operated on my tonsils [anginas], but...

D: Very well, allergic to some medication?

P: No.

D: Any food that brings out rashes?

P: No.

D: Clothing?

P: No.

D: Do you have a good sense of smell?

P: Yes.

D: Tumors?

P: Tumors? No, no.

D: Do you have all your teeth?

P: Yes.

D: Very well, your throat is okay now?

P: Sometimes it feels irritated.

D: Your ears don't fester?

P: No, but I hear noises and I hear a thunder, and sometimes it hurts.

D: Very well, go up on the cot and let's see your belly. Let's see the many animals you got there. (Examined by students, then by doctor, who looked at his feet.) Flat feet, it's bad. What about your genitals, normal, painful?

P: Yes.

D (Addressing the four students present): It is colitis, because, let's eliminate that there is a pathology, an abscess. (Addressing the patient): Let's see, you don't have a problem with stones? Very well, the heart area is normal.

Student: Do you have headaches?

(Doctor and students converse, and doctor instructs the students to explore the patient's thorax and two do so.)

D (to the students): You have all the data. Very well, what else? His feet are flat and that is his pathology. Nothing else. And a lordosis, discrete, but it is there, nothing else. And yes, there is a small curvature in the spine and that is what is.

P: Since I used to pick up very heavy things.

Student: and for the parasites?

D: Where?

Student: What medicine for the parasites?

D: Yes, my son, so that they [the parasites] go away.

P: And listen, can I do my exercises and lift heavy things, or should I suspend the exercises?

D: No, come in a week.

P: Yes.

The doctor referred Serge to Orthopedics, and wrote in the medical record and on the referral slip the diagnosis of unstable spinal column and flat feet.

D: Go there [Orthopedics] and he will tell you about exercise. You will take this [refers to the medication he prescribed, standard prescription for all patients] exactly as it says. Metrodinazol [antiamebiasis], Farmeban [antiamebiasis], and one analgesic.

D: You will take the third medication if there is pain.

P: You know what? Although I feel pain I don't take them. I don't like it.

D: Take one every twelve hours if there is pain.

(The doctor explained to him how to take the medication, one for three days, after each meal, and then to stop taking the first for ten days and then take the second medication [farmeban]).

Student: 6'3".

P: 6'5", but there are people even taller. (Patient repeated the name of the doctor he was supposed to see in Orthopedics.)

D: Please go and see Doctor So and So in Orthopedics.

P: Now? At this moment?

D: Yes, to see when they can see you.

P: Am I to ask him whether I am allowed to do exercises?

D: Yes he, he is the one that will tell you. And this medicine, take it now, all right?

(The patient was uncertain about hospital procedures, where he needed to go, and where to have the paperwork done. The doctor instructed Serge where to go for the blood and urinalysis that he ordered.)

P: And when do I return here?

D: In two weeks.

P: Okay. Thank you.

Physician 4 explained to me that the patient's principal problem was "an unstable spinal column and flat feet," which he had since childhood, and parasitic colitis. In Serge's context, the etiology of the spinal disorder, according to Physician 4 was muscular dysfunction.

Physician 4 had no confidence in most laboratory analyses, especially those for parasitic infections, because "technicians make mistakes" or because the "parasites do not appear in any one given sample." He observed that Serge's clinical symptoms, including pain in the belly, bowel movements with mucus (not mentioned by Serge), and rectal itching suggested parasitic infection. The medication he prescribed was a composite treatment for "all animals the patient may have in his belly."

The physician passed over Serge's presenting symptoms, his fears, pain in the "lungs," feelings of exhaustion, headaches, and high and low blood pressure, despite his customary, exhaustive history taking. Physician 4 did not respond to typical or other symptoms, inasmuch as his diagnoses were idiosyncratic, independent of patients' clinical symptoms.

Serge returned distraught a week later because he was feeling very sick. He was seen by the physician for seven minutes. He reported that he was in great pain and he had developed rashes on his skin.

The doctor concluded that Serge had an allergy, urticaria, for which he prescribed Flebocortid (antishock treatment), Avapena, and Chloromycetin (anti-inflammatory and antihistamine medications, respectively) to eliminate the itching. Serge was given another appointment, which he did not keep. The results of Serge's glucose analysis were negative (these were the only results in the medical record).

The patient's concern, on this and on the previous visit, that he was feeling depressed and sleepy, was not dealt with. He was being treated mechanically for parasites and the doctor even prescribed a medication that, according to the doctor, would make the patient sleepy.

Serge, unlike most patients, resisted medicalization of his symptoms when he told the physician that he would rather not take medication. As we will learn later, Serge read a lot of the sports journals emphasizing body building and natural diets, and he also recognized that his symptoms were not related to problems of the "belly."

Esperanza

Esperanza, who came to the hospital unaccompanied, was thirty-five years old, with three years of primary school education. She was seen by Physician 2, who attempted to make patients feel cheerful during the medical consultation. One sensed that he felt no distance between himself and his patients, whom he treated with a smile and a sense of deep concern. Nevertheless, he, like the other physicians, conducted the interviews following the model of the active physician and the passive patient. While Physician 2 was sensitive to his patients' life circumstances, we see in the case of Esperanza that he dealt with the patients' symptoms in a biomedical way, despite the fact that he recognized that their disorders were encompassed by socioeconomic causes. In addition to symptom exploration, medical history taking, and extensive physical examinations that included palpation and auscultation, Physician 2 relied on laboratory analysis to make his final diagnosis. He usually wrote as he interrogated patients, and addressed them in the formal "you." The consultation with Esperanza lasted twenty minutes.

Esperanza's case suggests the drama that is played out both in the doctor's struggle with himself and vis-a-vis the patient. Intuitively, he understood her sickness in a Mexican way, that Esperanza's condition embodied her life circumstances. Yet, as a physician he was locked into dealing with the patient in a biomedical manner, by administering medication and by referring her to Neurology, where her condition continued to be managed pharmacologically.

Esperanza (pressure 110/70, 115 pounds, 5'0") reported on the first interview that she came to seek help for terrible pains in her head that made her cry, for her pressure which got low, and for her hands which felt numb in the mornings. She feared that she might be going crazy and wondered who would take care of her children.

Doctor: How can I serve you? What is your problem?
Patient: My problem is that my head hurts a lot.
D: Since when?
P: Well, more than a year.
D: What other thing?
P: My pressure is low, and the ringing in the ears that enters my head.
D: Who told you your pressure was low?
P: The doctor that I saw in the Social Security Service, and he gave me drops.
D: Parisecon?
P: Aha.
D: What else?
P: And then I have a burning sensation in the soles of my feet, my hands get numb, and my feet... When I lay down on one side, it hurts a lot because it gets numb a lot. And my eyes get swollen, and when my head hurts, it seems as if it does like this [she hits her head and ears], and I hear a noise, and that is what is happening. I cannot go out or walk downtown because I am dying of pain. My head, and also I have some pain in my kidneys, and then when my arm goes numb it falls asleep constantly, and the pain in the head.
D: Is that what worries you most?
P: The head, and the tiredness I feel.
D: What medication have you received from doctors you have seen?
P: I will show you the medications. Well, I got this prescription for low blood pressure, and he told me that I had fever in my brain, and also animals [usually refers to parasites], and that I am losing my memory. I also have my clinical history here.

(She took out scraps of paper from her bag and the doctor recorded into the medical history the information on the slips. She had biometric analysis done in the Social Security Service two months earlier that indicated normal results, except that she had suffered from typhoid once, but she did not have it anymore. The papers also showed that she had been prescribed Effortil [antihypotension] to raise her pressure, Dolo-Tiaminal [analgesic and antineuritico], a vitamin, Kantrex [antibiotic], and an analgesic. Another physician had prescribed antibiotics, Beclysyl [?], a vitamin, A.S.Cor [antihypotension] to raise her pressure, and Sydolil [antimigraine], an analgesic. A private physician prescribed Bactrim F [antibiotic for respiratory infection] and Pentrexyl [antibiotic].)

D: Yes, you have it?

P: Yes, my clinical history.

D: And why are you telling me about your clinical history [she had been seen by physicians in Salud Hospital some years back], and where is your hospital ID card?

P: It burned. Well, our house burned down.

D: When did it burn down?

P: About three years ago.

D: Well, no matter. What can we do?

P: I can give you the date because I was interned here. I told them that and they told me to tell you to explain to you.

D: That is why they fill out papers--and they don't know what they are doing.

P: Well, yes, I can tell you what date I was here so you could look.

D: We will make do with this (clinical history). Any diabetics, cancer in the family?

P: Cancer, no.

D: Your father is diabetic?

P: Yes.

D: He is alive?

P: Yes.

D: Is he being treated for it?

P: Yes.

D: Anything else in the family?

P: My mother-in-law, but that has nothing to do.

D: No. Other family problems?

P: Of those that I know, no.

D: What do you eat?

P: A little.

D: Do you feel that you eat what you are supposed to?

P: No.

D: Have you been operated ever?

P: Yes, three times.

D: What?

P: Twice caesarian, and once gall bladder and pancreas.

D: Have you had a transfusion ever?

P: Yes, twice.

D: Allergic to any medication?

P: No.

D: Smoke?

P: No.

D: Drink?

P: No.

D: At what age did you begin menstruating?

P: At fifteen.

D: How often?

P: Every month.

D: How many days?

P: What?

D: How many days do you menstruate?

P: Three days.

D: How many times have you been pregnant?

P: Nine times.

D: Abortions, how many?

P: Four.

D: Three pregnancies?

P: Not including the....

D: Four abortions, two caesarean, and three normal births.

P: Yes.

D: Date of last menstruation?

P: Well, it's been three years that I have had my womb removed.

D: Three years then. Any problems on urination?

P: At night I urinate a lot. During the day not at all, but at night about five times.

D: Problems with bowel movements?

P: No. My stools are very hard.

D: Hard. You don't drink water with your meals?

P: I am not thirsty.

D: One should drink water.

P: Sometimes I forget. I am not thirsty.

D: Food does not get stuck. Go to the cot and lie down and uncover your belly with your head to the wall.

P: Yes.

D: Do you get tired when you run or something?

P: Yes.

(The doctor listened to her lungs with the stethoscope and asked her to breathe in and out.)

D: Let's see. What bothers you most are the headaches?

P: Yes.

D: You have had them for about one year?

P: Sometimes they are very strong. When I have pain in the head I feel that my eye is coming out.

D: You will do this, okay? Based on what you have told us, we will give you a treatment. We will continue and begin now with a medication so that your headaches diminish and stop.

P: Yes.

D: You will take the medication the way I tell you, and this is important, for the next time when you come I can judge if really the medicine had the effect we want.

P: Yes, of course.

D: Take one pill [Tonapan, antimigraine] every eight hours, one pill every eight hours only, when you have headaches. If you get better with one pill don't take any more. Don't take it every eight hours otherwise.

P: If I have no pain I don't take it.

D: If in one week, two weeks, you are without pain, don't take it. During the day take one pill, and if in six or seven hours the pain returns, take it in eight hours. We will also request these analyses. It looks like you still have your typhoid fever problem, and it is probably what is causing your headaches still. We will try to correct this. By means of the laboratory tests, we will see if you are still a carrier, and if you have animals, okay. And this is the treatment we will give you to eradicate the problem while you take the medication. Go to the front office, give them the information they request, and there they will tell you what you need to do.

P: Yes, doctor.

(The doctor gave Esperanza an appointment for two weeks later.)

P: And the tests, when will they tell me [the results]?

D: The results will be sent to me. All you need to do is have them done, and they will send the results to me.

P: Oh, good.

D: Take the pills.

P: There is a pharmacy here, true?

D: Only that it is already closed. Oh, if...

P: I will buy it outside [the hospital].

D: Yes, you can buy it outside. Actually this pharmacy does not have these pills.

P: Is that all? Thank you.

D: Take care.

The doctor ordered a fecal culture and urine and blood profiles; he diagnosed her condition as a parasite problem, "salmonellasis." He believed that Esperanza did not receive the proper treatment for typhoid fever, and therefore her headaches persisted. He also believed that she was a typhoid carrier. He wished to see the test results before prescribing any treatment.

In keeping with his socioeconomic etiological orientation, Physician 2 listed a series of causes that would explain Esperanza's headaches, including family problems, her children not eating, her lack of money, a drunken husband who beat her, her sick mother, sickness in the family, washing and ironing other people's clothing, too much sun, changed work, and changed living arrangements. According to Physician 2, all such difficulties could produce headaches because with such occurrences, messages are sent to the brain, stimulating the nervous system to respond. While Physician 2 was conscious of extrasomatic components of sickness, the script which he followed did not guide him to find out whether any or all of these factors he identified pertained to this patient.

Esperanza returned for the scheduled appointment, which lasted ten minutes. At this time, she reported that she continued to experience the same pains in her head even though she had taken the medication he had prescribed. She reported ringing in her ears, and that her eyes swelled. She further stated, "I feel something disturbing in the body." He again prescribed a medication for salmonella on the grounds that she had typhoid fever. "The medication we gave you first was because we thought that the headaches were produced by worry and stress, but it looks like your salmonella infection continues." He prescribed clorofenicol, and aspirin every eight hours for five days.

According to the doctor, Esperanza was a salmonella carrier; the medication he gave her last time was only for her anxiety. The clorofenicol he prescribed on this visit was to eliminate "the animals" (parasites). The test results he had received from the laboratory showed that her urine and stools were normal, but since there was some indication that she tested positive for salmonella, the physician added, "At least I considered it positive. "He was still waiting for the results of the blood examination.

Esperanza returned for her scheduled appointment two weeks later. The consultation lasted eight minutes.

He reviewed her record. He read, "The first time you came was when you had severe headaches. I prescribed a medicine that is called Tonapan, to take every eight hours." Esperanza reported that she continued to have headaches.

D: It seems that it didn't have much effect. Good, then I received the results of your analysis, and I tried to detect a problem of typhoid fever; it was positive, and I prescribed clorofenicol for ten days, salisilic acid [aspirin] 500 milligrams was the treatment; that's what I prescribed.

P: Yes, doctor.

D: And the headaches?

P: Yes, they stopped.... Well, so to say. I couldn't stay awake from eight in the morning till nine at night, and I couldn't go out to hang my laundry in the sun because I had such pain. Yes, this pain and the dizziness and pain in the eyes.... That is what doesn't let me go out in the sun.

(But as the consultation continued, Esperanza revealed that her headaches persisted, as did pain in "my feet. Consider me as if I were an old woman. I cannot coordinate, I cannot walk on my feet, and this ringing in the ears, think as if gas were coming out. The headaches make me vomit." He referred her to an ophthalmologist and suggested she take aspirin and return in two weeks.)

On her third visit she indicated that she had seen the ophthalmologist and she had no problems with her eyes, but the headaches continued. The aspirin and the original prescription for Tonapan did not alleviate her pain. He therefore referred her to Neurology and ordered that she stay on the Tonapan.

Physician 2 described to me his reasoning by recapitulating the steps that led him to assign the diagnosis. Initially he thought the headaches were due to stress, and the pain would be eliminated with the medication. Then, he interpreted one of the laboratory results as showing a "high count of antibodies," suggesting to him that the headaches were due to the persistence of the typhoid fever. But that did not seem to be the case. He thought they could be associated with an eye problem, but that was discarded. He referred her to Neurology to eliminate any possibility of a neurological problem, although he doubted that she may have had one because he believed her disturbance was due to stress, worry, and emotional difficulties with family and work. Esperanza did not return to see this physician. Two days later she was seen by a Neurologist who prescribed Cafergot tablets antimigraine and Evadyne antidepressant.

While Physician 2 was mindful in a stereotypic way that Esperanza must be having great difficulties, there was no attempt made to address them other than by medication. When she began referring to the possibility that the headaches were related to her problems with her husband, the physician was called away; he left the room and did not pursue the matter further. But it is important to emphasize that the patient did not expect the physician to deal with her life circumstances: She expected medication, which together with sleep, temporarily diminished her pain for a few hours.

Thelma

Physician 1's interview with Thelma, typical of his consultations, exemplifies the inherent drama of a clinical encounter when guided by the biomedical script. The doctor aimed at pinpointing the anatomical location of the patient's distress, which in Thelma, as in most instances, eludes the patient. Thelma's declaration of pain in her "lungs," which she relates to her hard work, was ignored. On the other hand, Thelma is indifferent to the temporal dimension of her sickness, an important datum for the doctor. Is she experiencing the symptoms before or after eating? how long has she had pain in her lungs?

Physician 1, unlike most of the other doctors, did not routinely give a diagnosis of parasites. Whereas theoretically his view of disease was informed by his epidemiological training and Marxist orientation, his diagnoses were strictly biomedical.

Physician 1 is soft-spoken and usually wrote copious notes as patients described their symptoms and as they responded to his queries. He saw Thelma for half an hour, during which time he also gave her a physical examination by auscultation and palpation. He addressed the patient in the formal "you."

Thelma (pressure 140/110, 127 pounds, 5'2") is forty-nine years old, with one year of primary school. She came to the hospital accompanied by her sister-in-law. Thelma's first language was Otomi, a native Indian language. In her slightly accented Spanish, she reported on the first interview that she could not walk because she was having terrible pains in her entire body, and she could not work to support her children. She thought she had a very serious illness.

Doctor: Good afternoon.
Patient: Good afternoon.
P: I have a pain.
D: Pain where?
P: In the stomach, in the back of the head [*cerebro*].
D: Yes, yes. But we are looking at your stomach.
P: The stomach, yes, the stomach.
D: We are interested in the stomach, yes? The abdomen?
P: Yes, well, the pain has calmed down a bit.
D: You are not interested that your stomach has grown a lot?
P: Well, yes, because I feel very bloated.
D: You have always been like this?
P: No.
D: Did it come suddenly or you have had it for long?
P: No, it's been five years but I have not felt that bad.
D: You have had five, six years pains in the stomach? You always had it that big?
P: Yes, there are times that it gets bloated and times when the bloating disappears. I don't know what I have but from here it hurts a lot. (pointing to the diaphragm down to the lower abdomen).
D: Yes, yes. Where does it hurt? In what part does it hurt?
P: It hurts. It hurts from here, all this and ends here (pointing to the same area).
D: How is the pain? It burns, it throbs like a jab, like a throbbing?
P: Yes, from here [pointing to the abdomen], it burns a bit.
D: Thank you.
P: The pain in the back of my head [*cerebro*]?
D: We are speaking about your stomach.
P: And that, stomach... Yes, it hurts.
D: Heartburn?
P: Sometimes.

D: A lot, do you belch a lot?

P: I have heartburn--like I repeat sour, nothing else.

D: Often or sometimes?

P: Sometimes.

D: You repeat a lot.

P: No.

D: Do you feel that you repeat the meal suddenly?

P: No.

D: Do you feel very full in your stomach?

P: Yes, I feel full.

D: Before or after eating?

P: Always.

D: Always what?

P: I always feel full.

D: Before or after eating? Whether you eat or don't eat in any event?

P: Even though I don't eat or eat a lot.

D: Does your gut grumble?

P: Well, very little.

D: No? A lot of gases in your belly?

P: Well, I feel gas but I don't let it go, and I only feel gas as a disturbance.

D: What disturbance? What disturbance?

P: Like a pain, like I have difficulty. The gas gets loose so that...

D: Normally, no?

P: No.

D: You have a problem moving your bowels?

P: What?

D: To make number two?

P: When the pain started I was constipated.

D: Now you are no longer constipated?

P: Very little.

D: What is very little? How often do you move your bowels?

P: Well, during the day, twice a day.

D: Are your stools with mucus, or with some blood, or that you need to make an effort?

P: Well, yes. I have had to force myself to move my bowels, but it's common.

D: When you finish moving your bowels you don't feel a desire to continue to be in the bathroom?

P: Yes.

D: You don't have problems on urination?

P: Yes. When I urinate, the urine gets ahead of me.

D: When you force yourself, the urine comes as well?

P: No.

D: When you laugh?

P (not understanding the question): What, do I laugh?

D: The urine does not come out even though you have no desire to go.

P: No.

D: Only when you walk, and if you don't go right away then the urine gets ahead of you?

P: Yes.

D: Burning on urination?

P: Whether I have burning sensation when I urinate? A little.

D: Since when?

P: Since it began, about fifteen days ago.

D: You urinate well, normally, or does it come every minute in spurts?

P: No, I am okay.

D: Tiredness.

P: Well, yes, when I walk, when I walk a lot, or when I wash a lot or when I do my chores.

D: Desire not to do anything?

P: Eh?

D: Desire not to do anything?

P: No... Yes, when I feel tired I lay down for ten minutes, five minutes, and I get up and I continue to work.

D: How is your appetite?

P: I, well, I have great desire to eat.

D: And, yes, you eat?

P: Yes, I eat whatever doesn't harm me, nothing, nor do I have pain in my stomach, I eat everything, but I have a desire to eat.

D: You have a desire to eat?

P: Yes, yes. Even though I am not hungry, I have desire to eat.

D: How many times do you urinate a day?

P: Bowel movement? Eat?

D: Urinate?

P: Urinate? Two, three times a day.

D: What other disturbance do you have, ringing in the ears?

P: No.

D: No? Dizzy?

P: Nothing.

D: Pain in the head?

P: The head yes, the *cerebro*.

D: The pain in the head is daily? Or only sometimes for a little while?

P: Well, all day and I feel a pain [diminutive] pain, but it goes away.

D: What other disturbance do you have?

P: My lungs, [back], they hurt and they burn a little.

D: Since when do they burn and since when have you had the pain in the lungs?

P: Since... It's been a while. The pain disappears.

D: How long? How long?

P: It will be, I don't know, something like six years.

D: It disappears by itself?

P: Yes, I rest and I lie down a bit and it goes away and I go back to work.

D: When do you feel that your back hurts most?

P: Well, only when, when I start working. When I wash I have pain in my lungs, in the back.

D: Any other thing?

P: The waist [*cintura*], I have a pain when I bend down. When I don't bend down fast it hurts a little, but when I bend down, the waist.

D: How does the *cintura* hurt?

P: Like it doesn't allow me to bend down fast nor does, nor does it allow me to turn around. I feel the back, the *cintura* as if it slipped.

D: It locks?

P: A little.

D: It burns? It throbs?

P: No, it does not burn. Only the pain.

D: Yes, yes, but it burns, it throbs like a jab, like a punch?

P: No, only the pain, the pain. And this foot, doctor, the joint, it hurts also, and inside the bone it hurts me also.

D: Very well.

P: And this arm, it hurts a little.

D: Since when?

P: Since when? About six months.

D: Anything else?

P: Like I have desire to give up, the stomach, and I don't go, well, no I don't vomit.

D: And that, why?

P: My mouth is dry as if there were a lot of heat in the stomach.

D: But you say that your stomach is well?

P: Yes, but I don't know why.

D: Since when have you had this disturbance?

P: A month.

D: A month?

P: Yes.

D: Nausea?

P: Yes, but sometimes.

D: Any member in the family have diabetes?

P: No.

D: Heart problems?

P: An uncle.

D: Tuberculosis, cancer, epileptic attacks?

P: Well, my father. The doctors said he was tubercular. He had a cough, but the truth is we didn't know what it was.

D: And he died from that?

P: Yes, because of the cough. He gave up phlegm but...

D: With blood?

P: No, pure phlegm, like nopal spittle [white secretion from the nopal plant].

D: At what age did you start menstruating?

P: I don't remember. It would be, I was about fourteen or fifteen.

D: Do you continue to menstruate?

P: No, since the second of November [three months earlier] no more, the menstruation has not come. Before that I was late two or three months. Now, no more.

D: No more.

P: It's been four months and it has not come.

D: At what age did you get married?

P: At nineteen.

D: How many times were you pregnant?

P: How many times? I was pregnant four times.

D: All in all?

P: Yes.

D: Your births were normal?

P: Yes.

D: All four?

P: All four.

D: Abortions?

P: Not one.

D: You didn't use contraceptive, true?

P: No. But sometimes, yes. After the last one, the fourth child. I was operated. I was tied.

D: When was that?

P: The tying? The boy is eight years old. He will be nine the sixteenth.

D: Smoke?

P: No, never, I don't like it.

D: Drink?

P: Nothing like that.

D: Nor *pulque*? (This is a local drink from her native region that comes from the maguey plant.)[2]

P: Before, when I was a little baby.

D: Were you ever operated?

P: No, never.

D: Have you had a blood transfusion?

P: Did I have a blood transfusion? No.

D: Did you ever break a bone on any occasion?

P: No.

D: Have you ever hit your head and lost consciousness?

P: Nothing like that.

D: Allergic to any medicine?

P: No.

D: Has any medicine caused you rashes?

P: No.

D: Any important sickness that you have suffered? The doctor mentioned typhoid, bronchitis, malaria, pneumonia, mumps, scarlet fever, and chicken pox. Nothing to date?

P: No. I haven't been sick till now.

D: Have you had measles?

P: Eh?

D: Have you had measles?

P: Well, yes, my mother told me that I had measles.

D: Whooping cough?

P: Whooping cough? When I don't have a cough?

D: Pain in the eyes [eye sockets]?

P: Well, very lightly.

D: Lightly, how lightly?

P: Very little.

D: And what does it consist of?

P: Well, well, sometimes because of the cold or because of the heat.

D: Where are you from?

P: I am from Hidalgo state.

D: You came from there?

P: No, I live here in Neza.

D: You want to go over there [he instructs her to lie down on the cot] and we will examine you.

P: Yes.

(The doctor examined the patient explored her abdomen, and asked her about her about the nature of her pain there.)

D: How does it hurt? It throbs, or like colics?

P: Throbs, yes, I don't know how it would be. I would like to know if it is because I am fat, or is it gas? Or it is bloated, doctor.

D: What?

P: I get very hungry.

D: What?

P: I get very hungry although I don't have a desire to eat.

D: You eat so much?

P: What do I do to lose?

D: You are very fat. I don't know if it is flesh or fat, I say it is fat.

P: It's flesh.

D: What do you eat? You are ten pounds overweight.

P: Oh, God.

D: You probably eat a lot of tortillas. Yes, true?

P: Yes, doctor, that is what I eat most. Tortillas.

D: How many tortillas?

P: Before, I ate about one and a half pounds and now not anymore, only three tortillas and hard ones, toasted bread, and vegetables.

D: Every day your stomach gets bloated?

P: Yes, daily yes, because I walk standing.

D: You want to walk sitting? (He laughs.)

P: Walk.

D: On foot you walk, well?

P: Yes, doctor.

D: Don't eat so many tortillas.

P: No, doctor, no more.

D: Because it will harm you.

P: Now that I feel sick in my stomach, not anymore. Three tortillas, toasted and bread.

(The doctor inquired about the patient's eating habits. In response, Thelma indicated that she ate eggs, white bread, beef or chicken soup, and vegetables daily, and that she consumed beefsteak twice or three times a week. Incredulously, he asked her if she did not eat beans. She said no.)

D: Like what vegetables do you eat?

P: Lettuce, squash, stringbeans, peas, mangos, spinach, carrots, potatoes, all this and...

D: Every day?

P: Every day.

D: You don't get bored?

P: No, because I cook them in different ways. I don't get bored. Similarly, fruit, not every week, but twice, sometimes three times a week.

D: The vegetables?

P: The fruit.

D: The fruit? What work does your husband do?

P: He helps, in the work.

D: In the work? What work?

P: Well, he works in a laboratory, as a helper.

D: And how much does he earn? You don't know?

P: Minimum wage, he says.

D: And how many are there in the family?

P: There is me, my husband, and four children. We are six.

D: And with this you eat twice or three times meat a week?

P: Well, yes, because then I was not sick [and] I went to work so that we would have enough. I used to work.

D: Do you drink milk?

P: Well, yes.

D: Yes? How many times a week?

P: Well, almost all week. Only in the morning. In the evening no more.

D: Why?

P: I buy it there, never in the stores, never, because it is very expensive, and I buy in the government store sometimes.

D: Sometimes?

P: Yes.

D: You have not felt on occasion that your heart jumps suddenly?

P: No.

D: As if you are short of breath?

P: No, doctor.

(The doctor ordered the standard laboratory tests.)

D: You will have these analyses done, daughter, please.

P: Yes, doctor.

D: You will have them done and I will see you on the next visit.

P: Yes, doctor.

D: If possible, have the analyses done tomorrow morning.

P: Yes. More or less at what time?

D: Well, at seven in the morning. Be here 7:30 so you can leave early.

P: Well, let's see if I can get here at that time because I live in Neza.

D: You have to come to have them done. There is no other way.

P: Yes.

D: Because it would be more expensive outside [privately].

P: Yes.

D: Do all that. It is possible to come early. We are up and around from five in the morning.

P: I came [today] five in the morning.

D: Why this early?

P: I came on a bus and then in the metro.

D: Good. You came by yourself?

P: I came with my sister-in-law. I spoke with my brother [and asked] if she could come with me because I didn't have anyone to accompany me.

D: Do you know how to read?

P: A little, doctor.

D: Good. Have the tests done, please. I will prescribe some pills so that your stomach does not get bloated.

P: Yes, doctor.

D: After every meal.

P: After every meal.

D: When we have the results we will prescribe what is necessary.

P: Yes, doctor. Thank you very much.

D: You will do your tests.

P: Is that all?

D: Yes, for the moment. Yes.

P: At what time do I need to be here?

D: You need to be here at seven in the morning.

P: At seven, to be here at that time.

D: Please.

P: Yes, thank you. What can I eat?

D: Now, whatever you can. When we see the results, then we will see. You need to lose weight. Please avoid soda pop.

P: Soda pop. No coffee?

D: Nothing more.

P: Coffee with milk?

D: Preferably. If you cannot drink milk, at least coffee with milk. Then I will give you another diet.

P: Yes, doctor, if you will do me the favor.

D: Well, since you like vegetables...

P: I love them more than meat.

D: Good.

P: Because frankly I am poor and I don't have, I don't have enough. I do everything possible. I help my husband. I work so that we can get ahead. My sons, I have four, and four are studying and I have to help them, with God's help. I am in yours and God's hands.

D: You will get better. You will have to listen to us, what we will tell you.

P: Yes, thank you very much. With your permission, doctor, we will see you next time.

D: Don't eat tortillas.

P: Yes, thank you very much, doctor. Very kind.

P: If I come tomorrow do I come to see you?

D: You will come to see me as indicated in your ID card. (He recorded the next appointment in the ID but did not tell her the date.) There is the next appointment when you come to see me.

P: Now, I am going to my house.

(He instructed her on where to go to have the paperwork done, and he gave her an appointment for two week later. He prescribed Onoton to assist the digestion.)

While he did not tell the patient anything about her condition, he explained to me that her arterial pressure was a little high, and she was a bit overweight from eating too many tortillas. Based upon her presenting symptoms, she had parasites and urinary problems. He prescribed urine and stool analyses, and Xray of the spine. He decided to wait until the results were in to give her antiparasitic treatment. He noted that it was likely that she had a spinal column disorder because her waist (*cintura*) hurt. He did not believe that she ate meat at all, as she said she did, given how little her husband earned.

Thelma kept her return appointment and she was seen by the doctor for twenty minutes. At this time she reported, "I have a little pain in the *cerebro*, in my head and in my vision." She had a burning sensation on urination. He concluded that she had a urinary tract infection and a problem with her spinal column.

This time the physician told me that her major problem was a "deviated spinal column, which also caused the headaches." She suffered from a urinary problem and her arterial pressure was normal, but she needed to lose weight in order to alleviate the problem with the spine. The doctor prescribed Nalidixico Briter (anti-urinary infections) for the urinary infection, which he treated on the basis of her symptoms, as he did other patients with similar symptoms. The Xray confirmed for him his original diagnosis of a problem with the spinal column.

To reiterate a point made earlier, for Physician 1 as for Physician 2, the medical diagnosis presented a particular struggle because both adhered to an ecological and socioeconomic explanation of sickness that conflicted with the traditional biomedical organic model of disease.

Poverty and ecology alone do not explain the patients' conditions or their perceived failure of recovery, as we will see in Chapter 11. Indeed, Thelma's pain in the "lung" tells us that she has worked arduously, but from the medical interview we cannot deduce that Thelma's sickness is not only related to her bodily condition and to her poverty, but also to the fact that she suffered from having been abandoned by her husband and from her problematic relationship with her sons. As we move our focus from the medical consultation and biomedical practice to the patients and their lives, we shall discover more specific phenomenological factors that combine with conditions on a macrolevel to explain these patients' sickness, as well as recovery, which will be discussed in Chapter 11.

Notes

1. Anderson and Helm 1979; Gill 1976; Hahn and Kleinman 1983; Haynes 1976; Pratt 1976.
2. See Finkler 1974.

PART THREE

Patients' Responses to Biomedical Practice

9

Patients and Their Complaints

We now turn to the patients, their complaints, their response to treatment, and the way they perceive their lives to deepen our understanding of sickness and biomedicine's role in the healing process.

Sociodemographic Profile

The sample population interviewed in Salud Hospital consisted of 205 women and 62 men between the ages of eighteen and sixty-five.

Table 9.1 summarizes selected sociodemographic characteristics of the hospital sample group.

The majority of the people in the sample were migrants to the capital. Only 48 percent of the men and 43 percent of the women were born in the Federal District, and 31.2 percent of the men and 17.1 percent of the women had lived in the Federal District for less than three years.

Most of the people were married, the majority in both a civil and religious ceremonies conforming to the most desired pattern of marriage for women in Mexico and according them legal protection and social approbation. Patients resided in households of four to seven people, with a mean household size of six. Of those that were married, about equal numbers of men and women (48 and 46 percent, respectively) have had four or fewer children, with the remainder having more than four.

The people in this study are usually referred to in Mexico as the "popular class." They stand at the base of the socioeconomic pyramid of Mexican society. The overwhelming majority lack permanent jobs, and only 12.6 percent of the men and 12.2 percent of the women had access to IMSS or ISSSTE, the national government health plans that cover the permanently employed and their dependents.

Table 9.1: Selected Characteristics of Sample Group by Sex

	Males	Females
Average age	30.0	33.5
Education (%)		
Primary	93.4	85.1
Secondary	48.3	33.6
College Preparatory	33.8	13.6
University[a]	19.3	5.3
Marital Status (%)		
Married	59.7	55.6
Single	37.1	28.8
Widowed	–	7.8
Separated	3.2	6.8
Divorced	–	1.0
	100.0	100.0
Employment Status (%)		
Unemployed two months prior to hospital interview	34.0	
Domestic and petty commerce[b]	22.0	32.0
Employed by others	24.0	
Students	17.0	11.0
Worked at odd jobs	3.0	
Housewives	57.0	
	100.0	100.0

[a] At least one year university, with one subject a university graduate.
[b] Street or market vendors; in the case of women also includes maids.

The people vary in access to economic resources and potential. Admittedly, various people were coy about disclosing their income, and some were unwilling, but most lacked fixed wages, so they were simply unable to list their financial resources. In the absence of a fixed and dependable income, poor people depend on a variety of sources that may include day work, petty commerce, having a child washing cars, and other such windfalls. In order to differentiate the population along economic lines, I ranked each household on a 1-5 point scale, with 1 representing the most and 5 the least affluent. This ranking was based on characteristics of the dwelling that I assessed during home visits.[1] Examples of people who comprise category 1 are a woman whose husband was a pharmacy proprietor, a vegetable merchant, a few women whose husbands were employed by multinational companies such as Ford Motors, and a woman who worked for her brother in his employment agency and had substantial economic resources. By and large those who make up category 5 were people displaced by the earthquake and women with alcoholic husbands. With two exceptions, all the participants in the study resided in the poorer neighborhoods of the city. Table 9.2 displays the economic assets of the group using the aforementioned criteria.

Table 9.2: Economic Status as Measured by Dwelling and Material Possessions (N=205)

Rank	N	%
1	12	5.9
2	30	14.6
3	62	30.2
4	67	32.7
5	14	6.8
Other[a]	20	9.8
	205	100.0

[a] Includes individuals who work as live-in maids who in effect lack any possessions, and who usually earn minimum or less than a minimum wage; individuals who were interviewed outside their dwellings and in one case a persons residing in an all-male hotel; and a few for which data were not recorded.

The rankings disclosed in Table 9.2 cut across renters and proprietors of the land on which their house stands, with the proportions of each divided equally.

In sum, the majority of the sample consists of women in their mid-thirties who were married in civil and religious ceremonies; they had at least a primary school education, about five children, and an impermanent source of income.

Health Characteristics and Patient Complaints

According to official statistics, the ten most common causes of morbidity in the Valley of Mexico include respiratory infections, followed by intestinal infections, helminthiasis, hypertension, diabetes mellitus, back problems and urinary infections, conjunctivitis, menstrual dysfunction, and gastritis and duodentitis.[2]

Patients whose presenting complaints included abdominal pain, chest pains, back pains, headaches, and general feelings of discomfort were channeled through the preconsultation procedures to Internal Medicine. The majority of patients were seen at least twice by the attending physician and a diagnosis was made on each visit. If we use the diagnoses provided by the attending physician for each patient at each visit, the most commonly diagnosed conditions for the 205 persons in the sample were infections and parasites (35.5 percent); specific etiology (30.6 percent); metabolic anomalies (10.7 percent); degenerative conditions (14.2 percent); psychological problems (6.5 percent); pregnancy (0.3 percent); the remainder were not diagnosed or were pronounced healthy.[3]

Table 9.3 displays the aforementioned categories in greater detail, showing the subgroups of the broader diagnosed entities.

Table 9.3: Medical Diagnoses for the Study Group (N=633)

Diagnosis	Number of Diagnoses	Percent
Infections and parasites	225	35.5
Digestive	113	17.9
Genitourinary	81	12.8
Respiratory	19	3.0
Other	11	1.8
Metabolic and/or systemic disorders	68	10.7
Diabetes Mellitus	7	1.1
Arterial Hypertension	20	3.2
Obesity	16	2.5
Anemia	25	3.9
Specific etiology	194	30.6
Degenerative traumatic/sequela	89	14.2
Psychological	41	6.5
Pregnancy	2	0.3
Healthy	3	0.5
No diagnosis	11	1.7
	633[a]	100.0

[a] Most people were given diagnoses in more than one category.

The degenerative category includes primarily scoliosis. "Specific etiology" represents single diagnoses and refers to a variety of conditions for which no one specific etiology could be given using biomedical criteria.

Conforming to the general morbidity trends, a large proportion of the diagnoses revolved around infections and parasites. Specific etiology, the second highest diagnostic grouping, corresponds to the overall morbidity trends of the population and includes conditions such as colitis for which the diagnosing physicians had not supplied a specific etiology, or fallen womb. The remaining diagnostic entities diverge from the overall pattern for the area; the degenerative grouping may represent individual physicians' diagnostic predilections.

The diagnostic entities shown in Table 9.3 represent objectifications of patients' bodily complaints. Generally speaking, patients report a litany of symptoms describing their bodily discomforts: "My feet get swollen," "I feel sourness," "I have pain when I finish urinating," "I feel constipated," "I sweat at night," "I wish to cry," "I have burning sensation in my skin." As we have seen in the previous chapter, they present the typical symptoms of pain in the abdominal region, such as pain in the ovaries, in the "mouth of the stomach," in the lungs (meaning upper back), or kidneys (referring to lower back or *cintura*), high and low blood pressure, chest pains, and more general bodily states.

Patients have their priorities in the symptoms they report to physicians. For most, headaches were more urgent than diarrhea. Based upon my observations, physicians by and large encourage patients to present symptoms by prodding them with "And what else?" A few patients were reluctant to report some disturbances such as urinary dysfunctions. However, many women openly discussed sexual problems, as, for example, Nomi. Occasionally, a patient would not divulge to physicians that she had had an abortion even when directly questioned. For example, a thirty-five-year-old woman reported she had problems with her ovaries, that she was menopausal and barren, and that she could not get pregnant. She never disclosed to the female physician, as she had done to me, that she had induced an abortion of a pregnancy resulting from an extramarital affair.

Diagnostic categories such as genitourinary dysfunction represent disease entities which patients do not present but which emerge during the physician's interrogation about vaginal discharges, for example. Women reported vaginal discharges infrequently, or as an afterthought, as they often took such signs for granted unless they were distressed by their offending odor. Not all physicians gave such discharges equal importance. One patient asked if it was not natural to have vaginal excretions. Even recurrent diarrheas were not spontaneously mentioned unless they were accompanied by severe abdominal cramps, which were the impetus to seek medical attention.

Despite the discomforts patients were experiencing, 53.1 percent of the women and 41.8 percent of the men chose to seek treatment on the particular day they did because "they had time"; only 22.6 percent of the men and 27.5 percent of the women came because "they were feeling sick or feeling worse than usual." The rest of the group, like Jose, came at that time because they accompanied someone else who had an appointment at Salud Hospital. This suggests that for many people, seeking treatment is independent of experiencing pain or discomforts. In fact, patients in the study group reported they had experienced their symptoms for an average of 2.2 years. Only 25.8 percent of the men and 14.1 percent of the women reported that they had been recently incapacitated by their illness to a degree that it impeded their daily functioning. In this study, as in my previous investigation (Finkler 1985), I found that day-to-day functioning was a poor measure of sickness in Mexico since people claim, and I observed, that they continue to carry on their daily chores irrespective of their professed state of ill health. Usually, only when people had a fever did they cease to carry out their daily obligations.

For the majority, pain was seen as the dominant problem of the sickness they were experiencing. Only 8 percent of the women and 14 percent of the men indicated that they became depressed and dejected by their illness; and 9.7

percent of the men and 12 percent of the women noted that they became nervous as a result of their impairments.

Many patients sought therapy at Salud Hospital as a last resort after they had sought help from private physicians or neighborhood health centers. If these modalities fail, then they may seek alternative treatments. To cite an extreme example, thirty-six year old Margaret kept a record of her health seeking trajectory so she could tell a doctor that she had already taken the medication he was prescribing even if "the doctor would not believe me, and with my record I could show him." She had seen ten physicians, including a veterinary doctor. She had had twenty electrocardiograms done within the past ten years. The treatment she received in Salud Hospital failed to alleviate her ongoing discomforts of sweating in her hands, breathing difficulties, numbness in her fingers, and jabbing in her heart and chest. (These were resolved a year later when she took karate lessons and also went to a Spiritualist healer.)

Generally speaking, patients seeking treatment at the hospital expected to receive technological management of their condition, including Xrays and laboratory analysis, but 35 percent of the men and 25 percent of the women had no specific expectations. Significantly, when patients were questioned on follow-up home interviews regarding what their treatment expectations were, their responses reflected reevaluations of their expectations. Table 9.4 displays patients' expectations before the medical consultation, and later at the home follow-up visit.

A comparison of patients' expectations in Table 9.4 reveals that a smaller percentage of people indicated they did not know what to expect after the doctor's visit. In fact, new expectations were voiced after the consultation, such as physical exploration and anticipation of a diagnosis. The fact that patients voiced their expectation of a diagnosis upon follow-up is especially noteworthy because whether a person was given a diagnosis or not significantly influenced his or her perceived response to treatment, regardless of whether the expectation was expressed. These data suggest too that expectations become fine-tuned, probably formulated in the medical consultation and redefined by its outcome. Similarly, the response "Don't know what to expect" decreased, while expectations for technological management and medications increased, expectations that are possibly promoted by biomedical practice itself.

In the next chapter we get an aggregate view of the people's responses to treatment that elucidate components of biomedical practice in Mexico influencing the healing process.

Table 9.4: Patients' Expectations of Treatment Before and After
Medical Consultation (in percent)

	Diagnostic and Treatment Expectation Before Medical Consultation (N=267)[a]	Diagnostic and Treatment Expectation After Medical Consultation (N=205)
Laboratory analysis	22.7	21.9
Xrays and ultrasounds	12.5	22.5
Medication	17.9	21.5
Operations	4.0	—
More than one of these (e.g lab analysis and Xrays, medication)	5.2	
To be given a diagnosis	—	12.7
Physical examination	—	11.2
Didn't know what to expect	30.4	10.2
Other (e.g., referral to specialist)	5.5	—
Missing data	1.8	—
	100.0	100.0

[a]Includes entire sample interviewed at the hospital.

Notes

1. 1=House includes concrete roof, indoor shower and bath, telephone, refrigerator, TV, stereo, videocasette players, and furnishings other than beds and table; 2=House with cement floor and roof, indoor bath, refrigerator, TV, videocassette player, and furnishings other than beds and table; 3=House with cement floor, and roof, indoor toilet, TV, and minimal furnishings; 4= House with cement floor tin or asbestos roofing, outdoor toilet, TV, and minimal furniture; 5= House without floor, with tin or asbestos roofing, barracks, and no furniture other than a bed and a table.

2. These data are based on 1985 statistical compilations by the Social Security Institute. There were no comparable figures available for patients of the Salud Hospital owing to the earthquake, when many of its statistical materials were destroyed and there were no reliable records available. Morbidity in Neza, from where a sizeable proportion of the study group

originated, largely conforms to the pattern encountered in the Valley of Mexico, according to the Neza district records. Their records also show that 19.34 out of every 1,000 inhabitants suffer from liver cirrhosis. Generally speaking, rates of alcoholism are high in the entire nation. According to some reports, 28 percent of the patients in one institution were diagnosed alcoholics (Hernandez 1988; Sesin 1987). However, in the study population there were no diagnosed alcoholics, although Physician 6 usually assumed that all her male patients were alcoholics. For a historical perspective on drinking patterns in Mexico see Taylor 1979.

3. The classification was done by Dr. Luis Martin Armendariz, School of Medicine at the National University of Mexico, based upon the individual diagnoses for each patient provided me by the attending physicians.

10

Patient-Perceived Therapeutic Outcomes: An Aggregate Analysis

This chapter examines patients' perceived responses to biomedical treatment. Analysis of patients' perceptions of their recovery illuminates various dimensions of human existence that impact on recovery requisites, including patients' reactions to biomedicine as practiced in Mexico. Not uncommonly, recovery responses are reduced to one set of variables. For example, prescribed medications, patient compliance with treatment, or patient satisfaction have been associated with the doctor-patient relationship and, by implication, with influencing outcome. I propose that patients' perceptions of recovery from similarly diagnosed *non-life-threatening subacute, sickness episodes* can only be understood when three levels of analysis are considered in tandem: objective conditions of the person's life, the medical consultation concomitant with the prescribed treatment, and the *subjective* elements of a person's being, their life's lesions. This proposition is developed in this and the following chapter.

Response to Treatment

To assess patients' responses to the treatment they received in Salud Hospital, I interviewed each one at home. This entailed visits with 205 (44 men and 161 women) of the original sample of 267 people whom I interviewed before they were seen by the physicians at Salud Hospital, or 76.7 percent of the entire sample.[1] Each patient was visited at home within thirty to fifty days of his or her last appointment with the doctor.[2] Fifty percent of the sample population was visited again between six and twelve months after the first home visit, and ten patients who resided in Neza were followed on a regular monthly basis, including those we have met in the previous chapters.

The data analyzed in this chapter were gathered during the first home visit, which usually lasted between three and eight hours, during which patients were engaged in open-ended discussion. They were interviewed using a fifty-two item interview schedule pertaining to their current health state, perception of the treatment they had received at the hospital, and sickness-management strategies since their last visit to the hospital. Included among the questions asked each patient at this time was: *"Do you consider your problem fully, partially, or not at all alleviated?"* On the basis of this question patients were placed in one of three categories: "Full Recovery," "Partial Recovery," or "None."

The "Full Recovery" category includes those individuals who stated that *all* the symptoms for which they had sought treatment at the hospital had been eliminated and their problem completely alleviated. The "Partial Recovery" category consists of individuals who said that *some* but not all of the symptoms for which they had sought treatment had been alleviated, and while they may have felt somewhat better, they regarded themselves as still being ill. Those in the "None" category reported that *none* of their symptoms had been alleviated and they continued to be sick. Only a small proportion of the sample (17.1 percent) reported full recovery. The majority (57.5 percent) reported partial recovery or some symptomatic relief. Over a fourth of the sample (25.4 percent) reported no recovery at all.

As we see in Table 10.1, this pattern holds for both men and women. As can be seen, there is no statistically significant difference in perception of recovery by sex.

Table 10.1: Patients' Perceived Recovery Along Sex Lines (in percent)

		Full	Partial	None	Total
Males	(N=44)	11.4	61.3	27.3	100.0
Females	(N=161)	19.3	56.5	24.8	100.0
Total	(N=205)	17.1	57.5	25.4	100.0

$X^2 = 1.452$ $df = 2$ $p = .10$

Emphasis was given to symptom alleviation for two compelling reasons. First, symptomatological expressions stimulated patients to seek treatment in Salud Hospital. As I suggested earlier, in the final analysis physicians must rely on patients' subjective reports of symptomatic relief (Spiro 1986). Second, presenting symptoms express through the body other facets of human existence. I propose that changes in symptomatic expression are associated with changes in aspects of a person's life which embody the sickness. I will return to the latter point in the next chapter.

Patients were also asked whether they were feeling *better*, the *same*, or *worse* since their visit to the hospital (Feinstein 1967) to assess whether there was a correspondence between how a person was currently feeling and alleviation of the sickness for which they had sought help at the hospital. A Pearson correlation between these two variables--degree of alleviation with whether patients were feeling "better," "same," or "worse"--was done and the result shows a high positive correlation (r=.60), significant at p=.0001 level, between those who reported alleviation and those who were also feeling better. This strong relationship between the way in which patients rated well-being at the time of the interview and their perception of recovery can further be seen in the data displayed in Table 10.2.

However, even among those who reported "feeling better", the vast majority still reported only partial recovery. The eleven people in the "None" group who indicated they were feeling better are especially interesting because while they attested to feeling better, they had not considered their problem at all alleviated, and they continued to experience the symptoms for which they had sought treatment.

Table 10.2: Patients' Perceived Recovery by Condition at Time of First Follow-up Interview (in percent)

		Full	Partial	None	Total
Better	(N = 150)	22.0	70.7	7.3	100.0
Same	(N = 47)	4.3	21.3	74.4	100.0
Worse	(N = 8)	----	25.0	75.0	100.0
Total	(N = 205)	17.1	57.5	25.4	100.0

X^2 = 96.417   df= 4   p=.001

One explanation for level of recovery might well be the nature of the sickness giving rise to the symptoms that led patients to seek treatment. Those with more serious conditions would not be expected to experience alleviation.

Patients' Diagnosed Conditions and Characteristics
as Related to Recovery

As discussed in Chapters 7 and 9, diagnoses were classified into eight broad categories. A comparative analysis was carried out on six categories, two of which, Infections/Parasites and Metabolic/Systemic, were further broken down into subcategories as displayed in Table 10.3. Since each individual might have received more than one diagnosis, perception of recovery for each category was examined in comparison with the entire sample's perception of recovery. It must be emphasized that none of the conditions in any of the categories was diagnosed by the physicians as grave. As is shown in Table 10.3, there is no statistically significant relationship between diagnosis and patients' perceptions of recovery. Importantly, when the physician diagnosed the patient as healthy or did not make a diagnosis, patients were significantly more likely to report that they had experienced no recovery. Not one patient in this category reported full recovery.

Table 10.3: Patients' Perceived Recovery by Diagnosis Category (in percent)

Diagnoses[a]	Full	Partial	None	Total	N	x^2	df	P
Infections/ Parasites	13.3	61.4	25.3	100.0	225	3.383	2	>.10
Digestive	17.7	58.4	23.9	100.0	113			
Genitourinary	11.1	64.2	24.7	100.0	81			
Respiratory	—	57.9	42.1	100.0	19			
Other	8.3	75.0	16.7	100.0	12			
Metabolic/ Systemic	22.1	55.8	22.1	100.0	68	1.273	2	>.10
Diabetes Mellitus	28.6	42.8	28.6	100.0	7			
Arterial Hypertension	10.0	75.0	15.0	100.0	20			
Obesity	31.3	56.2	12.5	100.0	16			
Anemia	24.0	44.0	32.0	100.0	25			
Degenerative/ Traumatic Sequela	13.5	62.9	23.6	100.0	89	2.152	2	>.10
Psychological	24.4	58.5	17.1	100.0	41	3.009	2	>.10
Pregnancy	50	50	—	100.0	2			
Healthy and/or no diagnosis	—	57.1	42.9	100.0	14	6.471	2	<.05

[a] Patients could and did have more than one diagnosis.

Table 10.4: Patients' Perceived Recovery by Number of
Diagnoses (in percent)

	Full	Partial	None	Total
0 (N=12)	——	50.0	50.0	100.0
1 (N=40)	30.0	50.0	20.0	100.0
2 (N=50)	22.0	54.0	24.0	100.0
3 (N=31)	9.7	54.8	35.5	100.0
4 (N=38)	10.5	63.2	26.3	100.0
5 or more (N=34)	14.7	67.7	17.6	100.0
(N=205)	17.1	57.5	25.4	100.0

x^2 = 16.940   df = 10   p = .10

The data in Table 10.4 show no statistically significant relationship between the number of diagnoses and patients' perception of recovery, though there is a tendency, except among those who were given no diagnosis, that the fewer the symptoms, the more likely the patient was to report full recovery. Certainly a large number of symptoms may make it more likely that the patient would continue to experience the disorder. For those with several diagnoses, it may be either that the patients' presenting symptoms were less well understood by the physician or that the patients' disease states were less discrete. Concomitantly, it may also suggest that the more diagnoses per patient, the more difficult it was for the physician to target an appropriate treatment, or that multiple diagnoses may have an adverse effect and influence patients' perception of recovery. It could also be argued that irrespective of the physicians' diagnoses, the patients reporting "Partial" or "None" were indeed experiencing diseases of greater gravity than those with "Full" recovery as measured by the results of routine laboratory analysis (blood profiles, urinalysis, stool cultures). While the majority of patients were ordered routine analysis (53.7 percent), the findings suggest that among those who had been ordered laboratory tests, there were no differences in perceived recovery and positive or negative results of laboratory tests, as is shown in Table 10.5.

Considering the lack of difference in the results of the analysis coupled with the similarities in the diagnostic categories for patients in each of the three groups, we can conclude that from a biomedical perspective, at least, patients in the three categories were not in a much different health state as measured by medical diagnostic techniques. It may, however, also be argued that the lack of variability in the conditions of the patients using these biomedical criteria is attributable to the idiosyncratic nature of clinical judgment rather than to the patients' condition based upon biomedical measurements.

Table 10.5: Patients' Perceived Recovery by Results of Laboratory
Analyses (in percent)

	Full	Partial	None	Total
Positive (N=68)	16.2	55.9	27.9	100.0
Negative (N=42)	16.7	61.9	21.4	100.0
Total (N=110)	16.4	58.2	25.4	100.0

$X^2 = .598$ df= 2   p=.10

In addition to the attending physicians' diagnoses, I used the Cornell Medical Index (CMI) to establish a standardized baseline measure of variability of self-perceived symptomatology among patients in the study. The CMI is an extensive questionnaire that focuses on all systems of the body and is available in Spanish.[3] The CMI was administered to patients at the initial interview and repeated on the first follow-up home visit to compare patients responses using this instrument before and after treatment.

While at the initial interviews, the "Full" group's average score was 38.4 percent "yes" responses, the "Partial" group's was 50.7 percent and the "None" group's was 56.8 percent. These differences were not statistically significant using the chi square test. On follow-up home interviews all people had lower CMI scores, but again there were no statistical differences among the second scores either.[4]

If we accept the lack of disease variability in the sample population using biomedical and standardized measures of self-perceived symptomatologies, how then do we explain differential patient-perceived recovery? To address this question we must look beyond biomedical diagnoses and presumably organic dysfunctions to explain the variation in patients' perceived responses to treatment. Only by exploring aspects of the medical consultation, including treatment, sickness management, sociodemographic variables, and phenomenological and existential factors within a cultural context that may influence perceived changes in health state, can we gain a full understanding of differential perceptions of recovery. In short, there is not one element, for example, medication or the doctor-patient relationship, but a concatenation of factors, that combine to explain differential patient responses to treatment. These factors are also closely linked to the onset of the illness episode.

The Medical Consultation and Patients' Perceived Recovery

The doctor-patient relationship within the context of the medical consultation is regarded as the essence of medicine and is crucial in the healing process. In his review of the literature on doctor-patient relationships from the 1930s to the 1980s, Armstrong (1982) observed that patients' dissatisfaction and noncompliance resulted directly from difficulties in doctor-patient communication, attributed by some to different types of literacies extant in complex societies (Cicourel 1983).

Perusal of the extensive literature on the role of the doctor-patient relationship reveals diverse components of the relationship as important in treatment satisfaction and patient compliance. Few studies examine the doctor-patient relationship and patient-perceived treatment outcome. Generally speaking, the focus rests on the physician's actions as being the major components that explain the successes and failures of the interaction and, by implication, outcome of treatment. While numerous scholars maintain that the doctor-patient relationship is the essential component for diagnosis and treatment, they fail to agree on the specific aspects of the interaction that are instrumental in effecting patient satisfaction, compliance, and positive outcome.[5] It is recognized that the physician exerts a degree of power over patients (Freidson 1970; Waitzkin 1979; Zola 1981), although researchers disagree about which aspects of the doctor-patient relationship aid in fostering satisfaction, compliance, and positive outcomes. Some have suggested shared understandings, especially regarding etiology (Kleinman 1980). Others have noted that physicians with the most faith in the efficacy of their treatment achieve the best results (Benson and Epstein 1975). Others have emphasized the importance of communication between doctor and patient, especially when the physician facilitates the patient's understanding of his or her impairment and what must be done to effect recovery (Haynes 1976). Pursuant to these considerations, Inui, et al. (1976) proposed that by informing patients of their condition, physicians foster patients' compliance and cure; Locker and Dunt (1978) suggested transmission of information about the illness and treatment, and awareness of patient concerns (Korsh and Negrete 1972), while others proposed an egalitarian relationship between patient and doctor (Anderson and Helm 1979; Pratt 1976). Some have advocated a relational model of mutual participation (Kushner 1981), and a patient-centered approach to treatment of the type Szasz and Hollander (1956) described as mutual participation to foster compliance and satisfaction (Stewart 1984). Fitzpatrick et al. (1983) have identified referral to a specialist and his or her reflected authority as important and possibly more significant than the physician demonstrating interest in patients' biographies, for example. However, these researchers as well as others (Stuart 1984) point out that while various factors promote compliance and satisfaction, their impact upon ultimate outcome, that is patients' health, remains unknown.

Earlier I proposed the view of the medical consultation as a dramaturgical event wrought with inherent conflicts emerging out of physicians' and patients' disparate experience of pain, for one. To resolve the drama requires a resolution of the patient's condition which gave the impetus to the interaction. The pain placed the patient in a new relation with the world, and to alleviate it the patient must be brought back to the habitual state prior to the onset of the pain. I postulated several aspects intrinsic to the medical encounter that would abet the resolution of the patient's condition and affect the patient's perception of therapeutic outcome. I have focused on variables derived from the verbatim transcripts by independent observers that are commonly regarded as relevant to the doctor-patient interaction. These center around the doctor communicating to the patient the nature of his or her sickness, the giving of a diagnosis, explaining its reasons, the patient agreeing with the physician concerning the diagnosis, meeting the patient's expectations of treatment, providing instructions about the prescribed medication, and giving reassurance. Also involved is how the physician addresses the patient, time spent with the patient, and the patient's participation in the consultation as marked by patients posing questions to the physician.[6]

An aggregate analysis of these variables highlights four statistically significant components of the medical consultation that influence patients perceptions of recovery.[7] These are: whether the doctor explained to the patient what was wrong; whether the doctor gave the patient a diagnosis, even when the diagnosis was unrelated to the patient's presenting symptoms, whether the patient agreed with the physician, and whether the patient had asked additional questions regarding his or her condition. These findings are displayed in Tables 10.6, 10.7, 10.8, and 10.9.

The results from this analysis further support the finding disclosed in Table 10.3 showing that when patients were not given a diagnosis or were diagnosed as healthy, they were significantly more likely to report that they had experienced no recovery.

Brody and Waters (1980) have put forward the proposition that the giving of a diagnosis acts as a placebo and is itself the treatment. My findings support this proposition. Within the parameters of the medical encounter, transmitting a diagnosis to the patient is highly significant in influencing patient-perceived positive outcome. The diagnostic process entails the *naming* of the condition and thereby giving it a reality, providing the patient with a handle on what may possibly be wrong with him or her, which then can be negotiated with oneself, also furnishing an interpretation of one's alien state. Contrary to Brody and Waters (1980), the diagnosis does not essentially give meaning to the patient's sickness because it does not necessarily purport that the patient understood its significance. In fact, when patients were asked on follow-up home visits what the doctor had told them, only 50 percent were able to restate the physician's diagnosis verbatim or in approximation; a somewhat higher percentage of people with full recovery exhibited a correspondence between the doctor's diagnosis and the patient's understanding of it. In response to the question "What did the doctor tell you was the problem?" a patient would report, for example, that the physician had told her there "was something wrong with my spine, it was crooked," when the diagnosis was scoliosis. On the other hand, one patient reported that the physician had told her she had worms on her brain when the diagnosis was parasitosis.

Table 10.6: Patients' Perceived Recovery by Whether or Not Physicians Explained to the Patients What Was Wrong (in percent)

Explanation	Full	Partial	None	Total
Explained What Was Wrong (N=122)	24.6	54.1	21.3	100.0
Did Not Explain What Was Wrong (N=75)	6.7	66.7	26.7	100.0
Total (N=197)[a]	17.8	58.9	23.3	100.0

$X^2 = 10.215$ df=2   p=.006
Wilcoxon $X^2 = 5.8687$ df=1   p=.0154

[a] Eight missing cases not included in analysis.

Table 10.7: Patients' Perceived Recovery by Physician Providing a Diagnosis (in percent)

	Full	Partial	None	Total
Provided Diagnosis (N=57)	28.2	54.1	17.7	100.0
Did Not Provide Diagnosis (N=140)	9.8	61.6	28.6	100.0
Total (N=197)[a]	17.8	58.9	23.3	100.0

$X^2 = 12.104$ df=2   p=.002
Wilcoxon $X^2 = 9.7623$ df=1   p=.0018

[a] Eight missing cases not included in this analysis.

Table 10.8: Patients' Perceived Recovery by Whether or Not Patients Agreed
with Physicians' Diagnoses at Time of First Follow-up Interview (in percent)

	Full	Partial	None	Total
Agreed (N=131)	19.8	61.1	19.1	100.0
Disagreed (N=53)	7.6	56.6	35.8	100.0
Total (N=184)[a]	16.3	59.8	23.9	100.0

X^2 = 8.062   df=2   p=.018
Wilcoxon X^2 = 8.0170   df=1   p=.0046

[a] One case was excluded because of missing data. Twenty cases were
excluded because the patient received neither a diagnosis nor a reason
for the disorder.

As could be gleaned from the consultations presented in Chapters 7 and
8, the medical encounter engages a passive patient with an active doctor.
Interestingly, however, when patients participate during the interview,
specifically by asking questions about their condition, it significantly
influences patients' perception of recovery. This finding is displayed in Table
10.9.

Table 10.9: Patients' Perceived Recovery by Whether or Not Patient Posed
Questions to the Physician (in percent)

	Full	Partial	None	Total
Patients asked questions (N=44)	27.3	61.4	11.4	100.0
Patients did not ask questions (N=153)	15.0	58.2	26.8	100.0
Total (N=197)[a]	17.8	58.9	23.3	100.0

X^2 = 6.427   df=2   p=.040
Wilcoxon X^2 = 6.3920   df=1   p=.0115

[a]Eight missing cases not included in this analysis.

In the final analysis, the significant variables associated with the medical
encounter differentiating persons with "Full," "Partial," or "No" recovery
revolve around the doctor giving the patient a diagnosis, explaining it, the
patient agreeing with it--even though the degree to which the patient may have

comprehended its meaning remains conjectural--and patient participation in the encounter as delineated by patients posing questions about their condition.

On follow-up home interviews, patients were asked whether the doctor had done what they had expected. As we saw in Chapter 9, patient expectations are often shaped by the medical encounter. Not surprisingly, while there is some difference, there is no statistically significant difference between perceived recovery and patients' expectations as met by physicians, as we see in Table 10.10. It is noteworthy that patients with no expectations were just as likely to experience "Full" recovery as those whose expectations were met.

Table 10.10: Patients' Perceived Recovery by Whether or Not
Patients' Expectations Were Met (in percent)

	Full	Partial	None	Total
Expectations Were Met (N=78)	20.5	57.7	21.8	100.0
Expectations Were Not Met (N=89)	12.4	58.4	29.2	100.0
No Expectations (N=38)	21.1	55.2	23.7	100.0
Total (N=205)	17.1	57.5	25.4	100.0

$X^2 = 3.052$ df= 4   p=.10

Patients averaged two visits with the physician. There was no difference in the time the physician spent with the patient during first and second visits. The average time spent with patients on the first visit was 21.5 minutes, and 8 minutes on the second visit. Physicians varied with regard to reassurance of patients. Some reassured patients "not to worry," while others were non-committal. There was no significant relationship between perceived recovery and the physician's reassurance as measured by the number of times a physician would tell a patient "Don't worry," "You will be cured," or "You will be made to feel better." The overwhelming majority of patients were not reassured using these markers.

Some physicians castigated patients, particularly if they had not brought their previous prescriptions with them. Some may have blamed patients for having "made angers" or for being nervous, especially when the physician attributed the sickness to the emotional states of the patient. In fact in 10 percent of the cases, and evenly distributed across the three categories, patients were scolded by the attending physician. One of the physicians was abrasive with her patients, whereas another one would frequently tell patients "Don't worry," but neither of these styles seems to have influenced the perceived treatment outcomes.

There was also no association between perceived recovery and mode of address, with the majority of patients having been addressed in the formal "you," marking the interaction with social distance and respect. But the paternalistic nature of the physician-patient encounter is most notable and underscored by the informal manner in which patients were addressed. Above and beyond the honorific plural "you" (*usted*), it was not uncommon for a thirty-year old physician to address a female patient of any age as "my daughter" ("*mi hija*"), a term of endearment used by a father or lover, while a female physician might have addressed a woman patient senior in age as "my queen" ("*mi reina*"), a term used by mothers speaking to daughters. When patients were questioned about the paternalistic posture of physicians as reflected in the informal modes of address, one patient's response summed up the general consensus: "I was treated the same by my parents." She did not seem to find it offensive to be addressed or treated as a child.

Consideration must be given to the role of medication. Medication includes pharmacological drugs and vitamins in capsules or injections, in which people have especially great faith. Generally speaking, many prescription drugs have become part of folk knowledge, including Terramicine (antibiotic), Naproxen (anti-inflammatory), Neurobrion (antineuritic), and people routinely purchase these in the pharmacies in Mexico where there have been no restrictions on their sale until recently.[8] Paradoxically, while people readily ingest medications, there is also a common belief that pharmaceutical drugs are harmful to the organism: In the words of one patient, "Medicines make me angry and I am an angry person already." It makes one "aggressive," and for these reasons, as well as fear of dependence upon drugs, people often prefer herbal remedies. Yet, despite the beliefs about the harmful effects of pharmacological drugs or that they act only as palliatives, people usually attributed recovery to the medication.

Compliance with a medication regimen is thus highly complex and related not only to availability of economic resources, as physicians often claim, but to more intricate and subtle reasons anchored in such paradoxes and related to etiological understandings. To illustrate, one hypertensive patient stopped her medication because, according to her, hypertension was a matter of nerves and she decided to control her nerves; therefore, she did not feel the need to take the medication.

An average of 3.3 medications were prescribed to all patients. There is no significant relationship between having had medication prescribed, having taken the drugs, and perception of recovery[9] as is disclosed by the findings displayed in Tables 10.11 and 10.12.

Table 10.11: Patients' Perceived Recovery by Whether Medication
Was or Was Not Prescribed (in percent)

	Full	Partial	None	Total
Medication was prescribed (N=184)	16.8	58.7	24.5	100.0
Medication was not prescribed (N=21)	19.0	47.7	33.3	100.0
Total (N=205)	17.1	57.5	25.4	100.0

$X^2 = 1.024$ df=2   p=.10

Table 10.12: Patients' Perceived Recovery by Whether or Not They
Reported Taking Prescribed Medication (in percent)

	Full	Partial	None	Total
Took prescribed medication (N=124)	20.1	58.1	21.8	100.0
Did not take prescribed medication (N=60)	10.0	60.0	30.0	100.0
Total (N=184)	16.8	58.7	24.5	100.0

$X^2 = 3.594$ df=2   p=.10

While there is wide variability among physicians concerning whether they explain how and when to take the prescribed medications, there is no statistically significant association between patients' perceived recovery and whether or not physicians explained how to administer the medication. Some physicians warned patients about the dire consequences of not following their treatment regimens. Others were cavalier about the medications they prescribed. Some explained in great detail how to take the medication they had prescribed while others mumbled pro forma instructions. None of these variants in style seems to have influenced the patients' perceived recovery response. My findings suggest that the physicians' instructions and explanations are not as significant as compared to whether physicians give patients a diagnosis, explain the reason for their sickness, and the patient concurs with it.

Individual approaches differ but it cannot be said that physicians' styles differentially influenced patient-perceived outcome. The highest percentage of patients who had perceived themselves fully recovered (25 percent) were treated by Physician 7, who also practiced homeopathy and acupuncture and who gave great importance to nerves. Characteristic of him, as we saw in Nomi's case, he prescribed mainly Maalox and he placed great stress on diet. On the other hand, the second highest percentage of patients with full recovery were treated by Physician 3, who was totally committed to the classical biomedical paradigm, minimized cultural explanations, tended to prescribe drugs, and gave short shrift to diet. However, Physician 7 gave the highest percentage of diagnosis to his patients (92 percent), explained the reason for the sickness (53 percent), and had the highest percentage of patients agree with him (76 percent). With the exception of Physician 5, who had the lowest patient compliance rate with prescribed medication (27 percent), the other physicians' compliance ranged between 50 and 90 percent. Physician 6, who was the oldest and most despotic of the physicians in the sample, had the third highest percentage of patients with "Full" recovery (15 percent), but also the second highest with "None" (20 percent).

Thus, we see that patient-perceived recovery is not significantly associated with number of visits, time spent with the physician, reassurances, and whether medication was prescribed and taken. We can thus conclude that in the study population, the major components of a biomedical consultation that are associated with differential responses to medical treatment converge around physicians furnishing a diagnosis and its elucidation, irrespective of the patients' comprehension of its meaning and for the patient's agreement with it, unless there was total misdiagnosis, as was the case with Nomi, whom we have met in Chapter 8.

Sickness Management

Aspects of the medical encounter alone do not sufficiently illuminate patients' perceptions of recovery. I now turn to examine hypothesized variables influencing perceived outcome that lie beyond the medical diagnoses and consultation by focusing on patients' sickness management and sociodemographic characteristics. A large percentage of people had not sought treatment for the sickness episode they were experiencing at the time prior to coming to the hospital, as was seen in Table 4.1. Of the 205 people who form part of the total sample, 37 people (18 percent) had sought treatment elsewhere during a thirty-to fifty-day period between the hospital and before the first follow-up home visit. Seeking treatment elsewhere is significantly related to perception of recovery in that those who sought other treatment were less likely to report full recovery and more likely to report no relief of symptoms, as shown in Table 10.13. However, in this case, it may be that failure to perceive recovery led to the search for alternate treatment.

Table 10.13: Patients' Perceived Recovery by Other Treatment Sought Between 30 and 50 Days Following Hospital Visit Before First Follow-up Home Visit (in percent)

	Full	Partial	None	Total
Sought other treatment (N=37)	5.4	56.8	37.8	100.0
Did not seek other treatment (N=168)	19.6	57.8	22.6	100.0

$X^2 = 6.374$ df=2   p=.05

Only two of those with full relief sought other treatment and only one attributed perceived recovery to the treatment received from another physician. Of those with partial relief, twenty-one had sought treatment from other physicians, twelve reported they felt some improvement but did not regard themselves as fully recovered, and three reported they felt worse as a result of the other treatment. The remaining seven felt no change in their health state as a result of additional therapy. Fourteen of the people with no recovery comprise the largest percentage who sought treatment elsewhere. Eight sought help from other physicians while six went to alternative healers. Of those fourteen, five reported some alleviation when they received additional treatment but at the time of the home visit continued to feel sick. These data suggest that whereas people who do not find relief from one health regimen source tend to seek out health care services from either another physician or alternative healers, they do not necessarily find them beneficial.

Importantly, a time dimension is significant in the management of sickness. Using one-way analysis of variance, there is a statistically significant difference regarding the length of time patients experienced the disorder before they sought treatment at Salud Hospital, as is shown in Table 10.14.

Table 10.14 establishes that whereas the people with full recovery experienced their sickness on the average less than a year prior to seeking help at the hospital, the people with no recovery felt sick an average of four years, and those with partial relief for about two and a half years. This finding suggests that chronicity is greatest among patients with no recovery and that

Table 10.14: Patients' Perceived Recovery by Number of Days Patients
Had Been Sick Before Seeking Treatment at Salud Hospital

Patient Category	Average No. of Days
Full recovery	304.7
Partial recovery	952.2
No recovery	1,510.0

F= 5.087 df = 2 p=.01

their condition tends to fail to respond to treatment readily, irrespective of the diagnosis.

There is an important subjective dimension of sickness management as measured by how patients perceived their overall health state, and how soon they anticipated improvement. Those who considered their general health state as poor were significantly less likely (p=.02) to experience perceived recovery as revealed by logistic regression analysis. In addition, when patients were asked how soon they expected to recover, 61.5 percent responded they didn't know. But of the remaining 38.5 percent, those who believed they would recover in less than a week as compared to months were significantly (p=.02) more likely to recover using logistic regression analysis.

Sociodemographic and Socioeconomic Variability

Of the sociodemographic variables postulated to impact on perceived recovery, including sex, age, education, economic resources, marital status, religion and degree of religiosity as measured by frequency of church attendance, number of people living in the household, age of children in the household, and place of birth, only the last two cited have a statistically significant relationship to perceived alleviation. The results of a logistic regression analysis reveal that having children in the home under the age of five had a statistically significant (p=.002) negative influence on perceived alleviation. Having children in the home above age five lacked similar impact. Not surprisingly, having children under the age of five at home alters health perception for many obvious reasons, not the least of which is the fact that with small children, women are heavily burdened in the home, especially when they lack assistance, impeding their perception of recovery.

Additionally, those born in Mexico City were more likely to experience alleviation than those who migrated to the city at a significant level (p=.05), according to the same logistic regression analysis. This finding, while unanticipated, is not surprising considering the fact that unlike well-ensconced natives of the city, migrants to the city may experience subjective and objective pressures that impact on their general health state and perceptions of recovery.

Using the ranking discussed in Chapter 9 as a tentative measure of economic status, based upon dwelling conditions and economic possessions, patients' perceived recovery was not associated significantly with this measure as can be seen in Table 10.15.

Table 10.15: Patients' Perceived Recovery by Ranking of
Socioeconomic Status (in percent)

Socioeconomic Ranking	Full	Partial	None	Total
1 (N=12)	8.3	50.0	41.7	100.0
2 (N=30)	13.3	60.0	26.7	100.0
3 (N=62)	17.7	63.0	19.3	100.0
4 (N=67)	23.9	53.7	22.4	100.0
5 (N=14)	7.1	57.2	35.7	100.0
Not Ranked (N=20)	10.0	55.0	35.0	100.0
(N=205)	17.1	57.5	25.4	100.0

$x^2 = 8.381$ $df = 10$ $p = .10$

I hypothesized that the more squalid the individuals' living conditions, as a measure of economic resources, the less likely they would perceive themselves recovered on the grounds of the long-established relationship between poverty and sickness. However, there was no statistically significant relationship between ranking of socioeconomic status and perceived recovery, as is suggested in Table 10.15. There is even a slight tendency for those with the highest status in terms of housing to be less likely to report full recovery. As will be recalled from our earlier discussion, while the sample as a whole forms part of the poorest segment of Mexican society within this large sector of the population, economic resources as measured by material possessions alone are insufficient to explain the differences in people's health state or its resolution. The commonly held view of a *direct* relationship between poverty and sickness lacks support using the findings displayed in Table 10.15.

Social Supports and Life Events

I hypothesized that patient-perceived improvement and recovery will be related to patients' perceived social supports and perceived stressful life events. Social supports refer to networks of relationships, upon which individuals may rely, including kinship relationships, and degree of perceived trust or reliance on others. The significance of social supports in mediating life stresses and health has been postulated by many scholars.[10]

People in Mexico generally enjoy a wide network of social relationships and social support. The natal family is the bulwark of human existence and all Mexicans can rely on their kin, especially their mothers, and even siblings for social support, even when dissension exists within the natal family. A social support instrument developed by Fleming (1982) measuring subjective dimensions of social support was administered to all patients on the first follow-up home interview. When aggregate scores were compared among patients in the three groups, there was no statistically significant difference between the three categories, indicating that the groups did not differ along this variable.

Stressful life events have been postulated by numerous investigators as influencing illness.[11] I postulated that life events experiences linger on not only to influence the onset of the illness but also its perceived outcome. To test this hypothesis, a life events inventory (Patrick 1982) was administered at the initial interview. Patients rated the degree to which a particular event may have affected them on a three-point scale: none at all, some, a lot.[12] Of the twenty-one possible events, patients averaged seven events. There was no association between perceived recovery and number of events experienced by individuals, with persons with no relief having experienced an average of eight, those with partial recovery an average of seven and with full recovery an average of six. This finding suggests that the number of events experienced during one's lifetime does not significantly influence perceived treatment outcome.

Moreover, when I examined perceived recovery in relation to specific events, only two, loss of a child and moving, significantly related to perception of recovery, as is disclosed in Table 10.16. (Because an individual

Table 10.16: Patients' Perceived Recovery by Life Events

	Full	Partial	None	Total	X^2	df	P
Death of a Child							
Yes (N=21)	—	52.4	47.6	100.0	8.675	2	< .05
No (N=184)	19.1	58.1	22.8	100.0			
Moved							
Yes (N=51)	7.8	56.9	35.3	100.0	6.037	2	< .05
No (N=154)	20.1	57.8	22.1	100.0			

could have experienced more than one of these life events, the distribution for each event was compared to the sample as a whole.)

When a given life event was correlated with how a person was affected by the life event, only the death of a child was highly correlated with the impact it had on the person. A logistic regression analysis showed that of all the life events, the death of a child had the only significant impact on perceived outcome of treatment. None of the individuals who had lost a child either at birth or during infancy experienced full recovery. As I have contended elsewhere (Finkler 1985a), loss of a child is especially traumatic to women in Mexico above and beyond the associated grief and demoralization because in the case of women, they are often blamed for the death.

Interestingly, only a small percentage of those who had moved reported full recovery; none in this category had been very much affected by the move, whereas 6 percent in the "No" recovery and 13 percent in the "Partial" recovery category indicated they had been strongly affected by moving. Logistic regression analyses reveal that although moving is related to perceived recovery at a statistically significant level (p=.05), the relationship is only indirect. When the other statistically significant variables are included in the analysis, its effect is no longer significant. Moving thus has an indirect effect depending on the circumstances and the impetus revolving around the experience of moving. Moving from one habitat to another may not play a consequential role in sickness or recovery, but its impact is felt when people become forcibly displaced and downwardly mobile. For instance, moving was traumatic especially for those who were displaced by the earthquake. Other traumatic moves included the case of Monica, who was forced to relocate to poor quarters because her husband had failed in his enterprises, or Esperanza, who was dislodged from her home by her husband's mistress and she was reduced to living in abysmal conditions, as we will see in Chapter 11.

In sum, in addition to specific elements of the doctor-patient encounter, through aggregate analysis I have identified several specific sickness management and sociodemographic variables, including specific life events, that impact significantly on perceived treatment outcomes.

Attributions for Recovery

To conclude the discussion of the variables associated with perceived treatment outcomes in aggregate terms, I present some important findings related to recovery attributions. The hypothesized variables bearing on the relationship between doctor-patient relationship and perceived outcome discussed earlier were derived from the transcripts of the medical consultation. The sociodemographic variables describe the objective conditions of a people's existence. When patients were questioned specifically to what *they* attributed their full or partial recovery, a variety of reasons were cited by the people in the "Partial" and "Full" categories. The prevailing first response was "The medications." It must be emphasized that people uniformly distinguish between treatment as palliative and treatment as cure. Palliatives are usually referred to when symptoms subside with the medication but return when the medication is stopped, whereas people regard themselves cured when their symptoms have been eliminated after they had stopped taking the medication.

Of those with full recovery, 51 percent attributed it to the medication. Other reasons cited were that they were "given confidence," were "made to feel tranquil," or "were given advice" (17 percent); laboratory analysis, Xrays, and other technological management (11 percent), and the remainder (17 percent) were unable to provide any attribution.

Of those in the "Partial" category, 28 percent attributed their partial improvement to medication. Additionally, they cited reasons such as "getting hope," "confidence," "advice," and "made to feel tranquil" (18 percent); the laboratory analysis, Xrays, and other technological management (9 percent); other reasons included physical examination (4 percent), having been well treated (3 percent), and referral to specialist (2 percent). The remaining 36 percent of the people in this category were unable to provide any attribution for partial improvement of their health state, suggesting that people often cannot verbalize their understandings and responses (Young 1981).

Importantly, many people responded with a combination of attributions. For example, physical examinations were frequently cited along with having been given advice, or having been told "that there was nothing wrong with me," or "the physician had asked a lot of questions." For the small percentage of people who were ordered Xrays and electrocardiograms (12 percent), the technological management was stressed, although there was no significant association between the doctor having ordered Xrays or ultrasounds and perceived recovery.

Significantly, other attributions emerged that revolved not around the medical consultation but around their own lives and thoughts. In ten cases people attributed their full or partial recovery to the unburdening of themselves through the questioning at the first interview conducted by the anthropologist prior to the medical consultation. This suggests that for these people, symptomatic expression was definitely associated in their own understanding with extrasomatic issues. Other reasons cited, distributed equally among the sexes, included "changes in my thinking," "not getting angry anymore," "being less worried," and change in situation. Examples of the latter include the husband leaving the household, the husband starting to work again, having less laundry to do, and changing social relations, particularly with a spouse or child.

As we saw in Chapter 3, there was some variation among men and women respecting etiological explanations. Interestingly, however, attributions do not vary along sex lines. While etiological explanations are culturally shaped, recovery attributions exhibit an international cast specifically as they refer to medication, especially the proverbial pills and injections, and technological apparatus.

Without diminishing the significance of other recovery attribution factors, the fact that there is among patients a preponderant emphasis on medication and technological management suggests that in the same way as expectations are molded by the medical consultation, biomedicine contributes to shaping a shared understanding of recovery attributions structured through the treatment it provides.

Besides the 10 patients with partial or no recovery whom I had followed on a regular basis, 90 of the 170 patients who reported partial or no recovery were followed up a second time between six and twelve months after the first visit. These patients were selected on the basis of the neighborhoods from which the largest concentration of patients in the sample were drawn, especially Neza. On the second follow-up home interview, patients were asked in open-ended discussion about how they were feeling, how they had managed their sickness since the previous home visit, and to what they attribute changes, if any. Based upon these visits patients were divided into groups that reported feeling "better," "same," or "worse."

Table 10.17: Patients' Stated Condition of How They Were Feeling at Time of Second Home Follow-up by Attribution and Treatment Sought (in percent)

Attribution/ or Treatment Sought	Better	Same	Worse	Total
Medical treatment only (N=37)	73.0	18.9	8.1	100.0
Change in emotional discharges and life situations (N=15)	86.6	6.7	6.7	100.0
Self treatment: home herbal remedies (N=10)	70.0	20.0	10.0	100.0
Alternative treatment (homeopath, naturalist sacred healer) (N=9)	77.8	22.2	—	100.0
None (N=19)	78.9	15.8	5.3	100.0
Total (N=90)	76.6	16.7	6.7	100.0

$X^2 =3.341$ df= 8   p=.10

Table 10.17 discloses that the overwhelming majority of those followed were feeling well on the second follow-up occurring within a year of the first interview. Patients attributed their improvement to changes in their lives and to emotional discharges, such as having stopped paying attention to the condition or having stopped making angers. Of those seeking medical treatment a few returned to Salud Hospital, while most sought treatment from private physicians. A significant percentage of those who were feeling better had done nothing and their improvement would seem to be a function of time.

On the second home follow-up, attributions bound to sickness management paralleled those of the first visit. Those who reported they were completely well and had sought other treatment modalities attributed recovery to them. For example, three individuals who had gone to sacred healers attributed recovery to the ministrations they had received there. Other reasons included statements such as "feeling more optimistic," "stopped eating food sold by street vendors," and stopped getting angry."

I postulated that if, after a year, an individual failed to improve, he or she would seek alternative treatment. Nine individuals sought alternative treatment of whom seven found it also beneficial. However, the hypothesis requires further testing. I expect that after two or three years, individuals who failed to gain alleviation of their conditions will seek alternative healers, such as Spiritualists, or other folk curers, especially when they begin to draw on the belief that their ailment was caused by witchcraft.

In this chapter we have examined the biomedical diagnostic categories, the medical consultation, sociodemographic and socioeconomic factors, and life events variables to explain patients' differential perceptions of recovery. First, we have seen that a series of factors must be examined in tandem to illuminate patients' contrasting responses to treatment. In examining these factors, I moved from hypothesized variables drawn from observations of the medical consultation--from which were derived such findings as those related to the physician giving a patient a diagnosis--even when patients failed to verbalize it to patients' subjective reports for attribution for recovery. Moreover, while much has been said about the importance of the doctor-patient encounter, I have identified specific variables that significantly influence perceived recovery, suggesting that not all aspects of the doctor-patient consultation are of *equal* importance to the healing process.

Upon long-term observation I found that for most of those who had a positive health outcome, some aspect of their life had changed. For many, improvement in their health state was associated not only with various treatments but with perceived changes in the conditions of their existence that reestablished in a familiar way their relationship to the life world, when life became as it "ought to be."

To comprehend, then, the healing process, we must resort to multilevel analyses, using direct observations, selectively devised instruments, and, most important, patients' subjective evaluations. In the next chapter, I probe indepth patients' narratives of their lives. My focus is on those individuals we have already met in the earlier chapters to weave together anthropological and patients' subjective understandings. To combine several levels of--analysis-in-depth scrutiny of the phenomenology of individual lives together with the more general factors discussed in this chapter--is to shed light on biomedical practice in its role in the healing process.

Notes

1. There was a 22.9 percent attrition rate upon follow-up. If after two visits, people were not found at home, either because they had moved or for other reasons, they were removed from the roster. Of those removed from the study, 27.9 percent were men and 72.1 percent were women. These percentages correspond to the male-female sample composition of 22.9 percent males and 77.1 percent females. Those who were not followed up on did not differ along the standard sociodemographic variables from the study population.

2. Preliminary discussions with physicians suggested that alleviation ought to take place between two and four weeks following treatment. For this reason follow-ups were begun thirty days after the last visit. However, due to the logistics of carrying out the home interviews in an urban center the size of Mexico City, it was impossible to adhere to a uniform and precise schedule. Patients who could not be found the first time were visited a week or two after the originally scheduled visit.

3. I have used the CMI in my previous investigations and demonstrated that the instrument measures patient-perceived symptomatologies (Finkler 1981b). As in the past, the standardized Spanish version was altered to accommodate to the local population's understandings. In the standardized version, only "yes" and "no" responses are solicited. People, however, had great difficulties in responding in discrete yes or no terms. Therefore, following a pretest, the option of "sometimes" was added. Responses of "sometimes" were calculated to equal half a "yes" point. For an extensive discussion of the CMI see Finkler 1981b, 1985.

4. There was a statistical difference at the $p = .005$ level of significance between the entire hospital sample population and a control group of healthy individuals. The mean score of "yes" and "sometimes" responses combined for healthy individuals was 39 and 51.7 for the sample group interviewed at the hospital.

5. The literature is extraordinarily rich on the subject and only a few selected references are noted: Almy 1980; Anderson and Helm 1979; Armstrong 1982; Ben Sira 1980; Brook 1977; Fabrega and Silver 1973; Fabrega and Manning 1979; Finkler 1984, 1985; Fitzpatrick 1983; Garrity 1981; Gill 1976; Golden and Johnston 1970; Hahn and Kleinman 1983; Hall and Dornan 1988; Haynes 1976; Helman 1985b; Kleinman 1980; Korsch et al. 1968; Korsch and Negrete 1972; Kushner 1981; Linn 1975; Locker and Dunt 1978; Mechanic 1968; Obeyesekere 1977; Parsons 1975; Pratt 1976; Quill 1983; Rosenberg 1979; Speedling and Rose 1985; Starfield et al. 1981; Waitzkin and Stoeckle 1972; Weinberger et al. 1981. A comprehensive review of the literature can be found in Hauser 1981; and Pendleton and Hasler 1983.

6. These included whether he explained to the patient the problem and also gave a diagnosis; explained the reason for the diagnosis; explained how to take the medication; indicated gravity non-gravity; did what the patient had requested; reassured the patient by linguistic markers such as "don't worry," "I will cure you," "I will make you better"; gave a return appointment whether the patient posed any questions to the doctor; whether the patient gave a self-diagnosis which the doctor affirmed or disconfirmed; doctor's mode of address (using the respectful plural or familiar singular).

7. The Wilcoxon and the Kruskal-Wallis that compare the means of the variables and the chi square tests were applied and these yielded statistically significant differences of the same variables.

8. Drugs prohibited in Britain and in the United States are sold freely in Mexico as well, including Neomelubrina, which contains dipirona, and Diadoquin, which are considered harmful to the nervous system (La Jornada 1987).

9. I checked the prescriptions in the *Diccionario de Especialidades Farmaceuticas* (1987) and most medications were appropriate for the diagnosis given.

10. See, for example, Antonovsky 1980; Berkman 1984; Berkman and Breslow 1983; Cassell 1974, 1976; Dean and Lin 1977; Eckenrode and Gore 1981; Fleming 1982; Holmes and Masuda 1974; Hyman 1972; Kaplan et al. 1979; Levy 1983; Margan et al. 1984; Mechanic 1974;) but Hyman (1972) notes that social isolation "can affect not merely the seeking of treatment but also its course and outcome" (85).

11. See for example, Barsky 1979; Birley and Connoly 1976; Brown 1974, 1974a; Cobb 1974; Day et al. 1987; Dohrenwend and Dohrenwend 1974; Eckenrode and Gore 1981; Finkler 1985a; Robkin and Streuning 1976.

12. The instrument included twenty-one life events that centered around failure in school, change of domicile, loss of spouse, divorce, separation, abortion, injury to loved one, business failure, lay-off, child leaving home, victim of crime, unemployed for over two months, jail term. The instrument was modified to include the earthquake and culturally identified stressors,

especially sudden fright and accusations of witchcraft. Initially patients were asked to identify events within the past twelve months. Significantly, however, people were unable to bracket the life event within a time frame, and would identify it irrespective of whether it took place a year or ten years earlier. A life event for a Mexican is an ongoing experience that transcends a time dimension. Consequently, life events were recorded no matter when they had taken place, and when they had taken place was asked separately. The life event identified most often was the earthquake.

11

Patient-Perceived Therapeutic Outcomes: A Phenomenological Perspective

In Chapters 7 and 8 individuals came into view during the medical consultation at the Salud Hospital as they presented their bodily ills to the physicians. In this chapter, we learn about their response to treatment, how they had managed their sickness, and about their life's lesions, which are not usually elicited by physicians in the course of a medical consultation. I propose that embodied sickness becomes alleviated not only through medical ministrations but through perceived existential changes in life's lesions that promoted sickness and gave impetus to the patient seeking treatment.

I examine perceived therapeutic outcomes within the context of patients' lives. Of the numerous patients about whose lives I gathered extensive materials and whom I got to know well, the case vignettes illustrate the ways in which differential response to treatment is related not only to the variables I discussed in the previous chapter but to lived experience. Owing to space limitations I present only abbreviated vignettes of a few whom we had met earlier from over 200 people's lives as they perceive and live it.

The people in this study share many characteristics, not the least of which is the poverty by which they are encompassed, and which dominates and shapes their survival. To explain their sickness *only* in terms of poverty, however, is to diminish the people's dignity as sentient beings whose bodies are extensions of their existence, and who engage in an ongoing evaluative process as social and moral beings. While they may or may not verbalize their evaluations, our task as anthropologists is to get at the ongoing appraisal, embedded in a cultural matrix, that people make of themselves and their lives, which forms a component part of the healing process.

If perceived response to treatment were solely an attribute of biomedical ministrations to the body, then all patients ought to have perceived themselves recovered within a short period of time, as stipulated by the physicians. This was not the case. To assign responsibility to physicians' ministrations and attribute failure to recover to faulty clinical judgment or to lack of compliance, as biomedical practitioners are wont to do, is to minimize the numerous dimensions of human existence that engender the healing process. In the vignettes that follow we see sickness and recovery being played out in multiple ways, as, for example, in Jose's and Arthur's residing with their in-laws, in Serge's height, and in Nomi's kidneys. In the same way as the onset of a sickness episode can only be comprehended in terms of an amalgam of embodied elements rather than in unicausal terms (Engel 1977), so too is its resolution. The recovery process takes place on several levels associated with transformations, effected separately or in tandem with treatment and alteration of perceived circumstance. This proposition comes into view in the case vignettes that follow.

Jose

Jose worked as a mechanic in his brother's car body shop and was the father of three girls. He resided with his in-laws in a large extended family. Jose, a short, powerful-looking man with shining eyes and an aquiline nose, suffered from intense pains in the lower back (*cintura*) that he feared may eventually render him a cripple. As we saw in Chapter 7, he was treated by two of the hospital physicians. His pains were temporarily alleviated with a muscle relaxant prescribed by the first physician and by a friend who gave him a powerful twist in the back. According to Jose, the medication was only a palliative.

After a few months he returned to the hospital. He was seen by a second physician, who recommended that Jose be treated in the orthopedic clinic, where he was diagnosed as having scoliosis. The ministrations he received there--muscle relaxants and an Xray--had not alleviated the pain until he went to a bonesetter, who gave him a massage, adjusting his "deviated spine" and "his whole body," for which he was charged about $25. He was completely recovered with the bonesetter's ministrations a year after his initial visit to the hospital.

Jose fell ill thirteen years before at age sixteen, when he said he was successfully treated by a specialist for a gastric ulcer and later with pure herbs and acupuncture treatments. At that time he experienced intense pain in the *cerebro*, and his nerves were disturbed "when everything made me angry because of the sickness." About five years earlier, when he moved to Mexico City, he started having the back pains that became intensified eight months prior to his first visit to the hospital.

Jose, the tenth of eleven children, born in a state neighboring Mexico City, shuttled back and forth between Mexico City and his native village where his elderly parents, about whom he worried a lot, resided. In Mexico

City, Jose lived with his wife's parents, her married brother and children, and an aunt who criticized him severely for permitting his wife to have a tubal ligation, particularly since Jose had only girls. His daughters were a source of great joy to him, but according to the aunt, contraceptive measures were used only by lazy people. This charge made both Jose and his wife angry because he felt "it was unjust" and assaulted his manhood.

Jose worked hard for his older brother, and he was satisfied with the work, for which he was paid a minimum wage. However, he disliked living in Mexico City, and that was why he traveled so often to his home village. But now they "don't have to beg" as they did when he got married, when they could not even maintain themselves.

During the span of a year and a half, from the time I knew Jose, he was building a room adjacent to the two rooms covered with tin that the entire extended family occupied. His move into his own dwelling coincided with his full recovery.

Jose attributed his sickness to his problems, which he associated with worries about his parents and other problems he claimed he was having, and his recovery to the bonesetter's treatment. Not coincidentally, Jose first began to feel the intense pains when he came to settle in Mexico City with his in-laws. His condition was completely alleviated when he finished building his little room and, in his words, he "became independent" from his in-laws when he no longer had to share his expenses with them. When I last met with Jose, a few months after he and his wife began living in their newly built quarters, Jose was beaming about how well he was feeling.

To grasp Jose's illness and full recovery is to understand not only the abysmal poverty in which he lived and continues to live, but also his cultural understandings that a man ought not to reside with his wife's family where the head of the household was his father-in-law, the eldest male, and where he was being criticized. It could be said that Jose's embodied pain had been alleviated by the prescribed medication or by the bonesetter; but more likely his recovery was related to the profound change that had taken place in his life when he moved 100 yards away from his in-laws and from the problems attendant on living with them, including the fact that he no longer had to contribute to the upkeep of a large household.

Arthur

Arthur did not have any such change in his life. He was experiencing high and low blood pressure and within the sixteen months that I knew him, he felt recovered only partially. Arthur lived in a large extended family with his in-laws in a poor section of the city.

A strikingly handsome young man with a soft smile and a wry sense of humor, Arthur had been married for three years and lived with his wife's parents, her unemployed married brother, and an unmarried sister with a child, in a two-story, well-constructed house that accommodated the household of eleven people. The house was situated in a lower-middle- class neighborhood populated by drug addicts and gangs but being from the neighborhood, Arthur did not feel threatened by them.

Living with his wife's family made Arthur very angry, and by his and his wife's accounts, he was a very angry person, especially because with his earnings he had to support his wife's brother, a ne'er-do-well. The wife's family originated from a small village, and in Arthur's estimation they had very little education and used foul language. He considered the wife's siblings slovenly, and lacking respect for him, for each other, and their parents. In fact, his overwhelming concern was that his three-year-old son would learn to behave like them.

Arthur was born in Mexico City, but when he was a year and a half old his mother died of a heart attack, leaving him, an older brother, and a newly born infant brother with their alcoholic father. The father left the children with his sisters who, Arthur recalled, beat the children, until they were removed and sent to live with another aunt, who sent them to school and brought them up very strictly. Arthur was, in his words, "deeply pained" that he had lost his mother and never had a happy home life.

When I first met Arthur he was studying accounting in a vocational school and was employed as an accountant in a small office. He regarded this as a dead-end job, paying him less than minimum wage and no social security that would have entitled him to health benefits. Arthur was especially disturbed that he was twenty-eight years old and he had not really achieved anything after all the effort he had put into studying in high school and preparatory school. He knew that even at his age it was already difficult to find a job because employers looked for people younger than he. He felt very pressured by his studies and concerned that he would fail his exams, scheduled for shortly after he first came to seek treatment at the hospital.

Arthur, who had a fiancee he loved, married his present wife under duress when he found out she was pregnant. Tears came to his eyes when he recounted that to his great regret he had to leave his fiancee. When his wife found out about the fiancee seven months earlier, she announced to all that she would have never married him had she known.

Arthur began feeling sick after he married, and he was afraid to participate in any sports. His symptoms intensified with the earthquake, when he fainted, and he began feeling desperate six months earlier. He developed high and low blood pressure and severe headaches, dizziness, jabbings in the chest, breathing problems, weakness, and his hands sweated. In his words, when his pressure was low or high "I feel I walk on air, float, and I can make a false step" and when he had pain in the *cerebro*, his body felt numb, "as if a liquid had been injected into it."

Soon after the earthquake he began seeking treatment from private physicians. One told him he had parasites, another indicated he had a tumor on his kidney, and a third that he may have been suffering from heart disease. The Salud Hospital physician confirmed that he was suffering from high and low blood pressure. Arthur feared cardiac arrest because his mother had died from a heart condition. He also considered that he might have a brain tumor because he felt something crawling inside and on his face after he got hit by a ball while playing soccer. His condition left him nervous and worried, and the medications he had been prescribed had not alleviated it.

Arthur tried to make sense of his condition. The results of the electrocardiogram and an ultrasound ordered by the Salud Hospital physician were all normal, but he didn't know what was wrong with him and the hospital physician never told him. He usually felt worse when he came home. When he left the city on an outing with his aunt, he felt fully recovered until he returned home. He would like to leave his in-laws' house, but he could not afford to do so. He wondered whether it could be "psychological," or perhaps "nerves," but then he dismissed these possibilities.

His wife did not believe he was sick because he had already seen so many doctors and, according to her, they all said there was nothing wrong with him. She maintained that the abandoned fiancee was bewitching him, since doctors were unable to cure him. At his workplace, a colleague suggested that he was being bewitched and that he was being envied, but he could not imagine why since he possessed nothing. Besides, he had a strong character, an angry character, which protected him against malfeasance; he also wore his underwear on the reverse side to safeguard him against witchcraft. Arthur went to a traditional curer, who he knew was not a charlatan because she had not charged him anything; but her treatments had not alleviated his condition and he had not kept his last appointment with her. He went to a social security doctor. There he was told that he had parasites and was given six medications. He took them briefly, but they made him sick and he stopped.

The last time I saw Arthur, he concluded that the "angers he was making" had made him sick because he was still living with his in-laws. Nevertheless, he had made a decision not to worry, and that was why he felt better. By then, sixteen months later, he also had landed a new and well-paying job, he was covered by social security, and he had completed his examinations successfully; he continued to live with his in-laws.

Arthur's case is instructive because a constellation of contradictions combine to impede his full recovery from what was clearly a state of depression. On the one hand, the new job not only relieved some of the economic pressures, but also helped to resolve the inconsistency of failed aspirations, of having worked hard, and not having had a decent job. On the other hand, like Jose, Arthur was trapped by having to reside with his in-laws, whom he clearly regarded as boors and who threatened the future of his son. Residing with them conflicted with cultural norms and engaged him in continuous conflicts with his wife's family. Unlike Jose, Arthur's loss of his own family with his mother's premature death had left him without a family substrate to anchor his being. Moreover, Arthur had not unraveled whether he was or was not being bewitched, which may have promoted his ill health and impeded his full recovery. Most likely, Arthur will not recover fully until his living situation changes and the paradoxes in his existence have become resolved.

Serge

Contradictions also enmeshed Serge, a young man who lived with relatives in Neza and whose unusual height in Mexico attracted people's attention. In fact, his height and athletic bearing were remarked upon by those present during the consultation.

Serge, like Arthur, suffered from high and low blood pressure, but he also presented jabbings in the chest and heart, dizziness, and feelings of desperation, tiredness, and pains in the "mouth of the stomach." He had been feeling this way and unable to do anything since he fell ill six months prior to seeking help in Salud Hospital, where he was diagnosed as having parasites, scoliosis, and flat feet. Because of the negative results of the laboratory analysis, he did not agree with the doctor that he had parasites, but he did accept the doctor's diagnosis that he may have a "sick spinal cord." Unlike Arthur, Serge felt no recovery after the first and second home visits. Not until two years after our initial meeting did he begin feeling a little better.

Serge had seen various physicians before attending Salud Hospital. They had ordered laboratory analyses and Xrays, all showing that "there was nothing wrong with me." Some told him he was suffering from high and low blood pressure, others that he had parasites. He was given a lot of medication and he felt he was being drugged. Neither the medications nor the teas that were usually taken for nerves and fright had any effect on his condition. He had also seen a psychologist, who told him that he needed to control himself.

Serge feared that he might have cancer, and to his disappointment he did not get a checkup "with machines" at the hospital, as he had hoped. He desired such an examination because the sickness caused great anxiety. He was suffering from nerves and he feared he might be going crazy, as his uncle had, by which he meant doing stupid things, losing his reason, and being unable to predominate over himself.

At the suggestion of an uncle, who was a practicing sorcerer, he went to a traditional healer, who told him that he had been bewitched when he was given something to eat.[1] But he felt that his strong character and being an angry person protected him from witchcraft. As he spoke, he remarked that his character was also bland. Besides, he did not really believe in witchcraft, and he wondered whether I did. His uncle, the sorcerer, had told him that there was a spirit that wished to kill him but that he was being shielded by the Angel of Death.

Serge is a devoted athlete who spent much of his time weight lifting, exercising, doing karate, and reading magazines about bodybuilding which instructed him to take a lot of vitamins and eat vegetarian foods. He read a lot about mind control to dominate his pain, as well as about natural therapy and acupuncture.

In his attempt to comprehend his condition, Serge attributed it to excessive exercise and vitamin ingestion (he drank thirty portions of brewer's yeast for breakfast), which made him tense; to the fact that he had not been doing anything except walking the streets (from one day to the next, he said, "I didn't have a sense of life, sometimes I would ask why am I here, what am I doing here, I look at the people as if they were a dream, and I lose reality"); and to the fact that when he was three years old he fell on his head and fainted.

Serge was born in Mexico City, a place he regarded as a "human zoological garden" and in total chaos. He lived in Neza in a well-constructed house that belonged to his paternal grandmother. The grandmother had moved in with her daughter shortly before Serge got sick and he remained in the house with an uncle and his family, a man he vehemently disliked because he had beaten Serge when he was a child.

Serge had been raised by his grandmother since he was two years old, after his mother abandoned him and left his drunken father, who had trouble with the police. All his life he had sought his mother. Only a year and a half earlier he was finally able to locate her. When he met his mother, she was indifferent to him, and he had little contact with his father. He, like Arthur, wished he would have had a mother and father, a "regular family."

Until he was about seventeen, Serge seldom left the house. When he did, he was laughed at and challenged to fights, especially by gangs in his neighborhood, groups he refused to join because he did not like to smoke any substance or drink. At first he would avoid fighting, but then he was accused of being a homosexual since he did not go out much and spent his time with his grandmother and aunts.

The gangs frightened him, but it was an emotion that made him "do spectacular things. Every time they challenged him, he defeated them and he feared that he would even kill somebody. In fact, the fear of killing a person during fights, to which Serge claimed he was constantly being challenged, was a recurrent theme in his discourse. He recounted that just before he got sick, as he came out of the subway a fellow attacked him and called him crazy; Serge warned him that he would hurt him. Before he hit the man he told him to remove his glasses. He knocked the man out and was terrified that the man was dead.

According to Serge, men challenged him because it made them feel manly to defeat him given his stature, but so far no one had. By his own account, he was embroiled in various fights and he always came out victorious.

Serge fell ill five days after he was mistakenly arrested, together with a group of boys in the neighborhood, who, unlike himself, were drunk. Their families came to bail them out the next day, but Serge was left in jail another day and he felt fear, the kind that did not make him "do spectacular things." Instead, it left him trembling and feeling alone "in an ugly way."

Serge finished a government preparatory school and wished to enter university, but he was unable to get the necessary documents from the school because he had a conflict with a teacher there. When he was seventeen he started training as a boxer, but he could not box professionally because there were no fighters in his weight range and the pay was small.

During a hiatus of about nine months when I did not see Serge, he had worked for the city police in a riot control squad. He resigned after six months because "I was being trained to kill people," but "We were not called out to fight." In fact, they were indoors most of the time. Joining the police force engaged Serge in a profound contradiction, one that did not escape him. He resigned, he said, because he was afraid he would kill somebody, but he also wanted to use his training in some way.

Serge supported himself with money his paternal grandfather, who lived in a rooming house, gave him and by working at odd jobs as a body guard and for his aunts in their curtain store. Working for the police gave him a larger income ($100 a month), but he wanted to attend the university and work in an office. When I saw him last he had joined a national soccer team, and at that point he reported he also began feeling somewhat better.

Serge, like Arthur, longed to be anchored in a family that he never had. Unlike Arthur, Serge's very body created a profound existential dilemma that may not ever be resolved for him. His body confers on him great powers in a society where most men are many inches shorter than he, but he is also regarded as a freak to be feared and conquered.

His body allows him to do "spectacular things" but it can also inflict death on others. With the unresolvable dilemmas, fears about his own death, coupled with the unresolved possibility that witchcraft may have been done on him since doctors could not help him, it is likely that Serge will continue to experience sickness and that he will continue to seek treatment for the sundry symptoms he experiences, particularly if he fails to secure work which challenges his physical and intellectual prowess.

Esperanza

Biomedicine has not alleviated Esperanza's condition either. She suffered from excruciating headaches, and like Serge, she feared she was going crazy. Esperanza, short, pug-nosed, and with bleached hair, had five children and was separated from her husband. She reported that for the past three years she was having screeching pains and ringing in the head and *cerebro* that made her want to vomit. She had no relief from the pain even when she fell asleep for a few hours. When her pressure was low, her heart stopped beating and her hands were numb. She forgot everything, walking in a zigzagging way, and felt dizzy. Esperanza was convinced that she was going mad like one of her brothers, who "used to take his shoes off and run in the street naked in the middle of the night." The diarrhea she experienced did not concern her, however. Subsequently, she also reported to me that she was having pains in the kidneys (that is, lower back) and her body was feeling swollen. Her nerves attacked her and she couldn't do anything; she felt lazy. Because of her sickness and nerves she could not work, yet when she worked she felt fine. The medicine the hospital physician prescribed alleviated the headaches intermittently, but she continued to feel sick when I saw her on the first home visit.

Esperanza had seen several physicians and a psychiatrist. None, including the Salud Hospital physician, succeeded in relieving her affliction. One doctor told her she had fever in her brain, while the Salud Hospital doctor did not tell her anything. He referred her to Neurology but there, too, they had not told her what was wrong since they had not ordered any studies and they could only guess what was the matter with her. All she was told was, "Some little thing was coming out of my head, and the blood was not flowing right in my head" because of nerves and because of her husband's beatings. The medication the hospital physician gave her had not helped her in the least, nor had the standard teas she took for nerves. She had no money to purchase the prescription ordered by the neurologist.

Prior to the hospital visit Esperanza was seen by a psychiatrist and also by a woman doctor. Both had told her that her problem was due to lack of sexual activity. Esperanza did not agree because she used to vomit as well and because she was not in the mood for having sex when she was this sick. Esperanza claimed she was given hormone injections to curb her sexual desires. After her visit to Salud Hospital, she went to a traditional healer, who instructed her to pray. He gave her some holy water to sprinkle in her house, but she continued to feel the same, perhaps because she lacked faith or because when she lived in her mother-in-law's house with her husband she had seen the devil. The devil, in a long cape, with hair standing on end, used to follow her when she went to work at a restaurant and it made her shiver and pray. She also had nightmares in which her sons were sinking and she could not rescue them; also, a dog wanted to bite her. Her heart "went tum tum" and then "I was back with my husband in the house and I woke up happy."

Esperanza tried hard to understand why she was sick. She gave various reasons for her malady: because her womb was removed three years earlier, because she had no money, because her husband's mistress was performing witchcraft on her, because of the beatings she had received from her ex-husband, because she saw the devil owing to her husband's running around with many women, because she was not working, and because she had no food to eat.

Esperanza, the fourth of eleven children, arrived in Mexico City with her parents when she was eight years old; at age seventeen she married and she went to live with her in-laws until three years earlier. She had a nice house and a car, and she worked in her husband's business as a cashier. Her husband, however, used to beat her, and she cried when she recounted how one time he kicked her in her vagina, and he and her mother-in-law called her a "whore." Six years before, her husband left her and her children for another woman. She was very angry, but she continued to live with her in-laws. Four years ago he returned and made her pregnant again, but he also brought another woman to live in the house. She was thrown out by the husband a year later. In any event, she could not bear watching the other woman coming and going in the house. She took four of her children, including the baby. She left her oldest son, then fourteen years old, with the husband. The boy was turned against her and she never saw him, adding to her woes.

At first she felt good when she left her in-laws' house and she no longer "made angers" as when her mother-in-law frightened and mortified her; but soon after she left, she fell ill and also started drinking. She stopped drinking soon after because the alcohol made her feel very sick.

Esperanza rented a two-room dwelling with a tin roof and earthen floor, set off from the outside courtyard by a piece of cloth. She shared the dwelling with another woman and her two small children. The house, located in Neza, was situated in a courtyard containing a pigsty, an outhouse, and a water faucet. On the day I visited her, there was no food in the house. Esperanza received a minimal subsidy for her children from the government (about 50 U.S. cents a day per child), and her father-in-law gave her a weekly allowance (about $5). After separating from her husband, she worked for her sister and then as a waitress on the midnight shift in a restaurant located three hours away from where she lived. She had made no attempt to find another man because she had young daughters (ages ten and eight) and she was afraid a strange man would molest them, as one of the teachers in the school had done.

Despite her terrible poverty Esperanza participated in a rotating savings club and the funds she received when her turn came provided her with a down payment on a piece of land in a newly developing district of Neza where electricity and water were still unavailable. She continued to participate in the savings club and built up sufficient cash in order to build a cinder block room on her land.

When I saw her a few months later she was feeling much better and looked extremely well. She had just returned from her waitressing job, for which she was being paid $10 a week. She also sold fancy clocks that her husband made and gave her to sell on commission. Esperanza reported that she was attending a Spiritualist temple, where she was told she had a gift for healing and was put into training to become a healer. She was feeling extremely happy. All her disturbances were gone, especially the headaches. A friend had introduced her to the temple and she acquired a spirit protector. She attended the temple once a week where she entered into a trance, which was like "getting an injection of anesthesia and the body becomes elevated and one sees a strong light."

Esperanza was at first very conflicted about joining the temple because it was against the Church's teachings and like her mother, she was an orthodox Catholic; however, since people who went to the temple believed in the Virgin Mary, she did not think it was wrong to go there.[2]

When I saw Esperanza two months later in her new dwelling on the outskirts of Neza, she was living in her newly constructed, doorless, cinder block room. She cooked outside with driftwood. She could not take a job because she could not leave her ten-year-old girl by herself since her "breasts were ripening and there were a lot of drug addicts who rape little girls." She supported herself and her four children by selling cake crumbs that she bought from a bakery for pennies and resold to children who usually ate them for their evening meal. She felt perfectly well. She attended a new temple in the neighborhood where she got "spiritual vitamins injected by spiritual intravenous injections." She had gone to doctors, but her disorder was not alleviated until she joined the temple. She no longer believed that her headaches were due to witchcraft, only to the fact that they were a sign from God for her to become a curer. She knew now that witchcraft did not exist. (Belief in witchcraft is usually against Spiritualist teachings.) Significantly, while Esperanza continued to live in extraordinary poverty, she nevertheless felt fully recovered because her life had been transformed by Spiritualist healing in ways that biomedicine was unequipped for and incapable of changing. She had been incorporated into a new group and given new dignity by becoming a healer herself.

Above and beyond her abysmal poverty, Esperanza's case suggests that her illness engaged her in constant anger, moral indignation about her husband's infidelity and abandonment, and the fear that she was a victim of witchcraft. The Spiritualists eliminated her anger and restructured her life and beliefs, including her conviction that she was being bewitched. In Esperanza's own words, "In the hospital all I got was pills and nobody tried to enter my head with Xrays to see what was there. Spiritualist had entered my head" by announcing to her that she had "a gift for healing" and she possessed a spirit protector, giving her a new dignity and self-esteem.

Thelma

Thelma had recovered only partially when I visited her at home. She had four sons and was separated from her husband. She was deeply pained by her estranged husband's conduct. Soft-spoken, with long braided hair and sad eyes, Thelma was experiencing pains in her whole body, head, and *cerebro*, and in the "lungs." She had a bloated stomach and she lacked energy.

Thelma fell ill four years earlier, when she "made a very strong anger" because her husband left her for another women. She had seen many private physicians and physicians at government health centers. She came to Salud Hospital so she would get an Xray to learn what was wrong with her. All the doctors had given her was a lot of medications, some of which had made her feel "just a little better," but then she felt sick again, especially when she "made an anger." She took teas for nerves because her husband told her she was suffering from nerves and that she was crazy. She kept searching for the right medicine, or the vitamins she knew would alleviate her ailment.

Thelma resided in Neza in a house that had two rooms and to which additional rooms were gradually being added for her twenty-four-year-old son, who recently came from her parents' home in her native village to live with Thelma.

Thelma, the second of three children, was born in a small village north of Mexico City, and not until she came to Mexico City, when she was twenty-one years old, had she learned to speak Spanish well. She was engaged to a man in her village and gave birth to a son, but the man beat her and she refused to marry him. She left her child with her parents and came to work as a maid in the city, but she missed her mother very much. She escaped three times from her job. When she was twenty-five years old, she married a man, who had asked for her hand, in civil and religious ceremonies, and she stopped working. For the first two years she was very happy with her husband.

Thelma had two teenaged sons and an eight-year-old boy, but she wished she had a daughter. She had stopped menstruating two years earlier. Four years earlier Thelma converted to the Seventh Day Adventist church because the priests in church never explained anything, the Virgin did not speak and she was not a Mexican; she was Spanish and the Spanish had killed many people when they came to Mexico. She also converted to give her children a better education, meaning that they would not drink or take drugs and be told to be afraid of evil spirits. She ceased going to the temple when her sons refused to attend it anymore.

Thelma tried hard to make some sense of her sickness, and in every conversation she stated that she would like to know why she was sick, why she had a pain in the *cerebro*, why she was feeling pain in her body, and why she had no energy. She attributed her infirmity to the fact that her children disobeyed her, to her husband not providing any support for her children, his preventing her from leaving the house to work, and to all the angers she had made, which caused dryness in her mouth, pain in the *cerebro*, and insomnia. She knew that her lungs hurt because she had worked hard all her life. It could also have been, she mused, because she was suffering from nerves following a tubal ligation. She did not agree with the doctor that she was sick because she had an infection and because her spine was deviated. One woman suggested that she was being bewitched, but she did not believe in witchcraft: "Only ignorant people believe in that but maybe a bad spirit had intruded on me."

Unlike her children, she always obeyed her parents. When they told her to go to the mill she did; when they sent her to pasture the animals she did. But her children would not listen to her. She could not understand why her children would not obey her since she knew that their disobedience was the real cause of her sickness, coupled with the angers that her husband had caused her to make because he beat her, and because of the sadness she felt. She had summoned her husband to the district's authorities on two occasions demanding support, which he finally gave her, but the money was insufficient to feed her and her sons.

According to Thelma, her husband wanted to remove her from the house in which she lived and it made her angry. She claimed that the plot of land was paid with money her father had given her and the land was hers and not her husband's. In fact, she asked what she ought to do about her husband, who also set her children against her. He gave them money, sided with them even when they did not obey her, and they drank and smoked. Everybody had advised her to leave her husband, but she knew that he had a responsibility to her because she was his legal wife inasmuch as they were married in a civil ceremony.

Thelma supported herself with the money her husband gave her ($15 a week) and by selling chewing gum and bread from house to house. Her oldest son helped her as well, but she could not work because of her sickness and she hardly had enough to feed herself and her family.

On the first follow-up visit, Thelma reported she was feeling partially better. She had stopped making angers and her husband and children recognized her plight. Their recognition of her sickness made her feel better even though she continued to experience most of the symptoms for which she had sought treatment. On a second visit five months later, she was feeling sick again, saying, "I am bleeding with pain." She had made an anger and she was in bed for several days. She vomited. She had pain in her stomach and *cerebro*. A private doctor came to her house, and he told her children that they were making her sick. Her husband stopped coming to the house.

Following this visit I passed her house on several occasions but she was not home. On my last visit two months later, Thelma was still feeling tired. She was having pain in her "lungs" and in the *cintura*, but otherwise she reported that she was feeling quite well. Her hair was cut and she looked well. She stopped getting angry because "I am not at home." She was working as a washer woman on a daily basis. Her widowed mother, whom she always missed, was visiting her, and her son had brought his wife to live in the rooms that by now were almost completed.

She summoned her husband to the authorities again and he was ordered to give her a weekly allowance ($25). She ordered her two teenaged sons, who were using drugs, to leave the house. About a month before, she stopped taking the various medications she had been prescribed, but when she had pain in the *cerebro*, she took vitamins and an analgesic.

Thelma had been treated for parasites, which no doubt were temporarily eliminated with the medicines she was prescribed by the various physicians. However, she regarded her disturbances as related to her family problems with her husband and children, which she did not relate to the physician, and not to the spinal column, as she was diagnosed. Thelma is a spunky woman, as evidenced by the number of times she had summoned her husband to the authorities. But her great poverty and her recalcitrant sons and husband presented her with a moral dilemma she was unable to reconcile. The sons disobeyed her and her husband failed to support her as her father had done her mother. She resolved the dilemma when she removed herself from the situation by working away from the home and ordering the sons out of the house. Thelma did not draw upon suspicions of witchcraft, in which she genuinely disbelieved, but she regarded her sickness as a test God gave her.

Thelma, like many other women in this study, was trapped in the belief that a man's prerogative was to dominate her; she as a woman was required to be submissive and her husband's duty was to financially take care of her and her children. Her husband, however, had not conformed to the tacit covenant. He did not take care of her, which unleashed angers that made her, like the other women, sick and impeded her recovery. In Thelma's case the local authorities rectified the situation in a just way by compelling the husband to give her financial support. Thelma gained a new self-respect that was visible in her bearing and which was also instrumental in the partial alleviation of her disturbances.

Nomi

Nomi, as we saw, was treated in Salud Hospital by the attending physician in his routine way with Maalox and a diet regimen based upon her symptomatology of abdominal and kidney pains, not unlike other patients in the study. Unlike the other women, who had embodied life's lesions in their "lungs," upper backs, heads, and in their entire bodies, Nomi's lesions became embodied in her kidneys, setting her on an extraordinary course in search of therapy that I will describe only briefly here.

Nomi whose mode of dress--a long skirt and scarf covering her graying long hair--signaled that she was a member of an Evangelical Protestant Church (Pentecostal), came to the hospital in order to have tests done so that she would know what was wrong with her. She reported that she had stomach problems and she had been told by one woman that amebas were dangerous "because they could enter my brain." She believed her stomach was upside down because her intestines hurt and she also experienced pain during sexual intercourse. She could not eat any food and the sickness did not permit her to attend to her children because she required sleep all the time.

Nomi's pains had begun fifteen years previously, immediately following the death of her grandmother, who had raised her, and the birth of her fifteen-year-old son. At that time she also took her husband to the authorities because he used to beat her terribly from the first night of their marriage. The disturbances, including pain in the kidneys and a burning sensation on urination, intensified five years before when she also experienced incessant diarrheas. She believed that she was ailing from a very serious condition, possibly cancer.

Prior to her visit to Salud Hospital, Nomi managed her condition by seeking treatment from numerous private physicians, health centers, and by administering herbal remedies. Physicians had diagnosed her disorder variously as anemia, kidney infection, animals in her stomach, hemorrhoids, vaginal ailment, and fallen bladder because she wet her pants when she coughed. Numerous medications, ovules, injections, and pills had been prescribed for her, none of which alleviated her disturbances and most of which had made her even more sick. To reposition her stomach in its right place she drank a mixture of garlic and milk on an empty stomach, but it did not make her feel better, nor did the bottle of olive oil (the customary remedy for "twisted intestines"), which only produced nausea.

A year before, a doctor from a health center had referred her to a psychiatrist because she had felt disoriented and depressed due to the fact that her husband had not given her any money for daily subsistence and she was feeling too much pain in her kidneys to enable her to work. When she told the psychiatrist that she had pain during sexual intercourse, the doctor told her that it was because she did not love her husband; she agreed that she might not love him, but she knew that she also had an infection. The female psychiatrist also told her that she was sick because she wished to attract her husband and mortify him and her children. She told the psychiatrist that her husband had caused her much suffering and that she worked very hard for her children. She said to herself that she did not need a psychiatrist.

Nomi and her family lived in their own four-room house in Neza, encircled by a courtyard cluttered with junk, together with her husband's two sisters and a sister's mute daughter. Nomi was raised by her paternal grandmother because she and her older brother were abandoned by their mother when Nomi was eight years old. When she was thirty years old, she met her mother for the first time. She explained to Nomi that the reason for her abandonment was that her father was a drunkard.

At sixteen Nomi married and on that day, "I regretted having been born because my husband beat me a lot and my sisters-in-law were very bad to me; they were always angry that I went to see my mother [her grandmother]." She bore seven children and, not wanting any more children despite the fact that "my husband wished to see me always pregnant," induced an abortion by lifting heavy crates and drinking various teas. The teas she had taken to "remove all the garbage from my insides" made her very sick, and she required medical treatment for this problem as well.

When I first met Nomi, she sold garlic in the markets and was able to keep her earnings for herself. Subsequently, her husband, who sold shirts in a market for a wholesale merchant, asked her to assist them; she could then no longer keep her earnings since she had to turn them over to her husband.

Nomi was born into the Pentecostal faith and she was a devout temple-goer. She did not believe in witchcraft. It was against the teachings of the Bible. The people in the temple helped her out financially when she was unable to go out selling because of her sickness. The only time she felt no pain was when she came before the alter of the temple and sang hymns, which "fill my soul with great joy. I forget my suffering and I have no pain then." She went to the temple daily to sing in the chorus.

While Nomi's husband did not drink and he was not a womanizer, he beat her. Her distressing relationship with her husband, who did not believe she was really sick and who would not give her any money to meet her household expenses, was a recurrent theme of Nomi's narrative. She found various means of getting money without her husband's knowledge, such as selling shirts for a higher price than what she reported to him and keeping the difference.

Five years earlier, Nomi had left her husband, after he beat her and she kicked him in return. She went to live with her brother, who called the authorities. They, together with her mother-in-law, intervened and she returned to her house with her children. Since then her husband had not beaten her.

Nomi variously attributed her sickness to the fact that as a child she used to carry heavy boxes with fruit and "we ate the rotten merchandize," to the dust in Neza, to the fact that she had to go out daily to the market to help her husband fold and sell shirts and carry heavy boxes, to her erratic eating schedule, to the bad spirits that roam around in the air and enter people's bodies when they are not prepared for God, and to her being like Job, upon whom God sent sickness to test her to see if she could endure the suffering.

While Nomi was feeling better on her second visit to the hospital, at the time of my first visit to her home she continued to feel sick. She did not agree with the doctor that she had animals in her body; she knew that her problem was with her urine because she had to run to the bathroom all the time and because one doctor had told her that she had a kidney dysfunction. Regardless of her disagreement with the Salud Hospital physician's diagnosis, she attempted to keep to the diet the doctor had prescribed. At first she began feeling better in her stomach; she even went back to work and "I could scold my children." However, she could not keep up the diet because it was too expensive and she could not afford to buy apples and fish with the allowance her husband gave her ($2 a day). Besides, the money she earned she needed for her children's school supplies. Furthermore, with that diet she lost more than 20 pounds in less than two months and she was beginning to look gaunt. She also worked very hard taking care of her children and doing laundry, and the diet did not sustain her energies.

A week after I saw her at home, she returned to the hospital for her scheduled appointment. However, two days earlier she had gotten very sick and, by chance, someone had referred her to a homeopathic doctor, who also treated her with "needles" (presumably acupuncture). To her relief the doctor told her that with the exception of chiles, she could eat everything. She terminated the diet and medication the Salud Hospital physician had prescribed because she had no confidence in that doctor. She wanted to have tests done on account of the foam that was coming out of her urine, but on the return visit the doctor ordered her to follow his original regimen of Maalox and the prescribed diet.

After weekly visits to her home, I found her in only four months after my last visit. As I arrived her husband was standing in front of the house and he immediately remarked to me smilingly that Nomi was going to die. She had a kidney removed two weeks earlier in a government hospital in Neza; she needed a transplant for her other kidney and he was not going to give her his. I found Nomi in bed accompanied by her mother-in-law who came to visit her from the village. Nomi recounted that she had improved briefly with three acupuncture treatments, but then she felt the pains in her kidneys again and she was treated in the health center in Neza, where she was diagnosed as having gastritis. An Xray was ordered that disclosed that she also had kidney stones.

Her entire kidney was removed. She showed me a jar containing the kidney stones that were removed. In her words, "My kidney was like a quarry pit." The operation was performed without her consent, however. She was told that her second kidney was equally laden with stones and she would need to have a kidney transplant; she would not consider it under any circumstance.

In fact, had she realized that her kidney would be totally removed she would never have consented to the operation.

She continued to have excruciating pain in her right side on urination, diarrhea, and difficulties breathing. She had been taking herbal medicine, including black radishes that were more costly than the medications, prescribed to her by a merchant in the market devoted to traditional medicinal cures. Subsequently, she embarked on an extraordinarily lengthy and poignant odyssey in search of a cure for the remaining kidney that took her to a Spiritualist healer, who failed to alleviate her condition. In her temple they prayed for her, and she also went to a health center where she was given capsules that made her urinate "six liters of water daily." She felt terrible. She gained access to a Social Security hospital with the help of her husband's boss, but there, too, the physicians were unable to do anything for her. She traveled to another state, where she was incorrectly informed that some foreigners had brought a machine that would "smash the stones" in her remaining kidney. She was referred to a private hospital in Mexico City, where she was told that there was a machine that "would crush the stones without an operation," but that the treatment would cost the peso equivalent of about $25,000, a sum that she could not even fathom. Finally, she was referred to yet another hospital, where she was charged $5,000, which she borrowed from her husband's boss, for "crushing her stones."

She had two treatments, and after each treatment she felt like vomiting. She wondered whether the treatment would not harm her because when they put these rays through her body, "All the doctors were protected by dark glass, behind screens." On these grounds, she reasoned the rays must be dangerous. She planned on continuing with the treatments nevertheless, and while she was still feeling sick she even traveled with her coreligionists to another city to celebrate Easter.

When I visited her two weeks later, one of her children informed me that she had gone to have some analyses done. A week later, she still was not home, but a neighbor informed me that Nomi had gone to work with her husband.

Just as life's lesions cannot be minimized embodied in Thelma's pain, so too Nomi's bodily lesions, by which her life was encompassed, cannot be played down. Nomi, like the other women, was besieged by angers emerging out of her constant struggle with her husband about support, and by the fact that her body was ravaged by him as well as by the physicians who had removed her kidney without her knowledge. The operation altered her body but it failed to alter the meaning of her experience of suffering. She was encircled by contradictions related to being an abused wife, which became imprinted in the lesions of her kidneys, and which in turn became aggravated by her quest to maintain her body intact. One cannot but wonder whether this indomitable woman will ever succeed in having her bodily lesions transformed by the treatment of "rays that were bombarding my body" or whether this treatment would also change the meaning of her existence, leading to full recovery.

Not all women's pains are embedded in contradictions engendered by oppressive marital relations. There are women whose husbands do not beat them and with whom they enjoy an egalitarian relationship, "the way it ought to be," but normative obligations of their roles are nevertheless oppressive to them, as was the case of Mary. Mary had a warm relationship with her husband but recovered from her bodily pains and headaches when she worked in the fields of California as an undocumented worker and she could do things for herself.

Sharon, whom we had met in Chapter 7, reported partial recovery. As Sharon's headaches embodied her isolation from her family that became aggravated when her closest friend left the city. She was relieved to learn from the physician that she was not suffering from anemia, which she took to be a very serious disorder. After numerous visits to the hospital the physician succeeded in alleviating her major concern, but his treatment model cannot alter Sharon's isolated existence, living locked in a house with a strange family with whom she has no exchanges other than about "what she would cook on a given day."

By way of conclusion, it is noteworthy that while patients associate their sickness with their lived experience, paradoxically and not uncommonly they associate positive treatment outcomes with the physician's management of their condition, as we saw in the last chapter. This is the case whether they have been prescribed medications, whether they have been questioned extensively by the physician, whether they have been ordered analysis and other technological tests, and whether they were referred to specialists. The patients' expectations of cure turn on the resolution of the drama in the medical consultation. In this sense, the medical consultation sets the recovery agenda for patients. As I pointed out previously, people clearly distinguish between treatment as palliatives and as cure when their pains merely subside on taking medication and when their pains have disappeared. When they have ceased to take the medication and their pains have been completely alleviated, they have been fully cured. What is not often recognized by physicians and patients is that a cure requires transformations of the body and the embodied conditions in life's lesions.

Similarly, while many physicians may recognize the role of life's lesions in producing sickness, they do not learn about the intricacies of the patient's suffering for which their armamentarium of remedies lacks cures. Physicians assume the responsibility for patients' recovery. Steered by the biomedical paradigm, the treatment outcome and the correctness of their diagnosis are attributed to the medication, divorced from the patient's life experience. If patients fail to recover, the blame falls on patients' noncompliance with the treatment or on an ontological state of nerves.

Paradoxically, both the power and the weakness of the biomedical model rest on the fact that it appropriates for itself the responsibility for a cure. By so doing, it exercises the power of structuring expectations for patients and attributing its failures to patients' psychophysiological attributes, such as nerves or somatization. Patients fail to perceive recovery because biomedicine ignores a major requisite for sickness resolution that is entrenched in the alterations of patients' day-to-day lives and in the resolution of contradictions in which patients are enmeshed, the very conditions that may have also precipitated the sickness episode.

In comparison, Spiritualist healers confer responsibility on the patient for his or her recovery, they resolve some profound contradictions for their patients, and in some cases they also transform their lives. In those instances they succeed in alleviating the patients' condition. A comparison between the two healing regimens is the concern of the next chapter.

Notes

1. There is a common belief that madness is caused by somebody giving the person food to eat and, in fact, people are frequently cautious about eating at others' homes.

2. Coincidentally, Esperanza joined the same movement I studied previously (1985); for a detailed discussion of the dilemmas people face when they join the Spiritualists, and how Spiritualist healers effect cures, see Finkler 1985, especially the case of Chucha.

PART FOUR

Two Systems of Healing

12

A Comparison Between Sacred Healing
and Biomedicine

The study of biomedical practice in Mexico ceded fresh insights into Spiritualist healing, which I had studied for many years. In turn, my work on Spiritualist healing illuminated biomedical practice in ways that I had not anticipated.

For the most part, physicians regard Spiritualist healers as "quacks," whereas Spiritualist healers see benefits in biomedicine and may refer patients to physicians. Yet, while the two regimens seem diametrically separated, they are joined by the people who resort to them, for, to reiterate a point made previously, when biomedicine fails to heal, patients often resort to alternatives, such as Spiritualist healing, setting the two regimens in a complementary relationship.

Because my study of Spiritualist healers and their patients was carried out in a rural sector and the present investigation was done in Mexico City, the two populations are not completely comparable.[1] They are situated in disparate ecological zones and differ along occupational lines; the rural population was primarily peasants supplementing their subsistence with wage work, while the Mexico City population was predominantly proletarian, or petty merchants dependent solely on cash for a livelihood.

Biophysicians are constantly compared to folk healers.[2] Because I was a participant and observer of both healing systems, using similar methodologies, my studies reveal similarities and dissimilarities between a secular and a sacred healing which broaden the grasp of the two and the differential impact they have on patients' responses to each and on the healing process. Such a comparison sheds light on the strengths and weaknesses of each.

On first glance, the reader may wonder if a comparison is even warranted considering the disparate epistemologies, practices, methods of recruitment, and nature of personnel. Even a synoptic view of Spiritualist healing reveals that the two regimens differ along most dimensions, especially since the former is embedded in a sacred context while the latter is sanctioned by secular science. Biomedicine is a professional system, staffed by professionals with many years of formal training and legitimized by the state. Spiritualist healers are folk practitioners, lacking any formal academies, academic preparation, and state legitimation. They are typically denigrated by the medical and academic establishment.

Spiritualist healing forms part of a widespread dissident religious movement (Finkler 1981, 1983, 1985, 1986). It recruits its membership largely by ministering to the sick. Generally speaking, healers are recruited into the healing role through their own sickness. The usual trajectory is for patients to seek biomedical treatment; when it fails to alleviate the disorder, they turn to a Spiritualist temple, usually on the recommendation of a person who had been treated in a Spiritualist temple. There, a healing spirit possessing the body of the healer informs some patients that they possess a gift. With this declaration the patient is in effect recruited into the Spiritualist movement. He or she is ordered into training for the role of healer or other temple functionary, depending upon God's designation.

Mexican Spiritualists tame spirit forces (spirits of the dead) roaming the universe and harness them for the good of mankind. They come to possess the bodies of the healers chosen to minister to the sick. Spiritualist curers heal in trance and they resort to a wide variety of healing techniques, including an extensive pharmacopoeia, ritual cleansings, purgatives, massages, baths, spiritual surgeries, trancing, religious ritual, and "passive catharsis." In some cases they transform the person's life when he or she is incorporated into a religious community (Finkler 1985), as in the case of Esperanza. In day-to-day practice, Spiritualist healers, like physicians, are not especially concerned with etiological explanations. Generally speaking, they subscribe to etiological beliefs shared by all Mexicans, with one notable exception. The group that I studied denounces the existence of witchcraft. It is believed that afflictions which stubbornly resist both biomedical and even Spiritualist ministrations must have been caused by the intrusion of a recalcitrant spirit that requires taming in the service of healing mankind, or must be removed from the body.

Putting aside some important differences between the two regimens that I will delineate shortly, I also note similarities. Patients seek symptom elimination from both. They present complaints to Spiritualist healers in much the same way as they do to physicians, and in the same way as biomedicine focuses on the body (Pellegrino and Thomasma 1979), so too Spiritualist healers address their ministrations to bodily discomforts, with one interesting exception. Biomedical consultations frequently focus on issues related to sexuality, whereas this subject is never addressed to or by Spiritualist healers, except for vaginal discharges. In the medical setting, marital relations often become expressed in problems of sexuality, as we saw in the case of Nomi, for instance. Patients confronting Spiritualist healers discuss male-female relations in terms of rights and obligations.

Both biophysicians and Spiritualist healers sustain a dualistic view of the body and its attendant disturbances, contrary to the culturally constructed holistic view of sickness. While the literature focuses on biomedical dualism, it is frequently overlooked that a similar dualism prevails between the body, "the material," and the spirit in sacred healing such as Spiritualism. The notion of dualism is basically contrary to the Mexican holistic conception of the body as an extension of one's day-to-day experience.[3] The distinction between corporeal (that is, "material") and "spiritual" is clearly delineated in Spiritualist diagnostic categories in much the same way as biophysicians distinguish between organic and psychological sickness, or nerves.

Moreover, there are structural, if not contextual, similarities between both Spiritualist healers and physicians in their encounters with patients. In both regimens the patient takes the role of a passive recipient of the healer/doctor's ministration. Both attend to the patient's bodily ills. It could be argued that in this instance Spiritualist healers replicate in a religious idiom biomedicine's secular practices, given biomedicine's hegemony.

But unlike in Salud Hospital, where consultations take place in relatively private surroundings, reflecting the individualist cast of biomedicine, in Spiritualist temples many healers sit in the same room, each receiving patients separately. Consequently, there is a cacophony of sounds in Spiritualist healing places that imparts a sense of a communal experience, unlike in the hospital, where the physician-patient interaction takes place either in isolation or with onlookers confined to students, nurses, and occasional visitors.

Both physicians and Spiritualist healers wear the same white robes which symbolically separate them from their patients. Spiritualist healers sit in trance with expressionless faces, eyes closed, holding or stroking the patient as he or she stands before the healer, briefly murmuring a description of his or her disorder. By contrast, during the medical consultation, the physician and patient sit facing each other, and their physical contact is limited to the physician's physical explorations by palpation and auscultation. Physicians' affective expressions vary. Some constantly smile at the patient, while others maintain a serious demeanor.

In their desire to know what is wrong with them, patients expect to have their bodies examined and their insides seen. Both physicians and healers attempt to look inside the patient's body, the former with technological apparatuses and the latter with the gaze of the spirits. According to Spiritualist healers and their patients, the healing spirits penetrate the body of their patients in order to ascertain what is wrong with them. The spirits proclaim their omniscience, and patients are not even required to say very much, often to the patients' relief. The spiritual gaze exerted by the healers' spirits parallels patients' expectations for technological management that enables physicians, in the words of various patients, "to look inside my body" in order to make a correct diagnosis. However, while the physician may often undergo a personal struggle and juggle available resources in deciding whether or not to utilize the technology, the spirit's gaze is routine and intrinsic to Spiritualist healing. As I suggest elsewhere (Finkler 1985), the patient experiences a "passive catharsis" as the healer tells the patient what the patient is experiencing, eliminating the need for the patient's active participation.

Like the medical gaze that extends its power beyond the patient's body, coming to dominate the life of members of a society and reinterpret their experience (Armstrong 1983; Foucault 1975; Turner 1984), Spiritualist healing encompasses the lives of those patients whom it succeeds in converting into adherents. For adherents, their bodies become extensions of the Spiritualist congregation upon which they become totally dependent (Finkler 1985, 1986), and this also forms part of the cure. Participation in the Spiritualist movement exerts power on the patient's existence because, as many patients readily admit, if they fail to attend to the various rituals and to heal others, they will revert to their morbid states.

Furthermore, patients respond positively to the physical examination given by the physician, as they do to the tactile communication in the Spiritualist healer-patient encounter, when the healer massages and cleanses the patient's body. This suggests that tactile communication between patient and healer has a therapeutic effect (Finkler 1985).

Within the physician- and healer-patient encounters there are individual differences among both with regard to the advice they each give to patients concerning life's problems. Some Spiritualist healers dismiss any social interaction problems, such as difficulties with a mate or child, while some physicians dispense advice in these domains.

Both Spiritualist healers and physicians in Salud Hospital "deworm" patients. The former almost always prescribed a purgative (Phillips Milk of Magnesia was especially favored in one temple) for all patients, and the latter frequently prescribed antiparasitic medication for a similar purpose.

Interestingly, Spiritualist healers do not necessarily devote more time to their patients than do physicians. Physicians may spend on an average about twenty-one minutes with a first-time patient, whereas the Spiritualist healer-patient interaction usually lasts less than half that time. The affective content of the interaction varies. Some Spiritualist healers and physicians were relatively brusque and indifferent to a patient's suffering, while others expressed concern and compassion. Folk healers are, nevertheless, frequently idealized in the literature. Their efficacy is regarded as residing in their relationship with the patient and their attributes of empathy, compassion, friendliness, and warmth; their personalistic and holistic approach to the patient is usually contrasted with the impersonal and disinterested biophysician.

It has been argued that the folk healer-patient relationship, in contrast to the doctor-patient interaction, is based upon shared etiological understandings and congruent explanatory models (Fabrega and Silver 1973). Mexican Spiritualists, however, do not always share their patients' explanatory models or etiological understandings. For instance, Spiritualist healers deny the existence of witchcraft, but by the time many patients come to seek treatment from Spiritualist healers, they are convinced that witchcraft has been performed on them. Similarly, most Mexicans do not believe that sickness is brought about by spirit possession, as Spiritualist healers do.

If folk healers of the Spiritualist kind are no more sympathetic to their patients than physicians; if they, like physicians, advance a dualism of body and mind that is contrary to the patients' etiological understandings, how do they differ from biomedical physicians? What makes them attractive as an alternative health care resource?

I have explored the psychological, cultural, physiological, and sociological levels by which Spiritualists succeed in healing patients elsewhere (Finkler 1985). The study of biomedicine illuminates some differences between biomedicine and alternative healing of the Spiritualist type that I postulate as significant in influencing people's great attraction to Spiritualist healing when biomedicine fails. Setting aside the fact that patients seeking Spiritualist healing avoid having to deal with bureaucratic hassles, most important, the Spiritualist healers' diagnostic repertoire and etiological explanations are relatively limited when compared with biomedicine's.

Spiritualist healers confer a coherent system of explanations usually reduced to environmental or spiritual assaults. Spiritualists eschew multiple diagnosis and there is usually a consistency among different healers regarding diagnosis, treatment, and etiology.[4] On the other hand, patients seeking treatment from physicians receive various diagnoses for the same symptoms from different physicians (Helman 1985; Koran 1975), giving rise, from the patient's perspective, to a lack of coherence. This leaves patients confused and befuddled about the nature of their disturbances, and wondering which physician's diagnosis is correct. Significantly, patients would often ask Spiritualist healers to verify physicians' diagnoses as a way of making sense out of them. Patients attempt to make sense of their sickness using both their own intuitive comprehensions and the diagnoses they had been given by various physicians, confounding their understanding of their condition.

The drama that entails the doctor-patient relationship is minimized in the healer-patient association. While clinical judgment often entails uncertainty and is grounded in a process of exclusion, spirit protectors treat patients with great *certainty*. Spiritualist healers are as sure of their diagnoses and courses of cure as patients are certain of their pain. Significantly, too, while the physician must cast the patient's sickness within a temporal frame, the omniscient and omnipotent spirits transcend time and space in the same way as the patient's sickness transcends time. The patient does not confine the onset of the affliction to a specific time but rather as he or she experiences it: timeless. The patient need not tell the healer very much for the healer to know everything, while the physician must question the patient, anchor the condition, and locate it in time and in a specific part of the body. Not unsurprisingly, patients welcome the physician's questioning, which assures them the physician will learn about their malady, a knowledge the spirits possessing the healers already have.

Moreover, while those recruited into the medical profession are usually particularly healthy individuals, those recruited into Spiritualist healing had experienced an affliction before becoming healers. The Spiritualist healer experienced pain, whereas the doctors, in most cases, had not. By converting the sick person to a health provider, Spiritualist healers furnish an example of the potentiality for recovery using Spiritualist ministrations and convincingly convey to the patient that they have grasped the patient's anguish through their experience. The person of the doctor cannot provide the patient with experiential evidence, as a Spiritualist healer does, that his ministrations induce a transformation from being sick to healing others.

Importantly too, the physician's treatment repertoire is relatively limited to medication, or in extreme cases, surgery. On the other hand, Spiritualist healers involve patients in various treatment activities that effectively engage them in their recovery. In keeping with this point, while physicians take full responsibility for the patient's successful cure, if not their failure to heal, Spiritualist healers assign responsibility to the patient for his or her cure, further involving the patient in his or her recovery; Spiritualist healers do not recognize failure.

Perhaps the most crucial difference between biomedicine and sacred healing is the fact that Spiritualist healers resolve contradictions for patients that biophysicians cannot if they are guided by the biomedical model. Patients seeking treatment from Spiritualist healers usually were led to consider the possibility that witchcraft had been performed on them. Spiritualist healers categorically denied this possibility. With the cleansings they provide a patient, they symbolically remove evil that may have befallen the patient, resolve the dilemma, and restore order into the patient's life, even if only temporarily.

While the technological management for which patients clamor carries a heavy symbolic load and no doubt aids in perceived recovery, the cleansings Spiritualist healers furnish are powerful symbols that address the profound contradictions in which the illness is embedded. Not surprisingly, of those patients who perceived themselves recovered as a result of Spiritualist healing, most attributed it to the cleansings they had received. Whereas patients may disagree with the treatment course proposed by physicians for medication, patients always agree with the Spiritualist treatment, especially when it involves ritual cleansings, coupled with herbal remedies and other ministrations.

There is yet another important dimension to the Spiritualists' denial of witchcraft: When they deny witchcraft as the source of affliction, they remove the blame for the patient's disorder from a neighbor, relative, or other persons with whom the patient interacts, and they place it squarely on the work of impersonal spirits for which the patient cannot be blamed.

On the other hand, biomedicine does not address the contradictions in which patients are enmeshed, nor can it help them. To explain sickness, the biomedical model may blame impersonal "animals" or pathogens having attacked the body, explaining the sickness in generalized terms rather than in terms of the patient's personal suffering. Or, it blames the patient himself or herself, especially poor habits (McKeown 1979). Biomedicine often requires patients to alter customary behavior such as diet, work, or drinking habits. It does not, however, attempt to transform the circumstances of a patient's life in the way Spiritualist healing does by incorporating the individual and sometimes even his or her family into new interpersonal networks or by placing the person in a new relationship with God. In the latter instance, relationships with other human beings become secondary to interaction with God, as was the case of Esperanza, for example. Biomedicine does not address the existential dilemmas. It does not reinterpret them, give them new meanings, or change the social relationships in which the patient is embedded, including those between husband and wife.

In the final analysis, Spiritualist healers, like biophysicians, fail to heal their patients (Finkler 1985) when they fail to attend to the patient's life world with the attendant contradictions and requisite transformations. We may thus conclude that to succeed in resolving non-life-threatening, subacute conditions, a healing system must address the patient's bodily ills and concurrently transform the patient's life's lesions by altering his or her perceived existence.

One last point merits noting. Much attention has been given to the doctor-patient relationship in biomedical practice. It has been assumed that the doctor-patient relationship, regarded as so important in biomedicine, is similarly significant between patient and sacred healer. Yet, as we have seen, only certain aspects of the doctor-patient relationship tend to influence the healing process in biomedical practice.

The proposition is advanced that the emphasis on the doctor-patient encounter in biomedicine represents a Western bias for several reasons (Finkler 1986a, 1986b). First, the emphasis placed on the role of the health practitioner, his or her personality, and expression of concern for patients may reflect the modern person's yearning for personalistic affective ties (Berger et al. 1974) and for compassion in an impersonal industrial world that, it is believed, seems to have existed and exists in nonindustrial societies. Second, the psychotherapeutic tradition has focused on the individual (Orlinsky and Howard

1975), fostering the notion that the therapeutic process is rooted in the physician-patient relationship itself (Haley 1963). The psychoanalytic model of the therapeutic relationship has been extended to biomedical practice. In fact, Wilson (1963) suggested that "although sensitive physicians have for centuries been alert to the importance of their interpersonal bond with the patient as an element in the course of illness and recovery, the self conscious examination of the bond is characteristically a modern concern" (285). According to Wilson this view emerged out of Freudian therapeutics, especially out of the notion of transference (Wilson 1963).

My argument is that biomedical practice relies greatly upon patient management during the therapeutic encounter because its healing techniques lack means to resolve the contradictions by which the patient is encompassed, to deal with the patient's subjective experience, or to reorder the patient's life. For this reason treatment hinges not only on healing techniques and underlying etiological understandings but on the encounter itself and the physician's personality.

In Spiritualist healing, the healer-patient encounter is secondary to the healer's techniques which aid patients in restructuring conflicts in which they may be entangled. For those patients who eventually become adherents, Spiritualist healing reorders their existence by incorporating them into a community of sufferers who share a satisfying religious reality and symbolic meanings. It also reorders the male macho role, promoting smoother marital relationships.

The emphasis on the role of the individual healer effecting a cure of the individual patient is modern Western society's bias, wherein the individual has become an atomistic unit. Fostering the drama of the consultation is the model of the doctor-patient relationship that reflects the prevailing ethos of the abstract, independent individual confronting a self-interested, autonomous physician during the encounter. The individual in Mexico is not solitary. He or she is embedded in a family and a moral order that engages the person with others in a continuing process of evaluating day-to-day existence, and in conflicts that must be resolved to influence perceived recovery. Spiritualist healing, for example, addresses issues of evil and witchcraft, and of culpability, and it reorders social relationships, especially those with one's mate (Finkler 1981), which biomedicine fails to do.

One last point needs to be made. Paradoxically, as a folk healing movement, Spiritualist beliefs exert little hegemonic force in Mexico on a national scale. But by transforming patients' existence through incorporation into a community of individuals spiritually healed, Spiritualist ministrations have promoted, on an aggregate level, religious pluralism in Mexico. Spiritualism thereby contributes to advancing social change by mobilizing a sizeable population and fomenting a growing movement that furnishes Mexicans with new options for religious participation. However, the

Spiritualist movement fails to restructure Mexican society in ways that could benefit its participants economically or politically (Finkler 1986). On the other hand, biomedicine, by treating individual bodies without transforming people's lives, fails to contribute to new social forms on an aggregate level. It succeeds only in maintaining its hegemony as the major authorized provider of health care with legitimation by the state.

Notes

1. For this reason I do not present the statistical findings comparing patient-perceived treatment outcomes.

2. For bibliography see Finkler 1985, 1986a, 1986b. Also see a formal economic analysis done by Lenihan (1990). She compared the cost-effectiveness of Spiritualist healers using the data reported in Finkler (1985) and in this book.

3. There is a profound conceptual difference between "mind" and "spirit" which, however, cannot be explored here.

4. I have demonstrated elsewhere (Finkler 1984) the high percentage of agreement among healers about etiology (85.7 percent) and prescribed remedies (61.1 percent).

13

Conclusion

The dual task of this endeavor has been to elucidate how a system of knowledge, specifically biomedicine, developed in one society becomes translated in another, and how patients respond to its treatment. We explored the history of biomedicine and its practice and explored the multifaceted aspects of Mexican existence in which sickness is played out. We saw that contrary to the commonly held canons, biomedicine is not uniformly practiced across cultures. I have proposed a model of biomedical practice which suggests that some biomedical domains are anchored in the culture in which they are embedded and in the individual practitioner's beliefs. Others retain an international cast. Biomedicine in Mexico is practiced along the lines of a worldwide biomedical model that focuses on the body and its anatomical lesions and depends chiefly upon pharmacological treatments. Diagnostic assessments employ international nosologies and nomenclatures. Importantly, we must conclude that since clinical reasoning is culturally and individually shaped, diagnoses fail to signify similar ailments universally. Hence, it must not be assumed that the labels physicians give to sickness experienced by patients in one society are analogous cross-culturally.

The materials I presented reveal that patients' perceived responses to treatment interventions are not solely dependent upon biomedical ministrations of bodily lesions or the medical encounter, but on a concatenation of factors that encompass an individual's life's lesions, ignored by the biomedical model. Biomedicine's comprehensions guide Mexican physicians to disregard a patient's life's lesions, of which they nevertheless are cognizant as private individuals. Biomedicine challenges biophysicians' traditional beliefs and intuitive knowledge as Mexicans and conflicts with their professional role as doctors. They must negotiate conflicts with themselves to accommodate to the biomedical paradigm that defines their identity as physicians. Biomedical practitioners draw upon cultural etiological understandings; concomitantly they are constrained by the biomedical model. They reinterpret the patient's suffering in a biomedical way by reducing it to physiological categories that are largely amoral evaluations of the individual's distress. In contrast, Mexican cultural etiological understandings encompass individual existential experiences that become especially manifested in typical presenting symptoms.

It would be erroneous and shortsighted to surmise that practitioners in other cultures are simply ill-prepared for their tasks because they do not practice medicine in the same way as we know it in the United States. The transplantation of biomedicine to Mexico creates a struggle for its practitioners between the doctor's intuitive knowledge as a Mexican and the pathophysiological model of disease that he or she has been taught. The doctor's sense of sickness, reinforced by his or her patients' understandings, carries a moral baggage, and is rooted in a cultural space. The result of the doctor's negotiated efforts reduces extrasomatic experience to biomedical categories such as the nervous system, psychosomatic problems, or stress. In so doing, the physician substitutes finely tuned existential meanings for meaningless, amoral, generalized categories such as stress, and concurrently accommodates to cultural beliefs that view experience as shaping the body's ailments. The structuration process emerging out of the physicians' struggle molds local beliefs that in turn also shape biomedical beliefs on a macrolevel within the cultural context of which it is part.

Several paradoxes encompass this conflict. Physicians in most industrially developing nations must confront the struggle between technological and clinical management of affliction as modern technology radiates throughout the world and human beings develop a commitment to it. Technological management of sickness gives rise to patients' expectations of clinical management; it also carries a symbolic load. However, with existing economic restraints, physicians rely upon clinical symptomatologies to make their diagnoses. In an industrialized society such as the United States, technological management of sickness is being questioned, but in industrially developing countries such as Mexico, patients clamor for it. Misplaced patients' expectations bear on patients' perceived outcome: Those patients who had received technological management tended to attribute recovery to it.

Moreover, reliance on diagnostic technology denies patients their unique symptomatologies with their attendant cultural and personal meanings. When the physician translates the patient's symptoms in biomedical terms, he or she transcends the patient's experience and his or her moral sensibilities, in which the sickness is embedded. Mexican physicians know that the patient is an extension of his or her family and that the anger and nerves patients experience are as much rooted in the body as they are in moral evaluations of the social and economic environment about which the physician, in his or her role as a physician, can do little, to the frustration of some doctors.

Related to this point, physicians must struggle with the recognition of failure. Kleinman has argued that traditional healers heal because they must; they cannot fail (Kleinman and Sung 1979). Arguably, the claim could be made for traditional healers, but it is more compelling for practitioners of biomedicine. The hegemonic belief permeating Mexican society is that biomedicine must work, and its aura of competence has taken on mythological proportions. Yet, while physicians cannot take full responsibility for either patients' perceived recovery or perceived failure to recuperate, biomedicine is accountable for promoting a model of sickness of the body torn away from space and time in which the patient and his or her sickness are entrenched.

Paradoxically, while Mexican physicians depend on patients' symptomatology to make their diagnoses, they are unwilling to accept patients' reports of unsuccessful treatment outcome. In fact, physicians insist to their patients, verbally or by intonation, that they are feeling better.

Besides, the Mexican physician, as an employee of the state, is in a structurally disadvantageous position; his or her authority as a physician is eroded by his or her subservience to the bureaucratic apparatus of the state. In fact, physicians and the various state institutions in which they work must compete amongst themselves for limited state resources. Such competition tends to splinter rather than foster professional identification, and the absence of such identification promotes idiosyncratic clinical judgments. The Mexican physician's status, flowing as it does from employment by the state, also opens the way for alternative systems to flourish when physicians' ministrations fail. My observations support the notion that physicians have less influence on their patients than do Spiritualist healers, for example.

While Spiritualist healing techniques utilize well-entrenched healing symbols and address moral issues of culpability, good, and evil, the physician must depend either on technological management or on his or her person encompassed by the doctor-patient relationship. Physicians are caught in the further dilemma that, lacking the technological tools to gaze inside the body of the patient, they lack the legitimacy of Spiritualist healers to see through the body by means of the spirits that possess the healers' bodies. Biomedical technology and the diagnostic process shoulder a symbolic load, yet they are new and alien symbols that fail to touch profoundly at the person's innards, as, for instance, Spiritualist healing does. Spiritualist healers confer responsibility on the patient for his or her recovery, rely on well-established symbols, resolve profound contradictions for their patients, and in some cases also transform their lives. In these ways they succeed in alleviating the patient's condition when biomedicine fails.

The findings of this study point to specific aspects of the doctor-patient encounter that influence the resolution of a sickness, such as those revolving around the physician's explanation of what is wrong with the patient. Yet we were left to wonder about the reasons why so much attention has been given to the doctor-patient relationship in biomedical practice. I addressed this question by suggesting that biomedicine, as practiced in contemporary times, is embedded in Western individualism. Its concern is with the solitary individual, as can be readily discerned from the dyadic relationship between the practitioner and the solitary patient who meet during the medical consultation. The dyadic relationship retains its international cast and physicians must depend on "managing" patients. When his or her technical armamentarium, in tandem with its symbolic significance and prescribed pharmacological treatments, fails to heal, physicians must nurture a personal relationship with the patient, if biomedicine is to retain its credibility.

But why does the drama of the medical encounter fail to have a successful resolution? Why do physicians fail to heal? I proposed that to understand sickness and the recovery process, it is necessary to simultaneously unravel sociodemographic and socioeconomic conditions, aspects of the doctor-patient relationship, and a person's lived experience. In this context it is essential to delve into the dilemmas a human being embodies in sickness (see also Helman 1987). To perceive him- or herself recovered, a human being must transmute his or her perceived existence. Spiritualist healers alter a patient's existence by incorporating them into a new community, removing the inconsistencies revolving around beliefs in witchcraft, and culpability, and by attributing sickness to impersonal spirit forces. The medical model fails to furnish the physician with techniques to alter the patient's extrasomatic existence or embodied contradictions, thereby heightening the drama of a medical consultation.

A Mexican physician lacks in his or her therapeutic kit a technology instrumental in changing a patient's life, other than through altering the symptoms, in the way Spiritualist healers do when they incorporate patients into their social environment and alter family dynamics. As I have argued elsewhere (Finkler 1985), Spiritualist healers are as helpless as physicians in successfully resolving a patient's sickness when the conditions of their patients' lives fail to change. The change, however, need not be implemented by a religious experience per se. It is not Spiritualism itself or any other religious movement but the process of changing the existential conditions and resolving contradictions with which the patient is confronted that is central to the healing process.

The paradoxes are a product of an amalgam of forces that include a society's history and socioeconomic conditions concomitant with its ideological beliefs. I have identified various extant contradictions in Mexico, such as those between belief and disbelief in witchcraft and between being an angry person, which at once protects against and makes one sick. Such complex conflicts are rooted not only in capitalism itself (Marx 1974; Wolf 1982), but in historical processes.[1] In Mexico, with the domination of Catholicism, and perhaps more important, with the hegemony of positivism imported from Europe during the nineteenth century, witchcraft beliefs were denigrated, as they are at present. Contemporarily, to believe in witchcraft is to be "primitive" and "ignorant," a characterization all Mexicans eschew. Yet, belief in malfeasance absolves the individual from culpability for his or her sickness.

Certainly, advances have been made by biomedicine in dealing with complex and life-threatening conditions, but on a day-to-day level they often fail to eliminate or even alleviate a patient's sickness. Scholars have recognized that "attempts to limit the scope of medicine to physical derangements fail to take into account psychological and psychosomatic illness" (Siegler 1981:630). To follow Siegler's assertion is to dichotomize the individual, separate his or her psychic from his or her physical ailments, and to overlook life's lesions, an inimical existential milieu, and the contradictions embodied in sickness.

It is frequently argued that in practical terms physicians cannot do their job as physicians and also ascertain and deal with transforming the patient's life's lesions. It is not incumbent upon a physician to carry out an anthropological analysis and get at a patient's anatomical and life's lesions for recovery to take place. Undoubtedly, a physician must know not only the physiology of the human body but also the anatomy and physiology of the "social body" that will give him insights to the nature of the contradictions a patient may be experiencing, contradictions promoted by social processes and cultural ideologies. Most important, it requires an understanding of the *unity* of anatomical and life's lesions, both of which are revealed by patients during the presentation of symptoms when they speak of bodily pain, typical symptoms, and etiology, such as "I have made an anger." Knowing that men and women are differentially confronted by contradictions and life's lesions, a physician can eschew the "just nerves" diagnosis that reduces the patient's suffering to a generalized entity such as "stress."

To know the cultural forms of symptomatic presentation and their attribution is to know that they communicate life's lesions. When patients in Mexico tell a physician that they have "made an anger," they inform the doctor that their lesions were shaped by an adverse interpersonal experience or moral indignation, as much as by any parasites which may have invaded their bodies. If these were incorporated into the medical history, it would facilitate a more accurate diagnosis and ease the physicians' goal to heal their patients.

As social scientists we must seek the universals of sickness and recovery by attending to their uniqueness. While sickness and recovery comprise a composite of sociodemographic and environmental conditions, aspects of the medical encounter, medication, and subjective meanings and contradictions generated by sociocultural and historical processes, the specific nature of these constituent elements will vary cross-culturally. Generally speaking, North Americans are not faced by contradictions bearing on beliefs in witchcraft, but they must, like Mexicans, resolve contradictions relevant to failure to achieve economic success in the face of an ideology of equal opportunity (Rubin

1976). Americans, like Mexicans and contemporary peoples the world over who recognize historicity and change, must confront generational conflicts, although the nature of parent-child relations differs between the two societies.

Our task then, is to develop models of universal processes of subjective meanings and extant and emerging contradictions, in much the same way as biomedicine has attempted to identify universal categories of disease entities, and to consolidate these into a model of human sickness, recovery, and medical practice to which this study has attempted to contribute.

Notes

1. It is even possible that contradictions form part of the human condition emerging as unintended consequences of social processes and human production of cultural forms (Finkler 1986).

Appendix

Methodology

The methodology employed in the study has been noted at various junctures relevant to the overall discussion. I described the ways in which the data were gathered for the investigation both in the hospital and in home interviews in the Preface and Part I of the book. We learned the ways in which subjects were selected for the study sample of physicians and patients, and the types of instruments used to get at the materials discussed.[1]

I selected Salud Hospital because it was one of the largest in Mexico City and it serviced a large and diverse patient population, which met with the sampling requirements. The Internal Medicine outpatient clinic was selected for study for several reasons, including the fact that it had the largest pool of patients from which to select the study sample. Moreover, after having sat with the preconsultation physicians for several weeks before patients were selected for interviews, I found that persons referred to the Internal/General Medicine service reported *non-life-threatening, sub-acute disorders*, and similar symptomatologies as those in the Spiritualist temple, allowing for comparison of patient-perceived response to treatment between the two populations.

I envisioned the initial interview with patients as brief so as not to detain them unnecessarily. As noted before, a specially designed interview schedule was administered during the first interview to get sociodemographic profile (sex, age, marital status, household composition, education, age of children, employment, explanatory models (Kleinman 1980), including patients' perceptions of their problems and causality, illness management, and a life events scale developed by Patrick (1982). Also, a health questionnaire was administered to get a standardized baseline of the study group's symptomatology.[2] These instruments were pretested on ten patients randomly selected in the hospital, and as a result they were modified in several ways. For example, to elicit the patient's understanding of the cause of the symptomatology, every time a patient responded that he or she was experiencing a particular symptom elicited by the CMI, the response was followed by the question, "Why do you believe you have it?"

As we began interviewing patients at the hospital, it quickly became apparent that with few exceptions, patients responded with extensive narratives to most questions. Consequently, first interviews were tape-recorded, yielding an unanticipated rich data base and allowing for validation of the information elicited by the interview schedule. For example, on both initial and home interviews, patients were asked about illness management prior to the hospital visit, and what had provoked the illness concomitant with etiological beliefs. In all cases there was full correspondence between the information given during the first and home interviews.

Patients were randomly assigned to the attending physicians. The seventeen physicians who treated the patients in the study sample were the focus of the study of medical practice. All physicians supplied the diagnosis, attributions, and results of analyses. In addition, hospital records for each patient were checked to verify the results of the various analyses ordered by the physicians and the diagnosis that was entered in the medical record.

Added to the fifty-two-item specially constructed interview schedule administered during the second interview, the CMI was administered again. When patients reported that they were no longer experiencing a symptom to which they had responded "yes" or "sometimes" on the first interview, they were asked to what they attributed alleviation or elimination of the symptoms. Also, a five-question social support instrument measuring perceived social supports developed by Fleming (1982) was administered.

It is noteworthy that some patients lacked explanations for attributions of sickness and recovery. In those instances more than any other, social scientists must resort to anthropologically informed analytical tools. A point that merits emphasis is that the use of multiple techniques, including ethnographic, phenomenological, and in-depth observation combined with quantitative analysis and hypothesis testing—in this instance, postulated variables influencing onset of a sickness episode and patient-perceived recovery—aids in offsetting deficiencies in any one type of methodology.

All my encounters with patients in the home, in the hospital, and during the medical consultations were taped and transcribed. All transcriptions were checked by two individuals independently. Data elicited from the first and home interviews and from the medical consultations were coded by two independent coders, checked by a third person, and spot-checked by me. All coded data were entered into a Lotus file and checked independently by two individuals. Frequencies were established using the Lotus program. The transcribed materials and intensive observation comprised the large corpus of materials for qualitative analysis.

Notes

1. Space does not permit me to report all the data gathered using the various instruments and traditional anthropological techniques, especially the 205 descriptions and narratives of patients. I recorded patients' life histories, which have led me to the conclusions presented in the book. Nor can I present 800 observations of medical consultations and the over 400 verbatim transcriptions of medical encounters with the patients who comprise the sample group.

2. The Cornell Medical Index was selected because I had used it previously (Finkler 1985) and it would permit me to compare the patterns of symptomatologies of the rural and patient population elsewhere.

References

Abramson, J.H.
1966 The Cornell Medical Index as an Epidemiological Tool. American Journal of Public Health 56(2):187-298.

Ackerknecht, Erwin H.
1967 Medicine at the Paris Hospital 1794-1848. Baltimore: The Johns Hopkins Press.

Acuña, Daniel López
1978 La Salud Desigual. Nexos 7:13-16.

Adams, Richard N., and Arthur Rubel
1967 Sickness and Social Relations. In Handbook of Middle American Indians, Vol. 6. Austin: University of Texas Press, pp. 333-356.

Aguirre Beltran, Gonzalo
1982 A Germàn Somolinàs d' Ardois. *In Memorium* In Historia de La Medicina en México. Tomo II by Francisco de Asis Flores y Troncoso, pp. VII-XXIX.

Almy, Thomas P.
1980 The Healing Bond. The American Journal of Gastroenterology 73(5):403-407.

Alvarez Cordero, Rafael
1986 La Red Hospitalaria Metropolitana. Uno Más Uno. September 19.

Alvarez, Ruben
1987 Abatida La Calidad De La Atención Médica: Oliva López. La Jornada. October 25.

Anderson, W. Timothy, and David Helm
1979 The Physician-Patient Encounter: A Process of Reality Negotiation In Patients, Physicians and Illness. E. Jaco (ed.). New York: Free Press, pp. 259-271.

Antonovsky, Aaron
1980 Health, Stress and Coping. San Francisco: Jossey-Bass.

Armon-Jones, Claire
1986 The Thesis of Constructionism. In The Social Construction of Emotions. Rom Harré (ed.). Oxford: Basil Blackwell, pp. 32-56.

Armstrong, David
1977 Clinical Sense and Clinical Science. Soc, Sci. and Med. 11:559-601.
_____1982 The Doctor-Patient Relationship: 1930-1980. In The Problem of Medical Knowledge. P. Wright and A. Treacher (eds.). Edinburgh: Edinburgh University Press, pp. 109-122.
_____1983 The Political Anatomy of the Body. Cambridge: Cambridge University Press.
_____1984 The Patient's View. Soc. Sci. and Med. 18:737-744.

Atkins, Paul
1975 Training for Certainty. Soc. Sci. and Med. 9:949-956.

Austin, Alfredo López
  1980 Cuerpo Humano E Ideologia. México: Universidad Nacional Autónoma De
  México.
Austin, Alfredo López, and Carlos Viescca Trevino
  1984 Historia General De La Medicina En México. Tomo I México Antiguo.
  Universidad Nacional Autónoma De México.
Báez, Guadalupe
  1988 Durante El Presente Sexenio Han Disminuido Cerca De 40 por Cento Los
  Gastos En Servicios De Salud. Uno Más Uno. June 13.
Balint, Michael
  1964 The Doctor, His Patient and the Illness. New York: International University
  Press.
Barragan Mercado, Lorenzo
  1968 Historia Del Hospital General De México. México: Edicion Lerner.
Barsky, Arthur J.
  1979 Patients Who Amplify Bodily Sensations. Annals of Internal Medicine
  91(1):63-70.
  _____1981 Hidden Reasons Some Patients Visit Doctors. Annals of Internal
  Medicine 94(Part I):492-498.
Battle, C., et al.
  1966 Target Complaints as Criteria for Improvement. American Journal of
  Psychotherapy 20:184-192.
Bedford, Errol
  1986 Emotions and Statements About Them. In The Social Construction of
  Emotions. Rom Harré (ed.). New York: Basil Blackwell, pp. 15-31.
Ben-Sira, Zeev
  1976 The Function of the Professional's Affective Behavior in Client Satisfaction: A
  Revised Approach to Social Interaction Theory. Journal of Health and Social
  Behavior 17:3-11.
  _____1980 Affective and Instrumental Components in the Physician-Patient
  Relationship: An Additional Dimension of Interaction Theory. Journal of Health and
  Social Behavior 21:170-180.
Benson, H., and Epstein. M.D.
  1975 The Placebo Effect: A Neglected Asset in the Care of Patients. Journal of the
  American Medical Association 232:1225-27.
Berger, Peter, et al.
  1974 The Homeless Mind. New York: Vintage Books.
Berkman, Lisa F.
  1984 Assessing the Physical Health Effects of Social Networks and Social Support.
  Annual Review Public Health 5:413-432.
Berkman, Lisa F., and Lester Breslow
  1983 Health and Ways of Living. New York: Oxford University Press.

Berliner, Howard
1975 A Larger Perspective on the Flexner Report. International Journal of Health Services 5:573-591.

Birley, J.C.T., and J. Connolly
1976 Life Events and Physical Illness. In Modern Trends in Psychosomatic Medicine. Oscar Hill (ed.). London: Butterworth.

Bizzarro, Salvatore
1981 Mexico's Poor. Current History 80:370-373, 393.

Blumer, Dietrich, et al.
1980 Systematic Treatment of Chronic Pain With Antidepressants. Henry Ford Hospital Medical Journal (Detroit) 28:15-21.

Bolton, Ralph, and Michel Sue
1981 Health and Wealth in a Peasant Community. In Health In the Andes. Joseph W. Bastien and John M. Donahue (eds.). Washington: American Anthropological Association, pp. 196-223.

Brady, Grace
1986 Medical Technology Policy. In The Adoption and Social Consequences of Medical Technology. Sociology of Health Care: Vol. 4. Greenwood: Jai Press, pp. 147-183.

Britton, Mona, et al.
1980 Patient Benefits from Medical Measures: Results in an Outpatient Clinic for Internal Medicine. Soc. Sci. and Med. 14A:481-484.

Brody, Howard
1987 Stories of Sickness. New Haven: Yale University Press.

Brody, Howard, and David B. Waters
1980 Diagnosis is Treatment. The Journal of Family Practice 10(3):445-449.

Brook, Robert
1977 Quality: Can We Measure It? New England Journal of Medicine 296:170-172.

Brown, George W.
1974 Life Events and the Onset of Depressive and Schizophrenic Conditions. In Life Stress and Illness. Springfield: Charles C. Thomas, pp. 163-188.
_____1974a Meaning, Measurement and Stress of Life Events. In Stressful Life Events. Barbara Snell Dohrenwend and Bruce P. Dohrenwend (eds.). New York: John Wiley and Sons, pp. 217-244.

Brudon, Pascale
1987 Medicamentos Para Todos En el Año 2000? México: Siglo Veintiuno Editores.

Calnan, Michael
1988 Lay Evaluation of Medicine and Medical Practice: Report of a Pilot Study. International Journal of Health Services 18(2):311-322.
_____1988a Toward a Conceptual Framework of Lay Evaluation of Health Care. Soc. Sci. and Med. 27(9):927-933.

Caplan, A.L., H.T. Englehardt, and J.J. McCartney
  1981 Concepts of Health and Disease: Interdisciplinary
  Perspectives. Reading, Mass.: Addison-Wesley.
Cardenas de la Peña, Enrique
  1976 Historia de la Medicina en la Ciudad de México. México: Coleccion
  Metropolitan.
Cassell, Eric J.
  1976 The Healer's Art. Philadelphia: J.B. Lippincott.
  _____1976a Disease as an "It": Concepts of Disease, Revealed by Patients'
  Presentation of Symptoms. Soc. Sci. and Med. 10:143-146.
  _____1982 The Nature of Suffering and the Goals of Medicine. The New
  England Journal of Medicine 36(11):639-645.
Chávez Rivera, Ignacio
  1984 La Atención a La Salud En México En El Campo De La Medicina Internal En
  Los Ultimos 40 Años. In La Evolución De La Medicina En México Durante Las
  Ultimas Cuatro Décadas. Ramon De La Fuente et al. (eds.). México: El Colegio
  Nacional, pp. 259-275.
  _____1987 México En La Cultura Médica México: Fondo De Cultura Economica.
Cicourel, Aaron V.
  1981 Notes on the Integration of Micro-and Macro-Levels of Analysis. In Advances
  in Social Theory and Methodology. K. Knorr-Cetina and A.V. Cicourel (eds.).
  Boston: Routledge and Kegan Paul, pp. 51-80.
  _____1983 Hearing Is Not Believing: Language and the Structure of Belief in
  Medical Communication. In the Social Organization of Doctor-Patient
  Communication. Sue Fisher and Alexander Dundes Todd (eds.). Washington, D.C.:
  Center for Applied Linguistics, pp 221-239.
Cleaves, Peter
  1987 Professions and the State: The Mexican Case. Tuscon: University of
  Arizona Press.
Cobb, Sidney
  1974 A Model for Life Events and Their Consequences. In Stressful Life Events.
  B.S. Dohrenwend and B.P. Dohrenwend (eds.). New York: John Wiley and Sons,
  pp. 151-156.
Comaroff, J.
  1978 Medicine and Culture: Some Anthropological Perspectives. Soc. Sci.
  and Med. 12B:247-254.
  _____1982 Medicine: Symbol and Ideology. In The Problem of Medical
  Knowledge. P. Wright and A. Treacher (eds.). Edinburgh: Edinburgh University
  Press, pp. 49-68.
Comaroff, Jean, and Peter Maguire
  1981 Ambiguity and the Search for Meaning: Childhood Leukemia in the Modern
  Clinical Context. Soc. Sci. and Med. 15B:115-123.

Córdova, Alejandro, et al.

1988 La Salud En Crisis: Un Balance Sexenal/L. Semanal 7 De Febrero: 5-8.

Cosío Villegas, Daniel

1956 Historia Moderna De México, Vol. 3. La Republica Restaurada, La Vida Politica. México City: Hermes.

Crosby, Alfred, Jr.

1972 The Columbian Exchange. Westport: Greenwood Press.

Davis, Dona, and Setha M. Low

1989 Gender, Health, and Illness. The Case of Nerves. New York: Hemisphere Publishing Corp.

Day, R., et al.

1987 Stressful Life Events Preceding the Acute Onset of Schizophrenia: A Cross-National Study from the World Health Organization. Culture, Medicine, and Psychiatry 11(2):123-205.

Dean, Alfred, and Nan Lin

1977 The Stress-Buffering Role of Social Support. Journal of Nervous and Mental Disease 165:403-417.

Díaz, Bernal

1963 The Conquest of Spain. Baltimore: Penguin Books.

1987 Diccionano de Especialidades Farmaceuticas. 33 Edicion Mexicana.

Dohrenwend, Barbara Snell, and Bruce P. Dohrenwend 1974 Stressful Life Events. New York: John Wiley and Sons.

Dossey, Larry

1982 Space, Time and Medicine. New York: Random House.

Dumont, Louis

1971 Religion, Politic and Society in the Individualistic Universe.Proceedings of the Royal Anthropological Institute of Great Britain and Ireland for 1970. London: Royal Anthropological Institute, pp. 31-41.

_____1977 From Mandeville to Marx. Chicago: University of Chicago Press.

Dunlop, Derrick, and R.S. Inch

1972 Variations in Pharmaceutical and Medical Practice in Europe. British Medical Journal 3:749-752.

Eckenrode, John, and Susan Gore

1981 Stressful Events and Social Supports. In Social Networks and Social Supports. B. Gottlieb (ed.). Beverly Hills: Sage Publishers, pp. 43-67.

Eisenberg, Leon

1977 Disease and Illness: Distinctions Between Professional and Popular Ideas of Sickness. Culture, Medicine and Psychiatry 1:9-23.

_____1980 What Makes Persons "Patients" and Patients "Well"? American Journal of Medicine 69:277-286.

Elstein, Arthur, et al.

1978 Medical Problem Solving. An Analysis of Clinical Reasoning. Cambridge: Harvard University Press.

Engel, George L.

1977 The Need for a New Medical Model: A Challenge for Biomedicine. Science 196:129-136.

Englehardt, H. Tristram, Jr.

1975 The Concepts of Health and Disease. In Evaluation and Explanation in the Biomedical Sciences. H.T. Englehardt, Jr., and S.F. Spiker (eds.). Dordrecht: D. Reidel Publishing., pp. 125-142.

_____1976 Ideology and Etiology. The Journal of Medicine and Philosophy 1(3):256-268.

Evans, John R., et al.

1981 Health Care in the Developing World. New England Journal of Medicine 305:1117-1127.

Fabrega, Horacio, Jr., and Peter K. Manning

1973 An Integrated Theory of Disease: Ladino-Mestizo Views of Disease in the Chiapas Highlands. Psychosomatic Medicine 35:223-239.

Fabrega, Horacio, Jr., and Daniel B. Silver

1973 Illness and Shamanistic Curing in Zinacantan. Stanford: Stanford University Press.

Feinstein, Alvan R.

1967 Clinical Judgement. Baltimore: Williams and Wilkins.

_____1973 An Analysis of Diagnostic Reasoning. Yale Journal of Biology and Medicine 46:212-232, 264-283.

_____1983 An Additional Basic Science for Clinical Medicine: 1. The Constraining Fundamental Paradigms. Annals of Internal Medicine 99:393-397.

Felix, David

1977 Income Inequality in México. Current History 72(425):111-114, 136.

Fernández De Castro, Hugo

1988 El Diagnostico Fisiopatológico. Uno Más Uno Mayo 31.

_____1988 El Diagnostico General O Integral. Uno Más Uno Junio 14.

_____1988a La Exactitud En La Medicina Y La Infinitesimalidad Homeopatica. Uno Más Uno Junio 6.

Field, Mark

1971 The Health Care System of Industrial Society: The Disappearance of the General Practitioner and Some Implications. In Human Aspects of Biomedical Innovation. E. Mendelson et al. (eds.). Cambridge: Harvard University Press, pp. 156-180.

_____1976 The Modern Medical System: The Soviet Variant. In Asian Medical Systems: A Comparative Study. Charles Leslie (ed.). Berkeley: University of California Press.

Figlio, Karl

1982 How Does Illness Mediate Social Relations? In Problems of Medical Knowledge. Peter Wright and Andrew Treacher (eds.). Edinburgh: Edinburgh University Press.

Finkler, Kaja

1974 Estudio Comparative De La Economia De Dos Comunidades De México. Mexico City: SEP Ini Series, Institut Nacional Indigenista.

_____1978 From Sharecroppers to Entrepreneurs: Peasant Household Production Strategies Under the *Ejido* System of Mexico. Economic Development and Cultural Change 27:103-120.

_____1980a Land Scarcity and Economic Development: When is a Landlord a Client and a Sharecropper His Patron? In Agricultural Decision Making. Peggy F. Bartlett (ed.). New York: Academic Press, pp. 265-286.

_____1981 Dissident Religious Movements in the Service of Women's Power. Sex Roles 7(5):481-495.

_____1981a A Comparative Study of Health Seekers: Or, Why Do Some People Go to Doctors Rather than to Spiritualist Healers? Medical Anthropology 5:383-424.

_____1983 Dissident Sectarian Movements, the Catholic Church, and Social Class in Mexico. Comparative Studies in Society and History. An International Quarterly 25(2):277-305.

_____1984 The Nonsharing of Medical Knowledge Among Spiritualist Healers and Their Patients: A Contribution to the Study of Intra-cultural Diversity and Practitioner-Patient Relationship. Medical Anthropology 8(3):195-209.

_____1985 Spiritualist Healers in Mexico. South Hadley, Mass.: Praeger, Bergin and Gravey Publishers.

_____1985a Symptomatic Differences Between the Sexes in Rural Mexico. Culture, Medicine and Psychiatry 9(1): 27-57.

_____1986 The Social Consequence of Wellness: A View of Healing Outcomes from Micro and Macro Perspectives. International Journal of Health Services 16(4):627-642.

_____1986a The Westernization of the Therapeutic Encounter. Paper prepared for the Joint Conference of British Medical Anthropology Society and the Society for Medical Anthropology, June 30-July 3.

_____1986b The Healer Patient Relationship in Sacred and Medical Contexts. Paper presented at Symposium on the Dialectic of Medical and Sacred Realities, organized by Thomas Csordas and Kaja Finkler. American Anthropological Association, Philadelphia, December 3-8.

_____1989 The Universality of Nerves. Health Care for Women International 8:115-123.

Fitzpatrick, Ray M., et al.

1983 Social Dimensions of Healing: A Longitudinal Study of Outcomes of Medical Management of Headaches. Soc. Sci. and Med. 17:501-510.

Fleming, Raymond, et al.

1982 Medical Influence on Several Key Points of Stress at Three Mile Island. Journal of Human Stress, September:14-21.

Flores Carbajal, Guillermo

1988 El Servicio Social En Facultad De Medicina. Seminario Diagnostico Facultad

De Medicina. Colegio Interdisciplinario De Profesionales y Academicos En Ciencias De La Salud.

Flores y Troncoso, Francisco De Asis
1982 Historia De La Medicina En México. México: Instituto Mexicano Del Seguro Social.

Foster, George M.
1953 Relationships Between Spanish and Spanish-American Folk Medicine. Journal of American Folklore 66:201-217.
_____1976 Disease Etiologies in Non-Western Medical Systems. American Anthropologist 78:773-782.

Foster, G.M., and B.G. Anderson
1978 Medical Anthropology. New York: John Wiley and Sons.

Foucault, Michel
1975 The Birth of the Clinic. New York: Vintage Books.

Fox, Renee C.
1980 The Evolution of Medical Uncertainty. Milbank Memorial Fund Quarterly/Health and Society 58(1):1-49.

Frankenberg, Ronald
1980 Medical Anthropology and Development: A Theoretical Perspective. Soc. Sci. and Med. 14B:197-207.
_____1986 Sickness as Cultural Performance: Drama, Trajectory, and Pilgrimage. Root Metaphors and the Making Social of Disease. International Journal of Health Services 16(4):603-626.

Freidson, Eliot
1962 Dilemmas in the Doctor-Patient Relationship. In Human Behavior and Social Process. Arnold Rose (ed.). Boston: Houghton Mifflin and Co., pp. 207-224.
_____1970 Profession of Medicine. New York: Harper and Row.

Frenk, Julio
1978 Cuadio Clinico De La Enseñanza Médica Mexicana. Nexos 1:21-24.

Fuente, Ramon, et al.
_____1984 La Evolución de la Medicina en México Durante las Ultimas Cuatro Décadas. México: El Colegio Nacional.

Gadow, Sally
1980 Body and Self: A Dialect. The Journal of Medicine and Philosophy 5(3):172-185.

Gaines, Atwood
1979 Definitions and Diagnoses. Culture, Medicine and Psychiatry 3:381-418.
_____1982 Cultural Definitions, Behavior and the Person in American Psychiatry. In Cultural Conceptions of Mental Health and Therapy. Anthony Marsela and Geoffrey M. White (eds.). Dordrecht: D. Reidel Publishing Co., pp. 162-192.

Garrity, Thomas
1981 Medical Compliance and the Clinician-Patient Relationship: A Review. Soc. Sci. and Med. 15E:215-222.

Geertz, Clifford
1973 The Interpretation of Cultures. New York: Basic Books.

Gereffi, Gary
1983 The Pharmaceutical Industry and Dependency in the Third World. Princeton: Princeton University Press.

Giddens, Anthony
1979 Central Problems in Social Theory: Action Structure and Contradictions in Social Analysis. Cambridge: Cambridge University Press.
_____1981 Agency, Institution and Time-Space Analysis. In Advances in Social Theory and Methodology. K. Knorr-Cetina and A.V. Cicourel (eds.). Boston: Routledge and Kegan Paul, pp. 161-174.

Gill, Derek G.
1976 Limitations Upon Choice and Constraints Over Decision Making in Doctor-Patient Exchanges. The Doctor-Patient Relationship in the Changing Health Scene. Eugene B. Gallagher (ed.). Washington, D.C.: U.S. Department of Health, Education and Welfare, Public Health Service, National Institute of Health. DHEW Publication No. (NIH) 78-183, pp. 141-154.

Glasser, Morton
1977 Psychiatric Cases in Family Practice: Analysis of Outcomes. Medical Anthropology 1:55-73.

Golden, Joshua, and George P. Johnston
1970 Problems of Distortion in Doctor-Patient Communication. Psychiatry in Medicine 1:127-149.

Gomez, Jaime Mendiola
1979 Historical Synthesis of Medical Education in Mexico. In Aspects of the History of Medicine in Latin America. J. Bowers and E. Purcell (eds.). New York: Josiah Macy, Jr. Foundation, pp. 88-96.

Gonzalez Casanova, Pablo
1980 The Economic Development of Mexico. Scientific American 243:192-204.

Good, Byron J., and Mary Joe D. Good
1981 The Meaning of Symptoms: A Cultural Hermeneutic Model for Clinical Practice. In The Relevance of Social Science for Medicine. Leon Eisenberg and Arthur Kleinman (eds.). Dordrecht: D. Reidel Publishing Co., pp. 165-196.

Gordon, Deborah
1988 Clinical Science and Clinical Expertise: Changing Boundaries Between Art and Science in Medicine. In Biomedicine Examined. M. Lock and D.R. Gordon (eds.). Dordrecht: Kluwer Academic Publishers.

Gorovitz, Samuel and Alasdair MacIntyre
1976 Toward a Theory of Medical Fallibility. Journal of Medicine and Philosophy 1:51-71.

Gortari, Elide
1980 La Ciencia En La Historia De México. México: Editorial Grijalbo.

Grady, Denise

  1988 Going Overboard on Medical Tests. Time. April 25:32-33.

Gutierrez, Gonzalo

  1986 Epidemiología Y Control De La Amibiasis En México. Archivos De Investigación Médica (Mexico) 17 (Suppl. 1):375-383.

————1987 Amibiasis Intestinal. Boletín Mensual Epidemiología 2(7):73-83

————1987a Personal communication.

Hahn, Robert, and Atwood Gaines

  1985 Physicians of Western Medicine: Anthropological Approaches to Theory and Practice. Dordrecht: Reidel Publishing.

Hahn, Robert A., and Arthur Kleinman

  1983 Biomedical Practice and Anthropological Theory: Frameworks and Directions. Annual Review of Anthropology 12:305-333.

Hahn, Steven R., et al.

  1988 The Doctor-Patient-Family Relationship: A Compensatory Alliance. Annals of Internal Medicine 109(11):884-889.

Haley, Jay

1963 Strategies of Psychotherapy. New York: Grune & Stratton.

Hall, Judith A., and Michael C. Dornan

  1988 What Patients Like About Their Medical Care and How Often They Are Asked: A Meta-Analysis of the Satisfaction Literature. Soc. Sci. and Med. 27(9):935-939.

Hampton, J.R., et al.

  1975 Relative Contributions of History-Taking, Physical Examination, and Laboratory Investigation to Diagnosis and Management of Medical Outpatients. British Medical Journal 2:486-489.

Harré, Rom

  1981 Philosophical Aspects of the Macro-Micro Problem. In Social Theory and Methodology. K. Knorr-Cetina and A.V. Cicourel (eds.). Boston: Routledge and Kegan Paul, pp. 140-160.

————1986 An Outline of the Social Constructionist Viewpoint. In The Social Construction of Emotions. Rom Harré (ed.). New York: Basil Blackwell, pp. 2-14.

————1986 The Social Construction of Emotions. New York: Basil Blackwell.

Hauser, Stuart T.

  1981 Physician-Patient Relationship. In Social Contexts of Health, Illness, and Patient Care. Elliot G. Mishler et al. (eds.). Cambridge: Cambridge University Press, pp. 104-135.

Haynes, Alfred M.

  1976 Medical Care and the Doctor-Patient Relationship. In the Doctor-Patient Relationship in the Changing Health Scene. Washington, D.C.: U.S. Department of Health, Education and Welfare, Public Health Service, National Institute of Health, DHEW Publication No. (NIH), pp. 78-183.

Helman, Cecil G.

1981 Observations from General Practice. Soc Sci. and Med. 15B:415-419.

_____1981 Observations from General Practice. Soc. Sci. and Med. 15B:415-419.

_____1985 Disease and Pseudo-Disease: A Case History of Pseudo Angina. In Physicians of Western Medicine. Robert Hahn and Atwood Gaines (eds.). Dordrecht: D. Reidel Publishing, pp. 293-332.

_____1985a Psyche, Soma, and Society: The Social Construction of Psychosomatic Disorders. Culture, Medicine and Psychiatry 9:1-26.

_____1985b Communication in Primary Care: The Role of Patient and Practitioner Explanatory Models. Soc. Sci. and Med. 20(9): 923-931.

_____1987 Heart Disease and the Cultural Construction of Time: The Type A Behaviour Pattern as a Western Culture-Bound Syndrome. Soc. Sci. and Med. 25:969-979

Henderson, Gail E., and Myron S. Cohen

1984 The Chinese Hospital: A Socialist Work Unit. New Haven: Yale University Press.

Hernandez, Rebeca Marin

1988 La Inasistencia Laboral Por Alcoholismo En 87 Causo Perdidas Por $400 Mil Millones. Uno Más Uno January 3:11.

Holmes, T., and M. Masuda

1974 Life Change and Illness Susceptibility. In Stressful Life Events. B.S. Dohrenwend and B.P. Dohrenwend (eds.). New York: John Wiley and Sons, pp. 45-72.

Horn, James

1983 The Mexican Revolution and Health Care, Or The Health of the Mexican Revolution. Latin American Perspectives 10:24-39.

Hyman, Martin

1972 Social Isolation and Performance in Rehabilitation. Journal of Chronic Diseases 25:85-97.

Idler, Ellen L.

1979 Definitions of Health and Illness and Medical Sociology. Soc. Sci. and Med. 13A:723-731.

Ingleby, David

1982 The Social Construction of Mental Illness. In The Problem of Medical Knowledge. P. Wright and A. Treacher (eds.). Edinburgh: Edinburgh University Press, pp. 123-143.

Ingman, Stanley, and A. Thomas

1975 Topics and Utopias in Health Policy Studies. The Hague: Mouton.

Inui, T., et al.

1976 Improved Outcomes in Hypertensions After Physician Tutorials. Annals of Internal Medicine 84:646-651.

Jennette, Bryan
  1986 High Technology Medicine: Benefits and Burdens. New York: Oxford
  University Press.
Jewson, N.D.
  1976 The Disappearance of the Sick-Man From Medical Cosmology, 1770-1870.
  Sociology 10:225-244.
Johnson, Mark
  1987 The Body in the Mind. Chicago: University of Chicago Press.
Jordan, Brigitte
  1983 Birth in Four Cultures. Montreal: Eden Press.
La Jornada. October 22, 1987 Medicinas Prohibidas En EU y Gran Bretana, De
  Libre Venta En México.
Kane, R.L., et al.
  1977 Relationship Between Process and Outcome in Ambulatory Care. Medical
  Care 15:961.
King, Lester S.
  1982 Medical Thinking. Princeton: Princeton University Press.
King, R.C.
  1987 Technology and the Doctor-Patient Relationship. International Journal of
  Technology Assessment in Health Care 3:11-18.
Kirmayer, Laurence J.
  1988 Mind and Body as Metaphors: Hidden Values in Biomedicine. In
  Biomedicine Examined. M. Lock and D. Gordon (eds.). Dordrecht: Kluwer
  Academic Publishers, pp. 79-93.
Kleinman, Arthur
  1978 Concepts and Models for the Comparison of Medical Systems as Cultural
  Systems. Soc. Sci. and Med. 12:85-93.
  _____1980 Patients and Healers in the Context of Culture. Berkeley: University
  of California Press.
  _____1986 Social Origins of Distress and Disease: Depression, Neurasthenia and
  Pain in Modern China. New Haven: Yale University Press.
  _____1988 The Illness Narratives. New York: Basic Books.
Kleinman, Arthur, and J. Gale
  1982 Patients Treated by Physicians and Folk Healers in Taiwan: A Comparative
  Outcome Study. Culture, Medicine and Psychiatry 6:405-423.
Kleinman, A., and L.H. Sung
  1979 Why Do Indigenous Practitioners Successfully Heal? Soc. Sci. and Med.
  13B:7-26.
Knorr-Cetina, Karin D.
  1981 Introduction: The Micro-Sociological Challenge of Macro-Sociology Towards
  a Reconstruction of Social Theory and Methodology. Advances in Social Theory and
  Methodology. K. Knorr-Cetina and A.V. Cicourel (eds.). Boston: Routledge and
  Kegan Paul, pp. 1-47.

Koran, Lorrin
1975 The Reliability of Clinical Methods, Data and Judgements. New England Journal of Medicine 293(13):642-646.

Korsch, Barbara, et al.
1968 Gaps in Doctor-Patient Communication. Pediatrics 612 (July-December):855-871.

Korsch, Barbara, and Vida Negrete
1972 Doctor-Patient Communication. Scientific American 227:66-74.

Kuhn, Thomas S.
1970 The Structure of Scientific Revolutions. Chicago: University of Chicago Press.

Kushner, Thomas
1981 Doctor-Patient Relationships in General Practice. A Different Model. Journal of Medical Ethics 7:128-131.

LaGuna, José
1984 La Enseñanza De Las Materias Basicas. In La Evolución De La Medicina En México Durante Las Ultimas Cuatro Decadas. Ramón De La Fuente et al. (eds.). México: El Colegio, pp. 65-72.

Laín Entralgo, P.
1982 Historia De La Medicina. Barcelona: Salvat Editores, S.A.

Lanning, John Tate
1985 The Royal ProtoMedicato: The Regulation of the Medical Profession in the Spanish Empire. Durham, N.C.: Duke University Press.

Latour, B., and S. Woolgar
1979 Laboratory Life: The Social Construction of Scientific Facts. Beverly Hills: Sage Publishers.

Leder, Drew
1985 Medicine and Paradigms of Embodiment. Journal of Medicine and Philosophy 9:29-43.
_____1990 The Absent Body. Chicago: The University of Chicago Press.

Lenihan, Bonnie J.
1990 The Economic Development Implications of Informal Sector Health Care. A Dissertation Presented for the Ph.D. The University of Tennessee, Knoxville.

Levi-Strauss, Claude
1967 The Effectiveness of Symbols. In Structural Anthropology. Garden City: Anchor Books, pp. 181-201.

Levy, Robert
1984 Emotion, Knowing and Culture. In Culture Theory. Richard A. Shweder and Robert A. LeVine (eds.). Cambridge: Cambridge University Press, pp. 214-237.

Levy, Rona
1983 Social Support and Compliance: A Selective Review and Critique of Treatment Integrity and Outcome Measurement. Soc. Sci. and Med. 17(18):1329-1338.

Lieban, Richard

1976 Cebuano Sorcery. Berkeley: University of California Press.

Lindsey, Malcolm I., et al.

1976 Quality-of-Care Assessment I: Out-Patient Management of Acute Bacterial Cystitis as a Model. Mayo Clinic Proceedings. SI:307-312.

Linn, Lawrence S.

1975 Factors Associated with Patient Evaluation of Health Care: Milbank Memorial Fund Quarterly/Health and Society 53:531-548.

Lock, Margaret M.

1977 An Examination of the Influence of Traditional Therapeutic Systems on the Practice of Western-Style Medicine in Contemporary Japan. Presented at the Annual Meeting of Asian Studies on the Pacific Coast. Eugene, Oregon. June.

_____1980 East Asian Medicine in Urban Japan. Berkeley: University of California Press.

_____1985 Models and Practice in Medicine. Menopause as Syndrome of Life Transition. In Physicians of Western Medicine. Robert Hahn and Atwood Gaines (eds.). Dordrecht: D. Reidel Publishing, pp. 115-140.

_____1986 The Anthropological Study of the American Medical System: Center and Periphery. Soc. Sci. and Med. 22(9):931-932.

Lock, M., and D. Gordon (eds.)

1988 Biomedicine Examined. Dordrecht: Kluwer Academic Publishers.

Locker, David, and David Dunt

1978 Theoretical and Methodological Issues in Sociological Studies of Consumer Satisfaction with Medical Care. Soc. Sci. and Med. 12:283-292.

Logan, Kathleen

1988 'Casi Como Doctor': Pharmacists and Their Clients in a Mexican Urban Context. In The Context of Medicines in Developing Countries. Sjaak van Der Geest and Susan Reynolds Whyte (eds). Dordrecht: Kluwer Academic Publishers, pp. 107-130.

Lominitz, Larissa Adler, and Marisol Perez-Lizaur

1987 A Mexican Elite Family 1820-1980. Princeton: Princeton University Press.

López Acuña, Daniel

1976 La Crisis De La Medicina Mexicana. Puebla: México Universidad Autónoma De Puebla.

_____1980 Health Service in Mexico. Journal of Public Health Policy 1:83-95.

Low, Setha M.

1981 The Meaning of *Nervios*: A Sociocultural Analysis of Symptom Presentation in San José, Costa Rica. Culture, Medicine and Psychiatry 5:25-48.

_____1982 Effects of Medical Institutions on Doctor-Patient Interaction in Costa Rica. Milbank Memorial Fund Quarterly 60:17-50.

_____1985 Culture, Politics, and Medicine in Costa Rica. New York: Redgrave Publishing Co.

Lozoya Thalmann, Emilio
1985 Social Security, Health and Social Solidarity in Mexico. In The Political Economy of Income Distribution in Mexico. Pedro Aspe and Paul E. Sigmund (eds.). New York: Holmes and Meier Publishing, Inc.

Lukes, Steven
1973 Individualism. New York: Harper and Row.

Lutz, Catherine
1985 Depression and the Translation of Emotional Worlds. In Culture and Depression. A. Kleinman and Byron Good (eds.). Berkeley: University of California Press, pp. 63-100.

MacCormack, Carol P., and Marilyn Strathern
1980 Nature, Culture and Gender. Cambridge: Cambridge University Press.

Maes, Urban
1951 The Lost Art of Clinical Diagnosis. American Journal of Surgery 82:102.

Mares, Marco
1986 La Reconstruccion De Servicios De Salud Costara Approximadamente 165 Mil Milliones De Pesos. Uno Más Uno. September 19.

Maretzki, Thomas
1985 Including the Physician in Healer-Centered Research: Retrospect and Prospect. In Physicians of Western Medicine. Anthropological Approaches to Theory and Practice. Robert Hahn and Atwood Gaines (eds.). Dordrecht: D. Reidel Publishing, pp. 23-50.
_____1989 Cultural Variations in Biomedicine: The *Kur* in West Germany. Medical Anthropology Quarterly 3(1):22-35.

Marsh, G.N., et al.
1976 Anglo-American Contrasts in General Practice. British Medical Journal 1:1321-1325.

Martínez Cortés, Fernando
1965 Las Ideas En La Medicina Nahuatl. México: La Prensa Medicana.
_____1979 Consulta Médica y Entrevista Clínica. México: Medicina Del Hombre En Su Totalidad.
_____1983 Enfermedad y Padecer. México: Medicina Del Hombre En Su Totalidad.
_____1987 La Medicina Científica y el Siglo XIX Mexicano. México: Fondo De Cultura Económica, S.A. De C.V.

Marx, Karl
1974 Capital. Vol. II. Frederick Engels (ed.). New York: International Publishers.

McAuliffe, William E.
1978 Studies of Process-Outcome Correlations in Medical Care Evaluations: A Critique. Medical Care 26:907-930.
_____1979 Measuring the Quality of Medical Care: Process Versus Outcome. Milbank Memorial Fund Quarterly/Health and Society 57:118-152.

McDermott, Walsh
    1977 Evaluating the Physician and His Technology. Daedalus 106:135-158.
McKeown, Thomas
    1979 The Role of Medicine. Princeton: Princeton University Press.
McVaugh, Michael
    1989 Personal communication.
Mechanic, David
    1968 Medical Sociology. New York: Free Press.
_____1974 Discussion of Research Programs and Relations Between Stressful Life
    Events and Episodes of Physical Illness. In Stressful Life Events. Barbara Snell
    Dohrenwend and Bruce P. Dohrenwend (eds.). New York: John Wiley and Sons,
    pp. 87-89.
_____1979 Correlates of Physician Utilization: Why Do Major Multivariate
    Studies of Physician Utilization Find Trivial Psychosocial and Organizational Effect?
    Journal of Health and Social Behavior 21:146-155.
Mendiola Quezada, Roberto
    1982 La Homeopatia Como Escuela Médica. Homeopatia Medicina Social
    Confedración Mexicana De Asociaciones Medico Homeopaticos, Organizaciones
    Conexas y Afines A.C. Abril-Junio (No. 3):16-20.
Merleau-Ponty, M.
    1963 The Structure of Behavior. Boston: Beacon Press.
Mishler, Elliot G.
    1984 The Discourse of Medicine: Dialects of Medical Interviews. Norwood,
    N.J.:Ablex Publishing Corporation.
Montagne, Michael
    1988 The Metaphorical Nature of Drugs and Drug Taking. Soc. Sci. and Med.
    26(4):417-424.
Munson, Ronald
    1981 Why Medicine Cannot Be a Science. Journal of Medicine and Philosophy
    6:183-208.
Navarro, Vincente
    1976 Social Class, Political Power and the State and Their Implications in Medicine.
    Soc. Sci. and Med. 10:437-457.
_____1986 Crisis, Health and Medicine. London: Tavistock.
Nichter, Mark
    1980 The Layperson's Perception as Perspective into the Utilization of Multiple
    Therapy Systems in the Indian Context. Soc. Sci. and Med. 14B:225-233.
Nobrega, Fred T., et al.
    1977 Quality Assessment in Hypertension: Analysis of Process and Outcome
    Methods. New England Journal of Medicine 296:145-148.
Obeyesekere, Gananath
    1977 The Theory and Practice. Psychological Medicine in Ayurvedic Tradition.
    Culture, Medicine and Psychiatry 1:155-81.

O'Brien, Bernie
1984 Patterns of European Diagnoses and Prescribing. London: Office of Health Economics.

O'Neil, C.W., and H.A. Selby
1968 Sex Differences in the Incidence of Susto in Two Zapotec Pueblos: An Analysis of the Relationships Between Sex Role Expectations and a Folk Illness. Ethnology 7:95-105.

Ordonez Plaja, A., et al.
1968 Communication Between Physician and Patients in Outpatient Clinics. Milbank Memorial Fund Quarterly 46:161-213.

Orlinsky, David E., and Kenneth I. Howard
1975 Varieties of Psychotherapeutic Experience. New York: Teachers College Press.

Orth-Gomer, K., et al.
1979 Quality of Care in an Outpatient Department: The Patient's View. Soc. Sci. and Med. 13A:347.

Ortiz De Montellano, Bernard
1975 Empirical Aztec Medicine. Science 188:215-220.
_____1989 Syncretism in Mexican and Mexican-American Folk Medicine. Manuscript prepared for 1992 Lecture Series Occasional Paper #6. Department of Spanish and Portuguese, University of Maryland.
_____1989a Personal communication.

Ortiz Monasterio, Fernando
1984 La Enseñanza Médica De Postgrado Durante Los Ultimos 40 Años. In La Evolución de la Medicina En México Durante Las Ultimas Cuatro Decadas, Ramón De La Fuente et al (eds.). Mexico: El Colegio, pp. 73-87.

Osherson, Samuel, and Lorna Amara Singham
1981 The Machine Metaphor in Medicine. In Social Contexts of Health, Illness and Patient Care. Elliot G. Mishler et al. (eds.). London: Cambridge University Press.

Palau, Gabriel Velazquez
1979 Medical Education in Latin America: A Brief Review. In Aspects of the History of Medicine in Latin America. J. Bowers and E. Purcell (eds.). New York: Josiah Macy, Jr. Foundation, pp. 124-131.

Parsons, Talcott
1975 The Sick Role and the Role of the Physician Reconsidered. Health and Society, Summer:257-278.

Patrick, Donald
1982 The Longitudinal Disability Interview Survey. Phase II Report. London: Department of Community Medicine. United Medical Schools of Guy's and St. Thomas's Hospitals.

Paz, Octavio
1961 The Labyrinth of Solitude. New York: Grove Press.

Pellegrino, Edmund D.
  1979 The Sociocultural Impact of Twentieth-Century Therapeutics. In The
  Therapeutic Revolution. Morris Vogel and Charles E. Rosenberg (eds.).
  Philadelphia: University of Pennsylvania Press, pp. 245-266.
Pellegrino, Edmund D., and David C. Thomasma
  1981 A Philosophical Basis of Medical Practice. New York: Oxford University
  Press.
Pendleton, David
  1983 Doctor-Patient Communication: A Review. In Doctor-Patient
  Communication. David Pendleton and John Hasler (eds.). New York: Academic
  Press.
Pendleton, David, and John Hasler
  1983 Doctor-Patient Communication. New York: Academic Press, pp. 5-52
Peña-Mohr, Jorge
  1987 Distributing and Transfering Medical Technology. International Journal of
  Technology Assessment in Health Care 3(2):281-292.
Perlman, Janice E.
  1976 The Myth of Marginality. Berkeley: University of California Press.
Piahaud, D.
  1979 The Diffusion of Medical Technology in Less Developed Countries.
  International Journal of Health Services 9:629-643.
Pinckney, Edward R., and Cathey Pinckney
  1989 Unnecessary Measures. The Sciences. January/February:20-27.
Plough, Alonzo
  1981 Medical Technology and the Crisis of Experience: The Cost of Clinical
  Legitimation. Soc. Sci. and Med. 15B:89-101.
Powles, John
  1973 On the Limitations of Modern Medicine. Soc. Sci. and Med. 1:1-30.
Pratt, Lois V.
  1976 Reshaping the Consumer's Posture in Health Care. In The Doctor-Patient
  Relationship in the Changing Health Science. Eugene B. Gallagher (ed.).
  Washington, D.C.: U.S. Department of Health, Education, and Welfare, Public
  Health Service, National Institute of Health, pp. 197-214.
Quill, Timothy
  1983 Partnership in Patient Care: A Contractual Approach. Annals of Internal
  Medicine 98:228-234.
  _____1985 Somatization Disorder. Journal of the American Medical Association
  254(21):3075-3079.
Rabkin, J.G., and E.L. Struening
  1976 Life Events, Stress and Illness. Science 194:1031-1020.
Reiser, David, and David H. Rosen
  1984 Medicine as a Human Experience. Baltimore: University Park Press.

Reiser, Stanley Joel
1978 Medicine and the Reign of Technology. Cambridge: Cambridge University Press.

Rice, Laura, and Leslie S. Greenberg
1984 The New Research Paradigm. In Pattern of Change. Laura N. Rice and Leslie S. Greenberg (eds.). New York: Guilford Press, pp. 7-26.

Richter, Maurice N., Jr.
1972 Science as a Cultural Process. Cambridge: Schenkman.

Robbins, James M., et al.
1982 Treatment for a Non-Disease: The Case of Low Blood Pressure. Soc. Sci. and Med. 16:27-33.

Rosaldo, Michelle Z.
1984 Toward an Anthropology of Self and Feeling. In Culture Theory. Richard A. Shweder and Robert A. LeVine (eds). New York: Cambridge University Press, pp. 139-157.

Rosaldo, Michelle Z., and Lousie Lamphere
1974 Woman, Culture and Society. Stanford: Stanford University Press.

Rosenberg, Charles E.
1974 The Bitter Fruit: Heredity, Disease, and Social Thought in Nineteenth-Century America. Perspectives in American History 8:189-235.
_____1979 The Therapeutic Revolution: Medicine, Meaning and Social Change in Nineteenth-Century America. In The Therapeutic Revolution. M.J. Vogel and Charles E. Rosenberg (eds.). Philadelphia: University of Pennsylvania Press, pp. 3-25.
_____1986 Disease and Social Order in America. Milbank Memorial Fund Quarterly 64 (Suppl. 1):34-55.

Rubel, Arthur
1964 The Epidemiology of a Folk Illness: Susto in Hispanic America. Ethnology 3:268-283.

Rubel, Arthur, et al.
1984 Susto. Berkeley: University of California Press.

Rubin, Lillian Breslow
1976 Worlds of Pain. New York: Basic Books.

Ruiz Torres, Francisco
1980 Diccionario De Términos Médicos Inglés-Español, Español-Inglés. Madrid: Alahambra Printing.

Sanday, Peggy Reeves
1974 Female Status in the Public Domain. In Woman, Culture and Society. M. Rosaldo and L. Lamphere (eds.). Stanford University Press, pp. 189-206.
_____1981 Female Power and Male Dominance. New York: Cambridge University Press.

Scarry, Elaine
1985 The Body in Pain. New York: Oxford University Press.

Selwyn, B.J., and M. Ruiz De Chavez
1985 Coverage and Patterns of Ambulatory Medical Care Use in Tlalpan, Mexico City. Soc. Sci. and Med. 21(1):77-86.

Sesín, Saide
1987 Bioquimíca en Terapias Contra El Alcoholismo. Uno Más Uno. December 17.

Shryock, Richard Harrison
1979 The Development of Modern Medicine. Madison: University of Wisconsin Press.

Shweder, R., and E. Bourne
1984 Does the Concept of the Person Vary Cross-Culturally? In Cultural Conceptions of Mental Health and Therapy. A.S. Marsella and G.M. White (eds.). Dordrecht: D. Reidel Publishing, pp. 97-140.

Sicherman, Barbara
1977 The Use of Diagnosis: Doctors, Patients and Neurasthenia. Journal of the History of Medicine and Allied Sciences 32(1):33-54.

Siegler, Mark
1981 The Doctor-Patient Encounter and its Relationship to Theories of Health and Disease. In Concepts of Health and Disease: Interdisciplinary Perspectives. A.L. Caplan et al. (eds.). Reading, Mass.: Addison-Wesley, pp. 627-644.

Simoni, Joseph J., and Richard A. Ball
1978 Institutionalized Exploitation: The Case of the Mexican Medicine Huckster. Sociological Symposium 23:27-40.

Soberón Acevedo, Guillermo
1984 La Investigación Biomédica Básica. In La Evolución De La Medicina en México Durante las Ultimas Cuatro Décadas. Ramón de la Fuente et al. (eds.). Mexico: El Colegio, pp. 111-134.

Soberón Acevedo, Guillermo, and José R. Narro
1984 El Perfil del Medico Mexicano. Cuadernos 8. Mexico City: Secretaria De Salubridad y Asistencia.

Solomon, Robert C.
1984 Getting Angry. In Culture Theory. Richard A. Shweder and Robert A. LeVine (eds.). New York: Cambridge University Press, pp. 238-254.

Solomons, Noel W., and Gerald T. Keusch
1981 Nutritional Implications of Parasite Infections. Nutrition Reviews 30:149-181.

Somolinos d'Ardois, Germán
1978 Capitulos De Historia Médica Mexicana I. Medicina en las Culturas Meso Americanas Anteriores A La Conquista. Mexico: Sociedad Mexicana De Historia y Filosofia de la Medicina.

_____1979 Capitulos De Historia Médica Mexicana II El Fenomeno De Fusion Cultural Y Su Trascendencia Médica. Mexico City: Dr. Juan Somolinos Palencia.

Sontag, Susan
1979 Illness as Metaphor. New York: Vintage Books.

Sox, H.C., et al.

1981 Psychologically Mediated Effects of Diagnostic Tests. Annals of Internal Medicine 95:680–685.

Speedling, Edward J., and David N. Rose

1985 Building an Effective Doctor-Patient Relationship: From Patient Satisfaction to Patient Participation. Soc. Sci. and Med. 21(2):115-120.

Spicker, Stuart F.

1984 Comments on Nordenfelt's 'On the Circle of Health.' In Health, Disease, and Causal Explanations in Medicine. L. Nordenfelt and B.I.B. Lindahl (eds.). Dordrecht: D. Reidel Publishing.

Spiro, H.

1986 Doctors, Patients and Placebos. New Haven: Yale University Press.

Starfield, Barbara

1974 Measurement of Outcome: A Proposed Scheme. Milbank Memorial Fund Quarterly 52:39-50.

Starfield, Barbara and David Scheff

1972 Effectiveness of Pediatric Care: The Relationship Between Process and Outcome. Pediatrics 49:547-552.

Starfield, Barbara, et al.

1979 Patient-Provider Agreement About Problems: Influences on Outcome of Care. Journal of American Medical Association 242:344-346.

Starfield, Barbara, et al.

1981 The Influence of Patient-Practitioner Agreement on Outcome of Care. American Journal of Public Health 2:127-131.

Starr, Paul

1982 The Social Transformation of American Medicine. New York: Basic Books.

Stebbins, Kenyon Rainer

1986 Curative Medicine, Preventive Medicine and Health Status: The Influence of Politics on Health Status in a Rural Mexican Village. Soc. Sci. and Med. 23(2):139-148.

Sternbach, Richard A.

1974 Pain Patients. New York: Academic Press.

Stewart, Moira A.

1984 What Is a Successful Doctor Patient Interview? A Study of Interactions and Outcomes. Soc. Sci and Med. 19(2):167-175.

Stewart, Moira, et al.

1979 The Doctor-Patient Relationship and Its Effect Upon Outcome. Journal of the Royal College of General Practitioners 29:77-82.

Sussman, Linda K.

1981 Unity in Diversity in a Polyethnic Society: The Maintenance of Medical Pluralism on Mauritius. Soc. Sci. and Med. 15B:247-260.

Szasz, Thomas S., and Marc H. Hollender
  1956 A Contribution to the Philosophy of Medicine. Archives of International Medicine 95:585-592.
Taylor, William B.
  1979 Drinking, Homicide and Rebellion in Colonial Mexican Villages. Stanford: Stanford University Press.
Thomas, Lewis
  1977 On the Science and Technology of Medicine. Daedalus 106:35-46.
Townsend, J.M.
  1978 Cultural Conceptions of Health and Illness: A Comparison of Germany and America. Chicago: University of Chicago Press.
Trostle, James, et al.
  1983 The Logic of Non-Compliance: Management of Epilepsy from the Patient's Point of View. Culture, Medicine and Psychiatry 7:35-56.
Tuckett, David, et al.
  1985 Meetings Between Experts. New York: Tavistock Publications.
Turner, Bryan S.
  1984 The Body and Society. New York: Basil Blackwell.
Turner, Victor
  1974 Dramas, Fields, and Metaphors. Ithaca: Cornell University Press.
Ugalde, Antonio
  1985 Health and Social Science in Latin America. Soc. Sci. and Med. 21(1):1-3.
Unschuld, Paul U.
  1980 The Issue of Structured Coexistence of Scientific and Alternative Medical Systems: A Comparison of East and West German Legislation. Soc. Sci. and Med. 14B:15-24.
Uzzell, Douglas
  1974 Susto Revisited: Illness as Strategic Role. American Ethnologist 1:369-378.
Vander Geest, Sjaak, and Susan Reynolds Whyte
  1988 The Context of Medicine in Developing Countries. Boston: Kluwer Academic Publishers.
Velez-Ibañez, Carlos G.
  1983 Rituals of Marginality: Politics, Process and Culture Change in Central Urban Mexico. Berkeley: University of California Press.
  _____1983a Bonds of Mutual Trust. New Brunswick, N.J.: Rutgers University Press.
Viesca, Carlos
  1986 Medicina Prehispánica de México. Mexico: Panorama Editorial, S.A.
Villanueva, Carlos Garcia, and Susana Perera Quintana
  1982 La Industria Farmacéutica En América Latina. Mexico: Instituto Mexicano Del Seguro Social.
Waitzkin, Howard
  1979 Medicine, Superstructure and Micropolitics. Soc. Sci. and Med. 13A:601-609.

_____1983 The Second Sickness. New York: Free Press.

Waitzkin, Howard and J.D. Stoeckle
1972 The Conceptualization and Measurement of Health for Adults in the Health Insurance Study. Vol. XI. Model of Health and Methodology. Published by the Rand Corporation R-1987/1 HEW.

Weinberger, Morris, et al.
1981 The Impact of Clinical Encounter Events on Patients and Physician Satisfaction. Soc. Sci. and Med. 15:329-344.

Weiner, Herbert
1978 The Illusion of Simplicity: The Medical Model Revisited. American Journal of Psychiatry 135:27-33.

Weisberg, Daniel
1984 Physician's Private Clinic in a Northern Thai Town -- Patient Healer Collaboration and the Shape of Biomedical Practice. Culture, Medicine and Psychiatry 8:165-186.

Whiting, Van R.
1984 The Politics of Technology Transfer in Mexico. La Jolla, Calif.: Center for U.S.-Mexican Studies, University of California, San Diego.

Willems, Emilio
1975 Latin American Culture. New York: Harper and Row.

Wilson, Robert N.
1963 Patient-Practitioner Relationships. In Handbook of Medical Sociology. Howard E. Greeman et al. (eds.). Englewood, N.J.: Prentice-Hall, pp. 273-298.

Wolf, Eric R.
1959 Sons of the Shaking Earth. Chicago: University of Chicago Press.
_____1982 Europe and the People Without History. Berkeley: University of California Press.

Woolley, F. Ross, et al.
1978 The Effects of Doctor-Patient Communication on Satisfaction and Outcome of Care. Soc. Sci. and Med. 12:123-128.

Wright, Peter, and Andrew Treacher
1982 The Problem of Medical Knowledge. Edinburgh: Edinburgh University Press.

Young, Allan
1980 The Discourse on Stress and the Reproduction of Conventional Knowledge. Soc. Sci. and Med. 14B:133-146.
_____1981 The Creation of Medical Knowledge: Some Problems in Interpretation. Soc. Sci. and Med. 15B:379-386.
_____1983 Rethinking Ideology. International Journal of Health Services 13:203-219.
_____1983a The Relevance of Traditional Medical Cultures to Modern Primary Health Care. Soc. Sci. and Med. 17(16):1205-1211.

Young, James Clay

1981 Medical Choice in a Mexican Village. New Brunswick, N.J.: Rutgers University Press.

Yoxen, E.J.

1982 Constructing Genetic Disease. In The Problem of Medical Knowledge. P. Wright and A. Treacher (eds.). Edinburgh: Edinburgh University Press, pp. 144-161.

Zborowski, Mark

1952 Cultural Components in Response to Pain. Journal of Social Issues 8:16-30.

Zola, I.K.

1966 Culture and Symptoms: An Analysis of Patients' Presenting Complaints. American Sociological Review 31:615-630.

_____1973 Pathways to the Doctor: From Person to Patient. Soc. Sci. and Med. 7:677-689.

_____1981 Structural Constraints in the Doctor-Patient Relationship: The Case of Non-Compliance. In The Relevance of Social Science and Medicine. Leon Eisenberg and Arthur Kleinman (eds.). Dordrecht: D. Reidel Publishing, pp. 241-252.

Glossary

Aire: A traditional sickness usually produced by tormented spirits possessing the body.

Anginas: Refers to a sore throat in general and to the tonsils in particular.

Baba de nopal: The white sap from prickly pear cacti.

Boca del estomago: Refers to the "mouth of the stomach, the area around the diaphragm between the lower front ribs and the upper abdomen.

Caida de mollera: Fallen fontanelle.

Cerebro: Pertains to the occipital-medula region of the head, down to the nuchal muscle.

Cintura: Refers to pain in the waist as well as the lower back. Women may also associate the pain in the waist with pain in the ovaries.

Cintura abierta: Open waist, also related to pain in the ovaries and fallen womb.

Curandera(f)/Curandeero (m): A folk curer.

Empacho: Bolus attached to the stomach, traditionally beleived to be experienced by children.

Loco: Crazy, characterizing persons "who do not know what they do", and "who have lost their five senses."

Medicos universitarios: Officially trained physicians in Colonial Mexico.

Novio: Fiance.

Ojo: Evil eye.

Piquetes: Refers to jabbing pain in the heart or chest, usually associated with emotional discharges such as anger or nerves.

Pulmon: Meaning lungs, refers to pains in the upper back and is usually associated with hard work.

Pulque: Undistilled alcoholic beverage extracted from **Agave** sp. widely used in rural Mexico. It had its origins in Preconquest times.

Susto: Cause of sickness associated with unexpected startle or fright.

Index

Abortion, folk methods used, 26, 167, 212. *See also* Women

Acupuncture, 51, 92, 94, 97, 198, 203, 213

Aire. See Typical symptoms

Anger (to make an)
embodied, 9
etiological belief, as an, 36, 78, 79, 81
and heredity, 40
and high and low blood pressure, 35, 82
and male-female relations, 37
and morality, 9, 37, 230, 233
and parent-child relations, 37
as protection against witchcraft, 42, 201, 202-203
provocation of, 37-38
and sickness, 38, 43, 44, 200, 201, 208, 209
and social relations, 9
symptoms resulting from, 32, 37, 39
and women, 10, 43

Anginas. See Typical symptoms

Antonovsky, A., 8, 194(n10)

Armstrong, D., 77, 78, 124, 177, 193(n5), 222

Arthur (patient), 23, 129-137, 199-202

Attributions for recovery. *See* Recovery attributions

Attributions of sickness. *See* Etiological explanations

Berliner, H., 1, 15(n1), 77

Bernard, Claude, 63

Bichat, Marie Francois Xavier, 63

Biomedical diagnoses, their meanings, 230. *See also* Clinical reasoning; Diagnoses; Diagnostic process

Biomedical education in Mexico, 64, 68, 73(n15)
criticism of, 68-69, 73(nn 10-12)
and the North American model, 66, 68-69
and specialization, 66, 73(n9)

Biomedical model, the, 216
and the doctor-patient encounter, 125
and life's lesions, 11. *See also* Life's lesions

Biomedical practice
International, cultural and idiosyncratic aspects of, 75-76, 229
in Mexico, 1
variability of, in Mexico, 91, 95-98

Biomedical technology, use of, by Mexican physicians, 84-85

Biomedical treatment regimen. *See* Treatment regimen

Biomedicine, 1, 2, 68-69
core characteristics of, 78
criticism of, 77
cross-cultural studies of, 4
and the family, 126
and the healing process, 192-193, 215
history of, 1,3,4,5,6
and individualism, 126, 221, 232
a model of its cultural transformations, 88-89

and pharmacological drugs, 77
and the structuration process, 5
See also Biomedical practice;
  Biomedicine in Mexico; Dualism;
  Health care delivery in Mexico;
  Physicians, individual; Physicians, in
  Mexico
Biomedicine and Spiritualist healing
  compared, 197-198, 223
  similarities between, 220. *See also*
  Diagnoses; Spiritualist healing
Biomedicine in Mexico, 8, 11, 65, 75,
  78, 229
  contrasted with North American
  medicine, 78
  and its influence on folk beliefs, 5
  North American influence on, 7, 65-67,
  69, 77
  patients' perceptions of, 2
  in the private sector, 47, and fees
  charged by private physicians, 54(n4)
  in the public sector, 45-46
  and the state, 45, 46, 47, 52, 65, 71,
  72, 227, 231
  See also Medicine in Mexico
Boca del estomago. See Typical
  symptoms
Brody, H., 10, 77, 178

Catholicism in Mexico. *See* Religion in
  Mexico
Cerebro. See Typical symptoms
Children, in Mexico, role of, 26
Chiropractic in Mexico, 92
Cicourel, A.V., 5, 45, 69, 70, 72, 123-
  124, 177
Cintura. See Typical symptoms
Cleaves, P., 45, 69, 70-71, 72
Clinical judgment. *See* Clinical
  reasoning
Clinical reasoning, 75, 76, 77, 84, 85-86,
  120-121, 231

variability, of as seen by individual
  physicians:
Physician 1, 92, 159
Physician 2, 92, 143, 147-149
Physician 3, 92-93, 104, 105-108
Physician 4, 93, 142-143
Physician 5, 93, 99
Physician 6, 93-94, 132-136
Physician 7, 94, 108, 114-115, 118,
  120
Physician 8, 94-95, 99-101
CMI. *See* Cornell Medical Index
Contraception, views on, 199
Cornell Medical Index (CMI), xv,
  90(n7), 176, 193(nn3, 4), 235-236,
  236(n2)

Davis, D., 16(n9)
Diagnoses, average number made by
  individual physicians, 96
  biomedical and Spiritualist compared,
  223-224
  role in the healing process, 178-179
  shaped by cultural and personal
  experience, 89
  validation of, 86
Diagnostic process, 76-77, 85
  of physicians, 84-86
  and the time dimension, 125-126
  variability among physicians, 95, 96,
  99-101, 101-121
  See also Clinical Reasoning
Disease, and environment in Mexico
  City, 17-18
  distinguished from illness, and
  sickness, 10
  and pollution, 79
  stress model of, 11-12
Disease in Mexico, introduced with the
  Conquest, 60
Doctor-patient encounter, 86-87, 232
  as drama, 123-125, 138-143

examples of, 98-101, 101-108, 108-121, 130-137, 143-149, 149-159
and the healing process, 123, 231
importance for micro- and macroanalysis, 123, 127
inherent conflicts of, 125
routine procedures of, 127-128
scripted by the biomedical model, 125
and the transmission of ideologies and morality, 88, 126-127, 129, 131, 132
universal characteristics of, 89
See also Medical consultation; physician-patient relationship; physician-sacred healer-patient encounter
Doctor-patient relationship. *See* Doctor-patient encounter
Dualism (mind-body)
in biomedicine, 66, 102-108, 109-121
in Mexican Spiritualism, 221
Dunt, D., 177, 194(n5)

Earthquake, in Mexico City (1985), 20-21
effects on government health care facilities, 30(n6), 47, 54(n3)
embodied, 40
and sickness, 38, 39, 40, 79, 200, 201
Economic crisis, in Mexico, 21-22, 30(n7), 30(n8)
effects on physicians, 21
and nerves, 38
Education in Mexico
demands for, 22
expectations of, 200
and symptomatologies, 22
See also Biomedical education
Emotional discharges
as moral judgments, 9
and the nervous system, 79
and sickness, 9, 11, 24, 25
and women, 43
Emotions, 9

Mexican view of, 67
Engel, G., 12, 66, 68, 89(n1), 124, 198
Englehard, T., 10, 76
Esperanza (patient), 12, 25, 92, 143-149, 189, 205-208, 216(n2), 220, 225
Etiological explanations, 31, 35-36, 199, 203, 206, 209, 212, 215
differences by sex, 43
folk, 6, 35-44, 78, 79, 111, 190, 216(n1)
physicians', 78, 79-83
Spiritualist and biomedical compared, 220, 223
See also Heredity
Evangelical movements in Mexico, 29, 212
effects on male-female relationships, 29
See also Religion in Mexico

Fallen womb. *See* Typical symptoms
Family, in Mexico, 23, 28, 67, 226
and the biomedical model, 126
conflicts in, 23
and physician management of patients, 87
relationships in, 24
and sickness, 23, 24, 108
and social support, 28, 188
See also Residence patterns
Feinstein, A., 75, 76, 78, 84, 173
Felix, D., 8, 21
Fieldwork
difficulties of, in Mexico City, xiv, xvi, 193(n2)
in a hospital, xii
in Spiritualist temple, xii
See also Methodology
Fitzpatrick, R., 3, 177, 194(n5)
Fleming, R., 188, 236
Flexner Report, 65, 69, 73(n7), 73(n13)
influence of, on biomedicine in Mexico, 65, 77
Flores Carbajal, G., 65, 68

Flores y Troncoso, F.,50, 51, 62, 64-65, 73(n1)
Folk beliefs
and biomedicine, 5
and pharmacological drugs, 182
and remedies, 211
Folk etiologies *See* Etiological explanations
Folk healers
Bonesetters, 198
Spiritualist healers, 219-227
Foster, G., 31, 60, 73(n1)
Foucault, M., 1, 15(n), 222
Frankenberg, R., 124
Frenk, J. 65, 68, 69
Fuente, R., 65, 66, 73(n8)

Gaines, A., 7, 16(n7), 76, 86, 91
Gereffi, G., xvii(n3), 81
Giddens, A., 5, 82
Good, B., 11, 31
Good, Mary Jo, 11, 31
Gutierrez, G., 86

Hahn, R., 15(n5), 16(n7), 26, 68, 91, 126, 159, 194(n5)
Harre, R., 9, 82
Headaches. *See* Typical symptoms
Healing process, 178-179
components of, 197-198, 199, 232
and therapeutic outcomes, 4
Health care delivery in Mexico
allocation of funds by the government for, 46
Institute for Social Security for State Workers (ISSSTE), 45-46, 47, 52, 71
Ministry of Health, 46, and population serviced by, 47
National Institute of Social Services (IMSS) 45-46, 65, 163, and physicians earnings in, 74(n16)
types of 45
See also Salud Hospital

Helman, C., 4, 8, 11, 129, 194(n5), 223, 232
Herbal remedies. *See* Medicinal Plants
Heredity
concepts of, 5-6, 41
as etiological belief, 40
physicians' emphasis on, 129
and symptomatology, 83
See also Medical history taking
High and low blood pressure, 34, 35, 41, 82, 199-200
medicalization of, 129-137
physicians' treatment of, 89(n3), 129, 201
symbolic meaning of, 82
symptomatology of, 129-138, 200, 202
See also Typical symptoms
Hollander, M., 177
Homeopathic medicine in Mexico, 50, 54(n5)
physicians views of, 92, 94, 97, 120
relationship with biomedicine, 71
type of treatment given by, 213
Hospitals, first established in Mexico, 62. *See also* Salud Hospital
Husband-wife relations. *See* Male-female relations

Individualism
and biomedicine, 221, 232
and the doctor-patient encounter, 126
Inheritability of disease. *See* Heredity
Institute for Social Security for State Workers (ISSSTE). *See* Health care delivery in Mexico
Intracultural variability in complex societies, 13
Inui, T., 177

Jabbing pain in chest (*piquetes*)
and young people, 34-35
See also Typical symptoms
Jewson, N.D., 2, 64, 125

Jose (patient), 23, 98-99, 99-101, 127, 167, 198-199, 202

Kidneys. *See* Typical symptoms
King, L.S., 64, 75, 76, 77, 78, 84, 89(n2)
Kleinman, A., xv, 4, 10, 15(n5), 31, 45, 68, 77, 90(n8), 177, 194(n5) 231, 235

Laennec, Rene, 64
LaGuna, J., 65-66
Leder, D., 11, 31
Lenihan, B., 227(n2)
Life events, 188-189
  and patients' perceived recovery, 188
  and symptomatology, 12
Life's lesions, 35, 171, 197, 215, 225, 229, 233
  and anatomical lesions, 11
  defined, 3
Lock, M., 4, 15(n5), 16(n7), 76
Locker, D., 177, 194(n5)
Lopez Acuna, D., 18, 45, 46, 53(n1)
Low, S., 15(nn5, 8, 9)
Lungs. *See* Typical symptoms

McVaugh, R., 5
Male-female relations, 24, 25, 26, 27, 111, 113, 201, 208, 210, 211 212, 213, 215, 221
  and anger, 37
  in control group, 30(n12)
  effects of evangelical groups on, 29
  and sickness, 24, 25, 26, 200, 205, 215
  and Spiritualist healing, 226
Maretzki, T., 15(n5), 76, 123
Marriage, 25, 163, 209. *See also* Male-female relations
Martinez Cortes, F., xvii, 63, 64, 68, 73(n1)
Medical consultation, 181-182, 183, 184
  average time spent with patients in, 181
  as drama, 7, 178, 232

literature on, 193-194(n5)
  and recovery attributions, 215
  significance of, 177
Medical encounter. *See* Medical consultation
Medical history taking, 6, 81, 83, 84, 85, 233
  and attraction for patients, 128
  and heredity, 128
Medicalization
  of existential conditions, 201
  by patients of their conditions, example of 129-137
Medication. *See* Pharmacological drugs
Medicinal plants, 51-52, 54(n7), 62, 198, 214
  and biomedical practice, 71, 93
  preference for, 182
  special market for, 54(n6)
  usage of, during the Preconquest, 59-60
Medicine, History of, in Mexico
  during the Colonial period, 60-62
  before the Conquest, 59-60
  during Independence, 63
  Spanish appropriation of native medicine, 61-62
Medicine in Mexico
  North American influences on, 65-67
  transformation of, 63-64
  Western European influences on, 63
  See also Biomedicine in Mexico
Men
  etiological beliefs of, 43
  and health-seeking trajectories of, 53
  and masculinity, 25, 203-204
  and sexuality, 26-27
  and sickness, 198-204
  social pressures on, 20, 23, 25, 27
  source of self-esteem, 26
Merleau-Ponty, M., 10
Methodology, xi-xii, xiii-xiv, xiv-xvi, 7-8, 13, 121(n1), 124, 127-128,

170(n3), 171-172, 176, 178, 188, 189, 191, 193(n1), 193(n2), 193(n3), 194(n6), 194(n7), 194-195(n12), 235-236

Mexico, economy of, 21. *See also* Economic crisis

Mexico City
description of 17-18, 19, 29(n1), 30(n4)
earthquake in, 20, and effects on health, 186-187
inhabitants' view of, 203
migration to and sickness, 198
pollution in, 17-18, 29(n2). *See also* Earthquake

Ministry of Health. *See* Health care delivery in Mexico; Salud Hospital

Mother-child bond in Mexico, 27, 28. *See also* Parent-children relations

National Institute of Social Service (IMSS). *See* Health care delivery in Mexico

Nerves, 9, 198, 201, 202, 205, 209
and the earthquake, 20, 38
and the economic crisis, 38
as etiological belief, 6, 19, 36, 78, 79
folk treatment of, 205, 208
and high and low blood pressure, 34, 82
meaning of, 39
as moral evaluation, 230
and the nervous system, 39
as a neurological disorder, 80
physicians' interpretations of, 6, 31, 79, 80, 92-94
symptomatology of, 38, 39, 44
and women, 10, 43

Nezahualcóyotl (Neza)
description of, 18-19, 206, 207
effects of earthquake on, 20
land prices in, 30(n4)
popular view of, 20

Nomi (patient), 25, 35, 80, 108, 121, 121(n4), 126, 127, 167, 184, 210-215, 220

Nonbiomedical treatment options, 50-52. *See also* Acupuncture; Homeopathic medicine; Medicinal plants

Ortiz de Montellano, B., xix, 5, 20, 60

Parasitic infections, 85, 86, 97
treatment of, 87, 210

Parent-child relations, 37, 43-44, 209, 234

Participant observation, the effects on the study population, xv

Patients
biomedical expectations and Spiritualist treatment compared, 221-222
description of, xiii, 19, 197
economic conditions, 22
and employment, 163
economic status, 164-165, 169(n), 187
expectations of treatment, 168-169, 181
health profile, 165-166, 169-170(n2)
interpretation of physicians' diagnosis, 107
perception of biomedicine, studies lacking of, 4
perception of sickness and recovery, 2-3
presenting symptoms, 166
reasons for seeking treatment, 167-168
religious profile, 29
residence patterns, 23
responses to physicians' explanations, 83-84
sociodemographic profile, 163, 164(Table 9.1)
treatment-seeking trajectories, 52-53, 53, 103, 105-108, 118, 119, 121, 220, by sex, 53. *See also* Doctor - patient encounter; Medical consultation

Patients' perceived recovery
and change in life circumstances, 199, 201
and expectations of treatment, 181, 230
and length of time patients were sick, 185-186
and life events, 188
and life's lesions, 171
measures used to assess, 172-173
and medical consultation, 171, 177
and medical diagnostic techniques, 175
and medication, 182
and migration to Mexico City, 186-187
and residence patterns, 199
and physicians' diagnoses, 173-174(Table 10.3)
on second follow-up, 191-192
by sex, 172(Table 10.1)
and sickness management, 184-185
and sociodemographic variables, 186
and socieconomic status, 187
and subjective evaluation of health status, 186
three categories of, 172
variables influencing, 178-181, 184, 229

Patrick, D., 188, 235

Pellegrino, E. 2, 3, 11, 75, 77, 123, 220

Pharmaceutical Industry in Mexico, xiii, 72, 76, 128
growth of, 81

Pharmacological drugs, 182
average number prescribed by physicians, 182, 183
and biomedicine, 77
as folk medicine, 182
and patients' perceived recovery, 182, 190, 201
and patients' response to, 208
prescribed by physicians 194(n8)
sold in Mexico 194(n8)

Physician-patient relationship, emphasis on, 225-226

Physicians, individual
Physician 1, description of, 91-92; treating patients, 149-159
Physician 2, description of, 92; treating patients, 143-149
Physician 3, description of, 92-93; treating patients, 101-108, 184
Physician 4, description of, 93, 96, 97, 98; treating patients, 138-143
Physician 5, description of, 93, 97,184; treating patients, 99-100
Physician 6, description of, 94, 98, 129; treating patients, 135-137, 184
Physician 7, description of, 94, 97, 98, 109; treating patients, 108-121, 114, 116-117, 129, 184
Physician 8, description of, 94-95, 97, treating patients, 99-101

Physicians, in Mexico
allegiance to the profession, 72
clinical reasoning, 85-86
competition for residencies, 73(n14)
conflicts of, 13, 76, 78, 92, 229-230, between technological and clinical medicine, 84
controlled by the state, 72
day celebrated, 73(n5)
diagnoses and patients' perceived recovery, 173-174
earnings of, 73-74(n16)
economic resources, 72
employment and underemployment among, 30(n9)
etiological beliefs, 78,79
folk etiological beliefs, 79-83
indications to patients, 99, 100, 105, 107, 114-116, 117, 119, 135, 136-137, 141-142, 147, 157-158
interpretations of typical symptoms, 32-33, 34-35, 39, 79-80, 81, 82-83
mode of addressing patients, 182
social status, 70-72

undifferentiated from other types of
healers by patients, 70. *See also*
Clinical reasoning; Doctor-patient
encounter; Medical consultation
Physician-sacred healer-patient encounter
compared, 221, 222-224, 226
Positivism in Mexico, 8, 63, 232
and Catholicism, 8
Psychiatrists, earnings of, 73(n11)
Psychiatry in Mexico, 66
in Salud Hospital 66-67
Pulque, 60, 64, 73(n2)

Recovery attributions, 182, 189-191,
199, 215
and the biomedical model, 216
Recruitment
into the biomedical profession, 67-68
into biomedicine and Spiritualism,
compared, 224
into Spiritualism, 220
Reiser, D., 15(n1), 63,64, 76, 77
Religion in Mexico
Catholicism, 208, 232
Evangelical movements, 28, 29, 208,
211, and membership in, 212, and
effects on male-female relationships,
29
Spiritualism, 226
Residence patterns, in Mexico, 18, 23,
206
and patients' perceived recovery, 199
and sickness, 199, 200, 201
Rosenberg, C., 2, 5, 6, 11, 194(n5)
Rubin, L., 233-234

Sacred healing. *See* Spiritualist healing
Salud Hospital
admissions procedures, xiii, 48
description of, 7, 46, 49
and earthquake, 20-21
fees charged by, 54(n2), 89(n5)
and Health Ministry, 46, 47

lack of diagnostic tools in, 78
physicians of, 72
preconsultations in, 48-50
psychiatry in, 66-67
reasons patients seek treatment from,
52, 168
services provided by, 46, 48
treatment expectations from, 168
treatment given by, 198, 201, 208
Serge (patient), 6, 138-143, 202-204
Sharon (patient), 93, 101-108, 126, 127,
215
Sickness
defined, 10-11, 12
and embodiment of day to day
existence, 10, 108, 120
and emotional discharges, 11
emotions producing, 9
and male-female relations, 200
management of, 184-185, 199, 201,
203, 205, 207, 208, 211, 213, 214-
215
Mexican view of, xv
and migration to Mexico City, 198, 199
and poverty, 81, 199, 197
and socioeconomic status, 187
and witchcraft beliefs, 202-203
and women, 10
Sickness attributions. *See* Etiological
beliefs
Siegler, M., 233
Spiritualism in Mexico, 29
Spiritualist healers, 192
Spiritualist healing, 216, 231
compared with biomedicine, xi, 1, 4,
197-198, 220, 221, 222, 223, 224,
225, 232
the gift of, 220
patient resort to, and biomedicine, 219
techniques of, 220
and social change, 226-227
Spiritualist temples, 207-208
Soberon, Acevedo, G., 48, 65, 68

Social supports, 28, 187-188
Somolinos d'Ardois, G., 59, 61, 73(n1)
Structuration process, 5, 82, 230
Study, aims of, xiv, 1, 2, 3, 4, 5, 7-8
Susto (fright)
  attributions to, 39
  and the earthquake, 20, 39
  and heredity, 40
  symptomatology of, 39
  See also Typical symptoms
Symptoms
  meanings of, 8, 11, 31, 32-35
  See also Typical symptoms
Szasz, T., 177

Thelma (patient), 149-159, 208-210
Therapeutic outcomes
  difficulties assessing, 3, 4
  defined, 3, 11
  See also Patients' perceived recovery
Therapeutic procedures. *See* Doctor-
  patient encounter; Medical
  consultation; Physicians, individual;
  Spiritualist healing compared with
  biomedicine
Treacher, A., 1, 7
Treatment expectations, patients', 202,
  205, 213
Treatment regimen, biomedical, 77, 78,
  86-88
  diet, 88
  pharmacological, 87, 89, 137
  referrals to specialists, 87. *See also*
  Medical consultation; Physicians,
  Individual
Treatment techniques. *See* Treatment
  regimen, biomedical; Spiritualist
  healing
Tuckett, D., 3, 125
Turner, B., 2, 8, 11, 222
Turner, V., 124
Typical symptoms
  Aire, 40

Anginas, 32
Boca del estomago, 33
cerebro, 32, 82, 198, 201, 205, 208,
  209
cintura, 33, 34, 198, 210
defined, 31, 32, 230, 233
headaches, 32
high and low blood pressure, 35
kidneys, 34, 82
pain in ovaries, and fallen womb, 33,
  125
physicians' interpretations of, 82-83,
  92-93
piquetes (jabbing in the chest), 34
pulmon (lungs), 34, 82
witchcraft, 40, 41
See also Anger; Emotional discharges;
  High and low blood pressure;
  Nerves; Physicians, Individual;
  Witchcraft

Valez-Ibañez, C., 18, 25
Viesca, C., xix, 59, 60, 73(n)
Vitamins, 87, 203, 210

Waitzkin, H., 5, 11, 69, 126, 177,
  194(n5)
Western medicine. *See* Biomedical
  Practice; Biomedicine
Wilson, R., 226
Witchcraft, 192, 206, 207, 209, 212,
  232-233
  accusations of, 25, 27
  and anger, 42
  and biomedicine, 41, 201
  as an etiological belief, 40, 41
  and Evangelicals, and Spiritualists, 29
  and the healing process 42, 202
  and one's personal character, 42
  problematic of believing in, 8-9, 42
  and sickness, 202-203
  and Spiritualism, 222, 223, 224-225
Wright, P. 1, 7

Wolf, E. 8, 60-61, 70, 232
Women, 210
  and abortions, 26, 167, 212
  and anger, 10, 43
  dietary deficiencies of, 43
  and education, 22-23
  etiological beliefs of, 43
  and emotional discharges, 43
  health seeking trajectories of, 53
  households headed by, 23
  infertility of, 26
  and loss of a child, 188-189
  and self-esteem, 26
  and sexuality, 26-27
  and typical symptoms, 33, 34
  and virginity, 24
Women's routine activities, 28

Young, A., 1, 10, 15(n6)

PHYSICIANS AT WORK, PATIENTS IN PAIN
Biomedical Practice and Patient Response in Mexico
Kaja Finkler

This ethnographic study offers a detailed and surprising picture of how modern biomedicine is altered when practiced in a developing country. Addressing the question of therapeutic outcome, Dr. Finkler examines various aspects of biomedicine that influence patient response, including specific components of the doctor-patient relationship. Her study sheds light on the ways in which biomedicine is molded by cultural context and distinguishes the universal, culturally specific, and idiosyncratic components of medical beliefs and practices. Although the focus is on biomedicine, this unique book also addresses the interplay between traditional healing and biomedical treatment.

Physicians and patients speak for themselves in interviews. Through the words and life narratives of the patients and through her own observations of doctor-patient encounters, the author shows that outcomes are strongly influenced by several factors, including the interaction with the doctor and the patients' own perceptions. Whether patients are cured depends less on the nature of the illness and the number of visits than on whether they are able to resolve certain contradictions in their lives and whether they are given and agree with the doctor's diagnosis.

Dr. Finkler concludes by discussing the significant problems for doctors in reconciling their training in biomedicine with the cultural dimensions of the society in which they practice.

Kaja Finkler is a professor of anthropology at the University of North Carolina.